Pocket Guide to Nursing Diagnoses

D1300114

The *Pocket Guide to Nursing Diagnoses* is available in the following foreign language editions:

Chinese, ed 5
French, ed 4
Italian, ed 3
Indonesian, ed 5 (forthcoming)
Japanese, ed 5
Spanish, ed 5

Pocket Guide to Nursing Diagnoses

Mi Ja Kim, RN, PhD, FAAN
Vice Chancellor for Research
Dean of Graduate College
University of Illinois at Chicago
Chicago, Illinois

Gertrude K. McFarland, RN, DNSc, FAAN
Health Scientist Administrator
Nursing Research Study Section
Division of Research Grants
National Institutes of Health
Bethesda, Maryland

Audrey M. McLane, RN, PhD
Professor Emerita
College of Nursing
Marquette University
Milwaukee, Wisconsin

SEVENTH EDITION

 Mosby

A Harcourt Health Sciences Company

St. Louis Baltimore Boston Carlsbad Chicago Naples New York Philadelphia Portland

London Madrid Mexico City Singapore Sydney Tokyo Toronto Wiesbaden

Mosby

Dedicated to Publishing Excellence

A Harcourt Health Sciences Company

Vice President and Publisher: Nancy L. Coon
Editor: Loren S. Wilson
Developmental Editor: Brian Dennison
Project Manager: Deborah L. Vogel
Production Editor: Mamata Reddy
Designer: Pati Pye
Manufacturing Manager: Don Carlisle

Seventh Edition
Copyright © 1997 by Mosby-Year Book, Inc.

Previous editions copyrighted 1984, 1987, 1989, 1991, 1993, 1995.

Printed in the United States of America

Mosby-Year Book, Inc.
11830 Westline Industrial Drive
St. Louis, Missouri 63146

Library of Congress Cataloging-in-Publication Data
Pocket guide to nursing diagnoses/[edited by] Mi Ja Kim, Gertrude K. McFarland,
    Audrey M. McLane.—7th ed.
        p.   cm.
    Includes index.
    ISBN 0-8151-4989-1
    1. Nursing diagnosis—Handbooks, manuals, etc.   2. Nursing care
plans—Handbooks, manuals, etc.   I. Kim, Mi Ja.   II. McFarland, Gertrude K.,
III. McLane, Audrey M.
    [DNLM: 1. Nursing Diagnosis—handbooks, 2. Patient Care
Planning—handbooks.   WY 49 P7395 1997]
RT48.6.P63   1997
616.07'5—dc21
DNLM/DLC   97-5479

00 01/9 8 7 6 5 4 3 2

Contributors

Kim Astroth, RN, MS
Clinical Instructor
Mennonite College of Nursing
Bloomington, Illinois

Sarah McNabb Badalamenti, RN, MSN
Clinical Nurse Specialist
St. Joseph's Hospital
Milwaukee, Wisconsin

Thelma I. Bates, RN, MSN, CS
Clinical Nurse Specialist
Washington Hospital Center
Washington, DC

Jean K. Berry, RN, PhD
Clinical Assistant Professor, Medical Surgical
University of Illinois at Chicago

Howard K. Butcher, RN, PhD, CS
Assistant Professor
Pacific Lutheran University
Takoma, Washington

Joan M. Caley, RN, MS, CS, CNAA*
Associate Chief Nurse/Long Term Care
Department of Veterans Affairs
Medical Center/Vancouver Division
Portland, Oregon

*The opinions expressed herein are those of the authors and do not necessarily reflect those of the National Institutes of Health, U.S. Public Health Service, U.S. Department of Health and Human Services, the Veterans Administration, or the Uniformed Services University of the Health Sciences.

Nancy S. Creason, BSN, MSN, PhD
School of Nursing and Health Sciences
University of Alaska-Anchorage
Anchorage, Alaska

Kathryn T. Czurylo, RN, MS, CS
Surgical Clinical Nurse Specialist
Alexian Brothers Medical Center
Elk Grove Village, Illinois

Donna M. Dixon, RN, MS
Instructor, Clinical Nursing
University of Missouri-Columbia
Columbia, Missouri

Susan Dudas, RN, MSN, FAAN
Associate Professor Emerita
University of Illinois at Chicago
Chicago, Illinois

Teresa Fadden, RN, MSN, CS
Clinical Nurse IV
St. Joseph's Hospital
Milwaukee, Wisconsin

Richard Fehring, RN, DNSc
Associate Professor
Marquette University
College of Nursing
Milwaukee, Wisconsin

Diane Marie Fesler, RN, MSN
Perioperative Clinical Specialist
Clinical Faculty
University of Illinois
Chicago, Illinois

Margaret I. Fitch, RN, PhD
Oncology Nurse Researcher
Comprehensive Cancer Program at
Toronto-Bayview Regional Cancer Centre/
Sunnybrook Health Sciences Centre
Faculty of Nursing, University of Toronto
Toronto, Ontario, Canada

Margie L. French, RN, MS, CS*
Clinical Nurse Specialist
Clinical Manager
Comprehensive Rehabilitation Unit
Veterans Health Administration Medical Center
Vancouver Division
Portland, Oregon

Michele Gattuso, RN, MS
Clinical Nurse Specialist
Maternal Child Health
Alexian Brothers Medical Center
Elk Grove Village, Illinois

Elizabeth Kelchner Gerety, RN, MS, CS, FAAN*
Clinical Nurse Specialist
Psychiatry Consultation
Portland Veterans Affairs Medical Center
Portland, Oregon

Wendy Goetter, RN, MS, CNRN
Neuroscience Clinical Specialist
University of Illinois Medical Center at Chicago
Adjunct Clinical Instructor, College of Nursing
Chicago, Illinois

Jane E. Graydon, PhD, RN
Associate Professor and Chair
University of Toronto
Toronto, Ontario, Canada

Terry Griffin, RN, BSN, MS, NNP
NNP
Rush Presbyterian St. Lukes Hospital
Chicago, Illinois

Mary V. Hanley, MA, RN*
Critical Care Nursing Instructor
DVA, VA Medical Center/Outpatient Clinics
Nursing Education
Boston, Massachusetts

Marilyn Harter, RN, MSN, CRRN
Clinical Nurse Specialist
Rehabilitation Services
St. Luke's Medical Center
Clinical Instructor
Marquette University, College of Nursing
Milwaukee, Wisconsin

Kathryn Hennessy, RN, MS, CNSN
Manager, Nursing Services
Clintec Nutrition Company
Deerfield, Illinois

Pamela D. Hill, RN, BSN, MS, PhD
Associate Professor
University of Illinois at Chicago
Quad-Cities Regional Program
Rock Island, Illinois

Karen E. Inaba, MS, RN, CS
Psychiatric Mental Health Nurse Practitioner
Multnomah County Health Department
Portland, Oregon

Joyce H. Johnson, RN, MSN, PhD
Associate Professor
University of Illinois at Chicago
College of Nursing
Chicago, Illinois

Karen Kavanaugh, RN, PhD
Assistant Professor
University of Illinois at Chicago
Chicago, Illinois

Jin H. Kim, RN, MSN, PhD
Assistant Professor
School of Nursing
Northern Illinois University
Dekalb, Illinois

Mi Ja Kim, RN, PhD, FAAN
Vice Chancellor for Research
Dean of Graduate College
University of Illinois at Chicago
Chicago, Illinois

Kristin M. Kleinschmidt, MS, RN
Clinical Nurse Specialist
Arrhythmia Center
Midwest Heart Specialists
Downers Grove, Illinois

Pamela Wolfe Kohlbry, RN, MSN
San Marcos, California

Patricia A. Koller, RN, MSN
Clinical Care Nurse III, Intensive Care
St. Joseph's Hospital
Milwaukee, Wisconsin

Candice S. Korb, RN, MSN
Staff Nurse
Cross Country Healthcare
Boca Raton, Florida

Carol E. Kupperberg, RN, BSN, MSN
Nurse Coordinator
Montgomery County Infants and Toddlers Program
Rockville, Maryland

Jane Lancour, RN, MSN
President
JML
Irvine, California

Janet L. Larson, PhD, RN, FAAN
Associate Professor
University of Illinois at Chicago
College of Nursing
Chicago, Illinois

Lorna A. Larson, RN, DNSc
Home Health-Mental Health Nurse
Adventist Home Health Services
Silver Spring, Maryland

Marie Maguire, RN, MSN, CNS
Director of Quality Management
Lakeland Nursing Home
Elkhorn, Wisconsin

Gertrude K. McFarland, RN, DNSc, FAAN*
Health Scientist Administrator
Nursing Research Study Section
Division of Research Grants
National Institutes of Health
Bethesda, Maryland

Audrey M. McLane, RN, PhD
Professor Emerita
College of Nursing
Marquette University
Milwaukee, Wisconsin

Ruth E. McShane, RN, PhD
Assistant Professor
University of Wisconsin at Milwaukee
School of Nursing
Milwaukee, Wisconsin

Karen McWhorter, RN, MN, CS*
Clinical Nurse Specialist
Adult Day Health Care Program
Veterans Health Administration Medical Center
Vancouver Division
Portland, Oregon

Judy Minton, RN, MS, FNP
Nurse Practitioner
Decatur, Illinois

Victoria L. Mock, RN, DNSc, OCN
Director of Nursing Research
The Johns Hopkins Oncology Center
Baltimore, Maryland

Martha M. Morris, RN, MSN, EdD
Associate Professor
School of Nursing
Saint Louis University Medical Center
St. Louis, Missouri

Charlotte E. Naschinski, RN, MS*
Deputy Director, Continuing Education for Health Professional
Uniformed University of the Health Sciences
Bethesda, Maryland

Emma B. Nemivant, RN, MSN, MEd
Clinical Instructor
Department of Maternal-Child Nursing
College of Nursing
University of Illinois at Chicago
Chicago, Illinois

Colleen M. O'Brien, MSN, RN
Clinical Educator
Bellin Hospital
Green Bay, Wisconsin

Linda O'Brien-Pallas, RN, PhD
Associate Professor and Career Scientist
Faculty of Nursing
University of Toronto
Toronto, Ontario, Canada

Annette O'Connor, RN, BScN, MScN, PhD
Associate Professor
University of Ottawa
School of Nursing
Ottawa, Ontario, Canada

Laura Pace Omer, BSN, MA*
Director of Continuing Education for Health Professionals
Uniform Services of University of the Health Sciences
Rockville, Maryland

Catherine J. Ryan, RN, MS, CCRN
Clinical Nurse Specialist–Critical Care
Alexian Brothers Medical Center
Elk Grove Village, Illinois

Karen V. Scipio-Skinner, MSN, RNC
Legislative/Practice Specialist
District of Columbia Nurses Association
Washington, DC

Maureen Shekleton, DNSc, RN
Satellite Site Coordinator
DuPage Community Clinic
Wheaton, Illinois
Adjunct Assistant Professor
University of Illinois at Chicago
College of Nursing
Chicago, Illinois

Kathleen C. Sheppard, RN, PhD
Director, Quality Improvement
University of Texas
M.D. Anderson Cancer Center
Houston, Texas

Margaret J. Stafford, RN, MSN, FAAN
Consultant/Lecturer in Cardiac Nursing/Professional Issues
Adjunct Assistant Professor, College of Nursing
University of Illinois at Chicago
Chicago, Illinois

Contributors—cont'd

Janet F. Stansberry, RN, MSN
Clinical Nurse Specialist, Infertility
University of Pennsylvania
Philadelphia, Pennsylvania

Rosemarie Suhayda, RN, PhD
Assistant Professor
Rush University
College of Nursing
Chicago, Illinois

Marie L. Talashek, RN, CS, EdD
Associate Professor
University of Illinois at Chicago
College of Nursing
Chicago, Illinois

Alice M. Tse, RN, PhD
Assistant Professor of Nursing and Medicine
University of Hawaii at Manoa
School of Nursing
Honolulu, Hawaii

Evelyn L. Wasli, RN, DNSc
Chief Nurse
Emergency Psychiatric Response Division
Commission of Mental Health Services
Washington, DC

Rosemary White-Traut, RN, DNSc
Associate Professor and Coordinator
Graduate Pediatric and Perinatal Programs
Department of Maternal-Child Nursing
University of Illinois at Chicago
Chicago, Illinois

Linda K. Young, RN, MSN
Assistant Professor
MSOE-School of Nursing
Milwaukee, Wisconsin

Contributors—cont'd

Preface

Since the first edition of the *Pocket Guide to Nursing Diagnoses* in 1984, nursing diagnoses have become integrated into nursing education, research, and practice in the United States. In addition, nursing diagnosis has gained acceptance in various countries and our *Pocket Guide* has so far been translated into six languages, including Japanese and French. Nursing students find nursing diagnoses to be a useful tool of learning. Both nursing students and practicing nurses find nursing diagnoses a useful way of conceptualizing nursing science and focusing on clinical decision making. Educators have adopted nursing diagnoses as an organizing framework for teaching and practice. Nurse researchers are using nursing diagnoses as a focus for research, while the North American Nursing Diagnoses Association (NANDA) taxonomy taken as a whole presents a challenge for systematic validation through research.

The nursing profession and its specialty organizations recognize the contribution of a nursing nosology to their ability to demonstrate the effectiveness of nursing practice and to influence health care policy. Given developments in the national health care agenda, nurses will have an expanded role as key health care providers, a trend in which nursing diagnosis can and will play a key role.

Finally, nursing diagnoses do and will continue to influence deliberations at the international level through such organizations as the International Council of Nurses (ICN). Currently an International Classification for Nursing Practice is being developed by nurse experts under the leadership of the ICN. Nursing diagnoses developed by NANDA played a significant role in the development of this work. The outcome of this work will most likely be submitted to the World Health Organization for the next edition of the *International Classification of Diseases—Clinical Modification (ICD-CM)*. This is significant progress at the international level and inclusion of a nursing taxonomy in such a standard classification system used worldwide will definitely improve nursing's ability to communicate more effectively, thereby stimulating the growth and dissemination of nursing's knowledge.

The major purposes of the *Pocket Guide* continue to be:

1. To present the most up-to-date information on NANDA nursing diagnoses terminology, definitions, related/risk factors, and defining characteristics
2. To present a prototype state-of-the-art care plan for each nursing diagnosis
3. To provide an easy-to-use guide for clinicians, faculty, and students in their daily practice
4. To stimulate critical thinking of practicing nurses, and
5. To facilitate the use of theory and research-based nursing interventions in the practice setting.

We are deeply indebted to the users of this book who generously provided their suggestions and who continue to endorse this book.

In keeping with the philosophy of the previous editions, every effort has been made to make this *Pocket Guide* easy to use while providing a theoretical and research base for each prototype care plan. We have chosen to present nursing diagnoses in alphabetical order because the conceptual framework for the organization of nursing diagnoses is still under development. The current NANDA taxonomy is presented in Appendix A for those who may want to know the taxonomic structure for these diagnoses. All NANDA-approved diagnoses are covered in this *Pocket Guide*, including the revisions approved in 1996.

Defining characteristics and related/risk factors presented are NANDA-approved, and the same is true for the majority of definitions. Definitions of nursing diagnoses approved by NANDA have been used to the extent they were developed. For completeness, we developed definitions for diagnoses that do not have definitions.

A concerted effort has been made to present nursing care plans as prototypes rather than standard care plans. By making the care plans prototypes, we have emphasized that they are for specific individuals or a group of patients with specified related/risk factors. Therefore in applying these plans to patients, practicing nurses will need to give specific consideration to individual patient requirements.

Each care plan was developed on the basis of a nursing diagnosis that comprises a diagnostic label and the term **"related to"** for related or risk factors. For example, if the nursing diagnosis for Risk for injury with a risk factor of "emotional lability," the nurse would record this as "Risk for injury related to emotional lability." We used the following guide for the development of the prototype care plans.

- The patient goals/expected outcomes reflect the desired health state of a patient and specify indicators addressing the extent of achievement of the patient goal(s).
- Scientific rationales are specified for interventions or cluster of interventions.
- Clinical conditions or medical diagnoses are specified for each care plan to emphasize the medical diagnosis/ nursing diagnosis link which make the care plans more focused for a specific type of patient.
- Nursing interventions are selected to address related facts or risk factors, to ameliorate/modify defining characteristics, and to assist patients in achieving their goals and optimal health state.
- Prevention is an important component of the care plans where possible.
- Nursing diagnosis and the selected nursing interventions reflect contributions the nurse can make within today's interdisciplinary environment and the importance of interdisciplinary teamwork.

The care plans were developed from a perspective of persons interacting with their environment in the pursuit of health. The use of nursing diagnoses and relevant nursing interventions are designed to meet patient goals and this has sharpened the focus of current practice and has demonstrated the usefulness of nursing diagnoses for contributing to quality health care.

Contributing authors of the *Pocket Guide* are clinical experts who reflect the state-of-the-art and science of nursing practice. We acknowledge substantive contributions made by practicing nurses to the development and refinement of nursing diagnoses. Practicing nurses are encouraged to engage in critical thinking while using the prototype care plans. Their participation in research on all nursing diagnoses is essential for the national and international development of nursing diagnoses taxonomy and a scientific base for nursing practice. There is also a critical need to comprehensively evaluate the nursing diagnostic terminology and taxonomy through ongoing nursing research. Advancements made in these areas are promising and we look forward to continuing our dialogue with all of you on the topic of nursing diagnosis through this book.

Mi Ja Kim
Gertrude K. McFarland
Audrey M. McLane

Practical tips for using the Pocket Guide

- If a nursing diagnosis is suggested by the assessment format you are using, look up the nursing diagnosis in Section One, "Nursing diagnoses: definitions, related/risk factors, and defining characteristics," and review the definition, defining characteristics, and the related/risk factors. Determine if the suggested nursing diagnosis is appropriate.

- Review the corresponding care plan for the chosen nursing diagnoses in Section Two, "Nursing diagnoses: prototype care plans." Determine which patient goals, expected outcomes, and nursing interventions are applicable to your patient.

- In Section Three, further nursing interventions along with their definitions are listed under each nursing diagnosis. This list supplies additional nursing interventions that may be applicable to your patient.

North American Nursing Diagnosis Association's (NANDA) Working Definition of Nursing Diagnosis

Nursing diagnosis is a clinical judgment about individual, family, or community responses to actual or potential health problems/life processes. Nursing diagnoses provide the basis for selection of nursing interventions to achieve outcomes for which the nurse is accountable.

Approved at the Ninth Conference on Classification of Nursing Diagnoses.

International Classification of Nursing Practice's (ICNP) Proposed Definition of Nursing Diagnosis

The description or label given by a nurse to the particular condition or human response which the nurse has identified as being the reason for a nursing intervention.

From *Nursing's Next Advance: An International Classification for Nursing Practice*, ICN Working Paper, April 1993, p. 11.

Contents

NURSING DIAGNOSES

Definitions, Related/Risk Factors, and Defining Characteristics

Activity intolerance

The state in which an individual has insufficient physiological or psychological energy to endure or complete required or desired daily activities.

Related factors
Generalized weakness
Sedentary lifestyle
Imbalance between oxygen supply and demand
Bed rest or immobility

Defining characteristics
Verbal report of fatigue or weakness
Abnormal heart rate or blood pressure response to
    activity
Exertional discomfort or dyspnea.
Electrocardiographic changes reflecting arrhythmias
    or ischemia

Activity intolerance, risk for

The state in which an individual is at risk of experiencing insufficient physiological or psychological energy to endure or complete required or desired daily activities.

Risk factors
History of previous intolerance
Deconditioned status
Presence of circulatory/respiratory problems
Inexperience with the activity

Adaptive capacity, decreased: intracranial

A clinical state in which intracranial fluid dynamic mechanisms that normally compensate for increases in intracranial volumes are compromised, resulting in repeated disproportionate increases in intracranial pressure (ICP) in response to a variety of noxious and non-noxious stimuli.

Related factors
Brain injuries
Sustained increase in ICP $\geq$ 10-15 mm Hg

Decreased cerebral perfusion pressure ≤ 50-60 mm Hg
Systemic hypotension with intracranial hypertension

Defining characteristics
Major
Repeated increases in ICP > 10 mm Hg for more
than 5 minutes following any of a variety of
external stimuli.
Minor
Disproportionate increase in ICP following single
environmental of nursing maneuver stimulus
Elevated P2 ICP waveform
Volume pressure response test variation (Volume-
pressure ratio >2, Pressure-volume index <10
Baseline ICP ≥ 10 mm Hg
Wide amplitude ICP waveform

Adjustment, impaired

The state in which an individual is unable to modify his/her
lifestyle behavior in a manner consistent with a change in health
status.

Related factors
Disability requiring change in lifestyle
Inadequate support systems
Impaired cognition
Sensory overload
Assault to self-esteem
Altered locus of control
Incomplete grieving

Defining characteristics
Verbalization of nonacceptance of health status
change
Nonexistent or unsuccessful ability to be involved in
problem solving or goal setting
Lack of movement toward independence
Extended period of shock, disbelief, or anger regard-
ing health status change
Lack of future-oriented thinking

Airway clearance, ineffective

The state in which an individual is unable to clear secretions or obstructions from the respiratory tract.

Related factors
Decreased energy
Tracheobronchial infection, obstruction, secretion
Perceptual/cognitive impairment
Trauma

Defining characteristics
Abnormal breath sounds (crackles, gurgles, wheezes)
Cough, ineffective or absent
Reports difficulty with sputum
Reports of chest congestion

Other possible defining characteristics
Change in rate and depth of respiration
Effective cough
Tenacious and copious sputum
Fatigue

Anxiety

A vague, uneasy feeling, the source of which is often nonspecific or unknown to the individual.

Related factors
Unconscious conflict about essential values and goals of life
Threat to self-concept
Threat of death
Threat to or change in health status
Threat to or change in socioeconomic status
Threat to or change in role functioning
Threat to or change in environment
Threat to or change in interaction patterns
Situational and maturational crises
Interpersonal transmission and contagion
Unmet needs

Defining characteristics
Subjective
Increased tension

Apprehension
Increased helplessness
Uncertainty
Fear
Feeling of being scared
Feeling of inadequacy
Shakiness
Fear of unspecific consequences
Regretfulness
Overexcitedness
Feeling of being rattled
Distress
Jitteriness

Objective
Sympathetic stimulation—cardiovascular excitation, superficial vasoconstriction, pupil dilation
Restlessness
Insomnia
Glancing about
Poor eye contact
Trembling; hand tremors
Extraneous movements—foot shuffling; hand, arm movements
Expressed concern regarding changes in life events
Worry
Anxiety
Facial tension
Voice quivering
Focus on self
Increased wariness
Increased perspiration

Aspiration, risk for

The state in which an individual is at risk for entry of gastric secretions, oropharyngeal secretions, or exogenous food or fluids into tracheobronchial passages due to dysfunction or absence of normal protective mechanisms.

Risk factors
Reduced level of consciousness
Depressed cough and gag reflexes

Presence of tracheotomy or endotracheal tube
Overinflated tracheotomy/endotracheal tube cuff
Inadequate tracheotomy/endotracheal tube cuff
    inflation
Gastrointestinal tubes
Bolus tube feedings/medication administration
Situations hindering elevation of upper body
Increased intragastric pressure
Increased gastric residual
Decreased gastrointestinal motility
Delayed gastric emptying
Impaired swallowing
Facial/oral/neck surgery or trauma
Wired jaws

Body image disturbance

Disruption in the way one perceives one's body image.

Related factors
Biophysical
Cognitive perceptual
Psychosocial
Cultural or spiritual

Defining characteristics
Either the following A or B must be present to justify
    the diagnosis of body image disturbance:
    A. Verbal response to actual or perceived change in
        structure and/or function
    B. Nonverbal response to actual or perceived
        change in structure and/or function
The following clinical manifestations may be used to
    validate the presence of A or B:
  Objective
  Missing body part
  Actual change in structure and/or function
  Not looking at body part
  Not touching body part
  Hiding or overexposing body part (intentional or
      unintentional)
  Trauma to nonfunctioning part

Change in social involvement
Negative feelings about body
Feelings of helplessness, hopelessness, or power-
lessness
Preoccupation with change or loss
Emphasis on remaining strengths, heightened
achievement
Extension of body boundary to incorporate envi-
ronmental objects
Personalization of part or loss by name
Depersonalization of part or loss by impersonal
pronouns
Refusal to verify actual change
It may be possible to identify high-risk pop-
ulations, such as those with the following
conditions:
Missing body part
Dependence on a machine
Significance of body part or functioning with
regard to age, gender, developmental level, or
basic human needs
Physical change caused by biochemical agents
(drugs)
Physical trauma or mutilation
Pregnancy and/or maturational changes

Body temperature, altered, risk for

The state in which an individual is at risk for failure to maintain
body temperature within normal range.

Risk factors
Extremes of age
Extremes of weight
Exposure to cold/cool or warm/hot environments
Dehydration
Inactivity or vigorous activity
Medications causing vasoconstriction/vasodilation,
altered metabolic rate, sedation
Inappropriate clothing for environmental tem-
perature
Illness or trauma affecting temperature regulation

Bowel incontinence

The state in which an individual experiences a change in normal bowel habits characterized by involuntary passage of stool.

Related factors
Neuromuscular involvement
Musculoskeletal involvement
Depression, severe anxiety
Perception or cognitive impairment

Defining characteristic
Involuntary passage of stool

Breastfeeding, effective

The state in which a mother-infant dyad/family exhibits adequate proficiency and satisfaction with breastfeeding process.

Related factors
Basic breastfeeding knowledge
Normal breast structure
Normal infant oral structure
Infant gestational age greater than 34 weeks
Support sources
Maternal confidence

Defining characteristics
Mother able to position infant at breast to promote a
    successful latch-on response
Infant is content after feeding
Regular and sustained suckling/swallowing at the
    breast
Appropriate infant weight patterns for age
Effective mother-infant communication patterns (in-
    fant cues, maternal interpretation and response)
Signs and/or symptoms of oxytocin release (let-down
    or milk ejection reflex)
Adequate infant elimination patterns for age
Eagerness of infant to nurse
Maternal verbalization of satisfaction with the breast-
    feeding process

Breastfeeding, ineffective

The state in which a mother, infant, and/or family experiences dissatisfaction or difficulty with the breastfeeding process.

Related factors
Prematurity
Infant anomaly
Maternal breast anomaly
Previous breast surgery
Previous history of breastfeeding failure
Infant receiving supplemental feedings with artificial nipple
Poor infant sucking reflex
Nonsupportive partner/family
Knowledge deficit
Interruption in breastfeeding

Defining characteristics
Unsatisfactory breastfeeding process
Actual or perceived inadequate milk supply
Infant's inability to attach on to maternal nipple correctly
No observable signs of oxytocin release
Observable signs of inadequate infant intake
Nonsustained suckling at breast
Nursing less than 7 times in 24 hours
Persistence of sore nipples beyond first week of infant's life
Maternal reluctance to put infant to breast as necessary
Infant exhibiting fussiness and crying within first hour after breastfeeding; unresponsive to other comfort measures
Infant arching and crying at breast; resisting latching on

Breastfeeding, interrupted

A break in the continuity of the breastfeeding process as a result of inability or inadvisability to put baby to breast for feeding.

Related factors
Maternal or infant illness

Prematurity

Maternal employment

Contraindications to breastfeeding (e.g., drugs, true breastmilk jaundice)

Need to abruptly wean infant

Defining characteristics

Major

Infant does not receive nourishment at the breast for some or all of feedings

Minor

Maternal desire to maintain lactation and provide (or eventually provide) her breastmilk for her infant's nutritional needs

Separation of mother and infant

Lack of knowledge about expression and storage of breastmilk

Breathing pattern, ineffective

A state in which the rate, depth, timing, rhythm or chest/abdominal wall excursion during inspiration, expiration, or both does not maintain optimum ventilation for the individual.

Related factors

Neuromuscular impairment

Pain, musculoskeletal impairment

Perception/cognitive impairment

Anxiety

Decreased energy/fatigue

Defining characteristics

Dyspnea, shortness of breath

Respiratory rate (adults [ages 14 or greater] < 11 or > 24, infants < 25 or > 60, ages 1 to 4 < 20 or > 30, ages 5 to 14 < 15 or > 25)

Depth of breathing (adults VT < 200 ml or > 500 ml at rest, infants 6 to 8 ml/kg)

Timing ratio of inspiration and expiration (if measured): inspiratory time < 1:2 or > 2:4), fractional inspiratory time < 0.36 or > 0.47, inspiration longer than expiration

Irregular breathing rhythm (e.g., apnea, frequent

signs, use of accessory muscles of breathing inappropriate to level of activity, asynchronous thoracoabdominal motion)
Grunting
Nasal flaring (infants)
Paradoxical breathing patterns
Use of accessory muscles
Altered chest excursion

Other possible defining characteristics
Fremitus
Abnormal arterial blood gas
Cyanosis
Cough
Assumption of three-point position
Pursed lip breathing
Prolonged expiratory phases
Increased anteroposterior diameter

Cardiac output, decreased

A state in which the blood pumped by the heart is inadequate to meet the metabolic demands of the body.

Related factors
To be developed

Defining characteristics
Variations in blood pressure (BP) readings
Arrhythmias
Fatigue
Jugular venous distention
Skin color changes
Rales
Oliguria
Decreased peripheral pulses
Cold, clammy skin
Dyspnea
Orthopnea/paroxysmal nocturnal dyspnea
Restlessness
Chest pain
Weight gain
Wheezing

Edema
Elevated pulmonary arterial (PA) pressures
Increased respiratory rate; use of accessory muscles
Electrocardiogram changes
Ejection fraction < 40%
Abnormal chest x-ray (pulmonary vascular congestion)
Abnormal cardiac enzymes
Altered mental status

Other possible defining characteristics
Decreased peripheral pulses
Decreased cardiac output (CO) by thermodilution method
Increased heart rate
S_3 or S_4, cough
Mixed venous O_2 (SaO_2)

Caregiver role strain

A caregiver's felt difficulty in performing the family caregiver role.

Related factors
  Pathophysiological/physiological
   Severity of illness of the care receiver
   Addiction or codependency
   Premature birth/congenital defect
   Discharge of family member with significant home healthcare needs
   Caregiver health impairment
   Unpredictable illness course or instability in the care receiver's health
   Gender of caregiver (female)
  Developmental
   Developmental inability to fulfill caregiver role (e.g., a young adult needing to provide care for a middle-aged parent)
   Developmental delay or retardation of the care receiver or caregiver
  Psychosocial
   Psychological or cognitive problems in care receiver

Marginal family adaption or dysfunction before caregiving became necessary

Marginal coping patterns of caregiver

History of poor relationship with care receiver

Spousal relationship to care receiver

Care receiver exhibits deviant, bizarre behavior

Situational

Presence of abuse or violence

Presence of situational stressors that normally affect families, such as significant loss, disaster or crisis, poverty or economic vulnerability, major life events (e.g., birth, hospitalization, leaving home, returning home, marriage, divorce, employment, retirement, and death)

Duration of caregiving required

Inadequate physical environment for providing care (e.g., housing, transportation, community services, equipment)

Isolation

Lack of respite and recreation

Inexperience with caregiving

Competing role commitments

Complexity/number of caregiving tasks

Defining characteristics

Not having enough resources to provide the care needed

Finding it hard to do specific caregiving activities

Worry about such things as the care receiver's health and emotional state, having to put the care receiver in an institution, and who will care for the care receiver if something should happen to the caregiver

Feeling that caregiving interferes with other important roles in caregiver's life

Feeling loss because the care receiver is like a different person as compared with before caregiving began or, in the case of a child, that the care receiver was never the child the caregiver expected

Family conflict around issues of providing care

Stress or nervousness in the relationship with the care receiver

Depression

Caregiver role strain, risk for

A caregiver is vulnerable for felt difficulty in performing the family caregiver role.

Risk factors
Pathophysiological
Severity of illness of the care receiver

Addiction or codependency

Premature birth/congenital defect

Discharge of family member with significant home healthcare needs

Caregiver health impairment

Unpredictable illness course or instability in the care receiver's health

Gender of caregiver (female)

Psychological or cognitive problems in care receiver

Developmental
Developmental inability to fulfill caregiver role (e.g., a young adult needing to provide care for middle-age parent)

Developmental delay or retardation of the care receiver or caregiver

Psychological
Marginal family adaptation or dysfunction before caregiving became necessary

Marginal coping patterns of caregiver

History of poor relationship with care receiver

Spousal relationship to care receiver

Care receiver exhibits deviant, bizarre behavior

Situational
Presence of abuse or violence

Presence of situational stressors that normally affect families, such as significant loss, disaster or crisis, poverty or economic vulnerability, major life events (e.g., birth, hospitalization, leaving home, returning home, marriage, divorce, employment, retirement, and death)

Duration of caregiving required
Inadequate physical environment for providing
    care (e.g., housing, transportation, community
    services, equipment)
Isolation
Lack of respite and recreation
Inexperience with caregiving
Competing role commitments
Complexity/number of caregiving tasks

Communication, impaired verbal

The state in which an individual experiences a decreased or
absent ability to use or understand language in human
interaction.

Related factors
Decrease in circulation to brain
Physical barrier, brain tumor, tracheostomy, intu-
    bation
Anatomic deficit, cleft palate
Psychological barriers, psychosis, lack of stimuli
Cultural difference
Developmental or age-related

Defining characteristics
Inability to speak dominant language
Refusal or inability to speak
Stuttering; slurring
Impaired articulation
Dyspnea
Disorientation
Inability to modulate speech
Inability to find words
Inability to name words
Inability to identify objects
Loose association of ideas
Flight of ideas
Incessant verbalization
Difficulty with phonation
Inability to speak in sentences

Community coping, potential for enhanced

A pattern of community activities for adaptation and problem solving that is satisfactory for meeting the demands or needs of the community but can be improved for management of current and future problems/stressors.

Related factors
Social supports available
Resources available for problem solving
Community has a sense of power to manage stressors

Defining characteristics
Major
Deficits in one or more characteristics that indicate effective coping
Minor
Active planning by community for predicted stressors
Active problem solving by community when faced with issues
Agreement that community is responsible for stress management
Positive communication among community members
Positive communication between community/ aggregates and larger community
Programs available for recreation and relaxation
Resources sufficient for managing stressors

Community coping, ineffective

A pattern of community activities for adaptation and problem solving that is unsatisfactory for meeting the demands or needs of the community.

Related factors
Deficits in social support
Inadequate resources for problem solving
Powerlessness

Defining characteristics
  Major
  None
  Minor
  Community does not meet its own expectations
  Deficits of community participation
  Deficits in communication methods
  Excessive community conflicts
  Expressed difficulty in meeting demands for
      change
  Expressed vulnerability
  High illness rates
  Stressors perceived as excessive

Confusion, acute

The abrupt onset of a cluster of global, transient changes and disturbances in attention, cognition, psychomotor activity level of consciousness, and/or sleep/wake cycle.

Related factors
Over 60 years of age
Dementia
Alcohol abuse
Drug abuse
Delirium

Defining characteristics
  Major
  Fluctuation in cognition
  Fluctuation in sleep-wake cycle
  Fluctuation in level of consciousness
  Fluctuation in psychomotor activity
  Increased agitation or restlessness
  Misperceptions
  Lack of motivation to initiate or follow through
      with goal-directed or purposeful behavior
  Minor
  Hallucinations

Confusion, chronic

An irreversible, long-standing and/or progressive deterioration of intellect and personality characterized by decreased ability to interpret environmental stimuli, decreased capacity for intellectual thought processes and manifested by disturbances of memory, orientation, and behavior.

Related factors
Alzheimer's disease
Korsakoff's psychosis
Multi-infarct dementia
Cerebrovascular accident
Head injury

Defining characteristics
  Major
    Clinical evidence of organic impairment
    Altered interpretation of or response to stimuli
    Progressive or long-standing cognitive impairment
  Minor
    No change in level of consciousness
    Impaired socialization
    Impaired memory (short term, long term)
    Altered personality

Constipation

The state in which an individual experiences a change in normal bowel habits characterized by a decrease in frequency and/or passage of hard, dry stools.

Related factors
Less than adequate intake
Less than adequate dietary intake and bulk
Less than adequate physical activity or immobility
Personal habits
Medications
Chronic use of medication and enemas
Gastrointestinal obstructive lesions
Neuromuscular impairment
Musculoskeletal impairment
Pain on defecation

Diagnostic procedures
Lack of privacy
Weak abdominal musculature
Pregnancy
Emotional status

Defining characteristics
Frequency less than usual pattern
Hard-formed stool
Palpable mass
Reported feeling of rectal fullness
Straining at stool
Decreased bowel sound
Reported feeling of abdominal or rectal fullness or
    pressure
Less than usual amount of stool
Nausea

Other possible defining characteristics
Abdominal pain
Back pain
Headache
Interference with daily living
Use of laxatives
Decreased appetite
Appetite impairment

Constipation, colonic

The state in which an individual's pattern of elimination is
characterized by hard, dry stool that results from a delay in
passage of food residue.

Related factors
Less than adequate fluid intake
Less than adequate dietary intake
Less than adequate fiber intake
Less than adequate physical activity
Immobility
Lack of privacy
Emotional disturbances
Chronic use of medication and enemas
Stress

Change in daily routine
Metabolic problems (e.g., hypothyroidism, hypocal-
cemia, hypokalemia)

Defining characteristics
Decreased frequency
Hard, dry stool
Straining at stool
Painful defecation
Abdominal distention
Palpable mass
Rectal pressure
Headache, appetite impairment
Abdominal pain

Constipation, perceived

The state in which an individual makes a self-diagnosis of
constipation and ensures a daily bowel movement through use
of laxatives, enemas, and suppositories.

Related factors
Cultural/family health beliefs
Faulty appraisal
Impaired thought processes

Defining characteristics
Expectation of a daily bowel movement with resulting
overuse of laxatives, enemas, and suppositories
Expected passage of stool at same time every day

Coping, defensive

The state in which an individual experiences falsely positive self-
evaluation based on a self-protective pattern that defends
against underlying perceived threats to positive self-regard.

Related factors
To be developed

Defining characteristics
Denial (of obvious problems, weaknesses)
Projection (of blame/responsibility)
Rationalization of failures

Defensiveness (hypersensitivity to criticism)
Grandiosity
Superior attitude toward others
Difficulty establishing/maintaining relationships
Hostile laughter or ridicule of others
Difficulty in reality testing of perceptions
Lack of follow-through or participation in treatment
    or therapy

Coping, family: potential for growth

Effective managing of adaptive tasks by family member involved
with the patient's health challenge, who now is exhibiting desire
and readiness for enhanced health and growth in regard to self
and in relation to the patient.

Related factors
Needs sufficiently gratified and adaptive tasks effec-
    tively addressed to enable goals of self-actualiza-
    tion to surface

Defining characteristics
Family members attempt to describe growth impact
    of crisis on their own values, priorities, goals, or
    relationships
Family member is moving in direction of health-
    promoting and enriching lifestyle that supports
    and monitors maturational processes, audits and
    negotiates treatment programs, and generally
    chooses experiences that optimize wellness
Individual expresses interest in making contact on a
    one-to-one basis or on a mutual-aid group basis
    with another person who has experienced a similar
    situation

Coping, ineffective family: compromised

A usually supportive primary person (family member or close
friend) is providing insufficient, ineffective, or compromised
support, comfort, assistance, or encouragement which may be
needed by the client to manage or master adaptive tasks related
to his or her health challenge.

Related factors
Inadequate or incorrect information or understanding by a primary person
Temporary preoccupation by a significant person who is trying to manage emotional conflicts and personal suffering and is unable to perceive or act effectively in regard to needs
Temporary family disorganization and role changes
Other situational or developmental crises or situations the significant person may be facing
Little support provided by client, in turn, for primary person
Prolonged disease or disability progression that exhausts supportive capacity of significant people

Defining characteristics
Subjective
Patient expresses or confirms a concern or complaint about significant other's response to his or her health problem
Significant person describes preoccupation with personal reaction (e.g., fear, anticipatory grief, guilt, anxiety to illness, disability, or to other situational or developmental crises)
Significant person describes or confirms an inadequate understanding or knowledge base that interferes with effective assistive or supportive behaviors
Objective
Significant person attempts assistive or supportive behaviors with less than satisfactory results
Significant person withdraws or enters into limited or temporary personal communication with the client at the time of need
Significant person displays protective behavior disproportionate (too little or too much) to the abilities or need for autonomy

Coping, ineffective family: disabling

Behavior of significant person (family member or other primary person) that disables his or her own capacities and the capacity to effectively address tasks essential to either person's adaptation to the health challenge.

Related factors

Significant person with chronically unexpressed feelings of guilt, anxiety, hostility, despair, etc.

Dissonant discrepancy of coping styles for dealing with adaptive tasks by the significant person and patient or among significant people

Highly ambivalent family relationships

Arbitrary handling of family's resistance to treatment, which tends to solidify defensiveness, as it fails to deal adequately with underlying anxiety

Defining characteristics

Neglectful care of the patient in regard to basic human needs and/or illness treatment

Distortion of reality regarding the health problem, including extreme denial about its existence or severity

Intolerance

Rejection

Abandonment

Desertion

Carrying on usual routines, disregarding needs

Psychosomaticism

Taking on illness signs of client

Decisions and actions by family that are detrimental to economic or social well-being

Agitation, depression, aggression, hostility

Impaired restructuring of a meaningful life for self

Impaired individualization, prolonged over concern for patient

Neglectful relationships with other family members

Patient's development of helpless, inactive dependence

Coping, ineffective individual

Impairment of adaptive behaviors and abilities of a person in meeting life's demands and roles.

Related factors

Situational crises

Maturational crises
Vulnerability

Defining characteristics
Verbalization of inability to cope or inability to ask
    for help*
Inability to meet role expectations
Inability to meet basic needs
Inability to problem solve*
Alteration in societal participation
Destructive behavior toward self or others
Inappropriate use of defense mechanisms
Change in usual communication patterns
Verbal manipulation
High illness rate
High rate of accidents
Expression of anxiety, depression, fear, impatience,
    frustration, irritability, discouragement, and life
    stress

Decisional conflict (specify)

A state of uncertainty about the course of action to be taken
when choice among competing actions involves risk, loss, or
challenge to personal life values. (Specify focus of conflict; e.g.,
choices regarding health, family relationships, career, finances,
or other life events).

Related factors
Unclear personal values/beliefs
Perceived threat to value system
Lack of experience or interference with decision making
Lack of relevant information
Support system deficit

Defining characteristics
Verbalized feeling of distress related to uncertainty
    about choices
Verbalization of undesired consequences of alterna-
    tive actions being considered
Vacillation between alternative choices
Delayed decision making

*Critical

Self-focusing

Physical signs of distress or tension (increased heart rate, increased muscle tension, restlessness, etc.)

Questioning personal values and beliefs while attempting to make a decision

Denial, ineffective

A conscious or unconscious attempt to disavow the knowledge or meaning of an event to reduce anxiety/fear to the detriment of health.

Related factors
To be developed

Defining characteristics
Delay in seeking or refusal of medical attention to the detriment of health

Does not perceive personal relevance of symptoms or danger

Use of home remedies (self-treatment) to relieve symptoms

Does not admit fear of death or invalidism

Minimization of symptoms

Displacing source of symptoms to other organs

Inability to admit impact of disease on life pattern

Presence of dismissive gestures or comments when speaking of distressing events

Displacing fear of impact of condition

Inappropriate affect

Diarrhea

The state in which an individual experiences a change in normal bowel habits characterized by the frequent passage of loose, fluid, unformed stools.

Related factors
Stress and anxiety
Dietary intake
Medications
Inflammation, irritation, or malabsorption of bowel
Toxins

Contaminants
Radiation

Defining characteristics
Abdominal pain
Cramping
Increased frequency of bowel movements
Increased frequency of bowel sounds
Loose, liquid stools
Urgency
Changes in color

Disuse syndrome, risk for

The state in which an individual is at risk for deterioration of body systems as the result of prescribed or unavoidable inactivity.

Risk factors
Paralysis
Mechanical immobilization
Prescribed immobilization
Severe pain
Altered level of consciousness

Diversional activity deficit

The state in which an individual experiences a decreased stimulation from or interest or engagement in recreational or leisure activities.

Related factors
Environmental lack of diversional activity
Long-term hospitalization
Frequent, lengthy treatments

Defining characteristics
Boredom
Desire for something to do, to read, etc.
Usual hobbies cannot be undertaken in hospital

Dysreflexia

The state in which an individual with a spinal cord injury at T7 or above experiences or is at risk of experiencing a life-threatening uninhibited sympathetic response of the nervous system attributable to a noxious stimulus.

Related factors

Bladder distention

Bowel distention

Skin irritation

Lack of patient and caregiver knowledge

Defining characteristics

Individual with spinal cord injury (T7 or above) with the following:

Paroxysmal hypertension (sudden periodic elevated blood pressure where systolic pressure is over 140 mm Hg and diastolic pressure is above 90 mm Hg)

Bradycardia or tachycardia (pulse rate of less than 60 or over 100 beats per minute)

Diaphoresis (above injury)

Red splotches on skin (above injury)

Pallor (below injury)

Headache (diffuse pain in different portions of head and not confined to any nerve distribution area)

Chilling (shivering accompanied by sensation of coldness or pallor of skin)

Conjunctival congestion (excessive amount of blood/tissue fluid in conjunctivae)

Horner's syndrome (contraction of pupil, partial ptosis of eyelid, enophthalmos, and sometimes loss of sweating over affected side of face due to paralysis of cervical sympathetic nerve trunk)

Paresthesia (abnormal sensation, such as numbness, prickling, or tingling; increased sensitivity)

Pilomotor reflex (gooseflesh formation when skin is cooled)

Blurred vision

Chest pain

Metallic taste in mouth

Nasal congestion

Energy field disturbance

A disruption of the flow of energy surrounding a person's being, which results in a disharmony of the body, mind, or spirit.

Defining characteristics
Temperature change (warmth or coolness)
Visual changes (image or color)
Disruption of the field (vacant/hold/spike/bulge)
Movement (wave/spike/tingling/dense/flowing)
Sounds (tone or words)

Environmental interpretation syndrome, impaired

Consistent lack of orientation to person, place, time, or circumstances more than from 3 to 6 months, necessitating a protective environment.

Related factors
Dementia (Alzheimer's disease, multi-infarct dementia, Pick's disease, AIDS dementia)
Parkinson's disease
Huntington's disease
Depression
Alcoholism

Defining characteristics
  Major
  Consistent disorientation in known and unknown environments
  Chronic confusional states
  Minor
  Loss of occupation or social functioning from memory decline
  Inability to follow simple directions or instructions
  Inability to reason
  Inability to concentrate
  Slowness in responding to questions

Family processes, altered: alcoholism

The state in which the psychosocial, spiritual, and physiological functions of the family unit are chronically disorganized, leading to conflict, denial of problems, resistance to change, ineffective problem solving, and a series of self-perpetuating crises.

Related factors
Abuses of alcohol
Family history of alcoholism, resistance to treatment
Inadequate coping skills
Genetic predisposition
Addictive personality
Lack of problem-solving skills
Biochemical influences

Defining characteristics
Major
Feelings
Decreased self-esteem or sense of worthlessness
Anger or suppressed rage
Frustration
Powerlessness
Anxiety
Tension
Distress
Insecurity
Repressed emotions
Responsibility for alcoholic's behavior
Lingering resentment
Shame or embarrassment
Hurt
Unhappiness
Guilt
Emotional isolation and loneliness
Vulnerability
Mistrust
Hopelessness
Rejection
Roles and relationships
Deterioration in family relationships or disturbed family dynamics

Ineffective spouse communication or marital problems

Altered role function or disruption of family roles

Inconsistent parenting or low perception of parental support

Family denial

Intimacy dysfunction

Chronic family problems

Closed communication systems

Behaviors

Expression of anger inappropriately

Difficulty with intimate relationships

Loss of control of drinking

Impaired communication

Ineffective problem-solving skills

Enabling alcoholic to maintain drinking

Inability to meet emotional needs of its members

Manipulation

Dependency

Criticizing

Alcohol abuse

Broken promises

Rationalization or denial of problems

Refusal to get help or inability to accept and receive help appropriately

Blaming

Inadequate understanding or knowledge or alcoholism

Minor

Feelings

Being different from other people

Depression

Hostility

Fear

Emotional control by others

Confusion

Dissatisfaction

Loss

Misunderstood

Abandonment

Confused love and pity

Moodiness

Failure
Being unloved
Lack of identity
Roles and relationships
Triangulating family relationships
Reduced ability of family members to relate to each
other for mutual growth and maturation
Lack of skills necessary for relationships
Lack of cohesiveness
Disrupted family rituals
Family unable to meet security needs of its
members
Family does not demonstrate respect for individu-
ality and autonomy of its members
Pattern of rejection
Economic problems
Neglected obligations
Behaviors
Inability to meet spiritual needs of its members
Inability to express or accept wide range of feelings
Orientation toward tension relief rather than
achievement of goals
Family special occasions are alcohol centered
Escalating conflict
Lying
Contradictory, paradoxical communication
Lack of dealing with conflict
Harsh self-judgment
Isolation
Nicotine addiction
Difficulty having fun
Self-blaming
Unresolved grief
Controlling communication and power struggles
Inability to adapt to change
Immaturity
Stress-related physical illnesses
Inability to deal with traumatic experiences con-
structively
Seeking approval and affirmation
Lack of reliability
Disturbances in academic performance in children

Disturbances in concentration
Chaos
Substance abuse other than alcohol
Failure to accomplish current or past developmental tasks or difficulty with life cycle transitions
Verbal abuse of spouse or parent
Agitation
Diminished physical contact

Family processes, altered

The state in which a family that normally functions effectively experiences a dysfunction.

Related factors
Situational transition and/or crises
Developmental transition and/or crises

Defining characteristics*
Family system unable to meet physical needs of its members
Family system unable to meet emotional needs of its members
Family system unable to meet spiritual needs of its members
Parents do not demonstrate respect for each other's views on child-rearing practices
Inability to express or accept wide range of feelings
Inability to express or accept feelings of members
Family unable to meet security needs of its members
Inability of family members to relate to each other for mutual growth and maturation
Family uninvolved in community activities
Inability to accept or receive help appropriately
Rigidity in function and roles
Family does not demonstrate respect for individuality and autonomy of its members
Family unable to adapt to change or to deal with traumatic experiences constructively

*The first 13 defining characteristics are specifically from Otto H: Criteria for assessing family strengths, *Fam Process* 2:329-338, Sept 1963.

Family fails to accomplish current or past developmental task
Ineffective family decision-making process
Failure to send and receive clear messages
Inappropriate boundary maintenance
Inappropriate or poorly communicated family rules, rituals, symbols
Unexamined family myths
Inappropriate level and direction of energy

Fatigue

An overwhelming sense of exhaustion and decreased capacity for physical and mental work.

Related factors
Overwhelming psychological or emotional demands
Increased energy requirements to perform activities of daily living
Excessive social/role demands
States of discomfort
Decreased metabolic energy production
Altered body chemistry (e.g., medications, drug withdrawal)

Defining characteristics
Verbalization of fatigue/lack of energy
Inability to maintain usual routines
Perceived need for additional energy to accomplish routine tasks
Increase in physical complaints
Emotional lability or irritability
Impaired ability to concentrate
Decreased performance
Lethargy or listlessness
Disinterest in surroundings/introspection
Decreased libido
Accident proneness

Fear

Feeling of dread related to an identifiable source that the person validates.

Related factors

Natural or innate origins—sudden noise, loss of physical support, height, pain

Learned response—conditioning, modeling from or identification with others

Separation from support system in a potentially threatening situation (hospitalization, treatments, etc.)

Knowledge deficit or unfamiliarity

Language barrier

Sensory impairment

Phobic stimulus or phobia

Environmental stimuli

Defining characteristics

Subjective

Increased tension

Apprehension

Impulsiveness

Decreased self-assurance

Afraid

Scared

Terrified

Panicked

Frightened

Jittery

Objective

Increased alertness

Concentration on source

Wide-eyed

Attack behavior

Focus on "it, out there"

Fight behavior—aggressive

Flight behavior—withdrawal

Sympathetic stimulation—cardiovascular excitation, superficial vasoconstriction, pupil dilation

Fluid volume deficit

The state in which an individual experiences decreased intravascular, interstitial and/or intracellular fluid. This refers to dehydration, water loss alone without change in sodium.

Related factors
(1) Failure of regulatory mechanisms
(2) Active fluid volume loss

Defining characteristics
Decreased urine output
Increased urine concentration
Sudden weight loss
Decreased venous filling
Increased hematocrit
Decreased skin/tongue turgor
Decreased BP
Dry skin/mucous membranes

Other possible defining characteristics
Thirst
Increased pulse rate
Decreased pulse volume/pressure
Change in mental state
Increased body temperature
Weakness

Fluid volume deficit, risk for

The state in which an individual is at risk for experiencing vascular, cellular, or intracellular dehydration.

Risk factors
Extremes of age
Extremes of weight
Excessive losses through normal routes (e.g., diarrhea)
Loss of fluid through abnormal routes (e.g., in-dwelling tubes)
Deviations affecting access to, intake of, or absorption of fluids (e.g., physical immobility)
Factors influencing fluid needs (e.g., hypermetabolic states)
Knowledge deficiency related to fluid volume
Medications (e.g., diuretics)
Increased fluid output
Urinary frequency
Thirst
Altered intake

Fluid volume excess

The state in which an individual experiences increased isotonic fluid retention.

Related factors
Compromised regulatory mechanism
Excess fluid intake
Excess sodium intake

Defining characteristics
Edema
Effusion
Anasarca
Weight gain
Shortness of breath
Intake greater than output
Abnormal breath sounds, rales (crackles)
Decreased hemoglobin and hematocrit
Increased central venous pressure*
Jugular vein distention*
Positive hepatojugular reflex

Other possible defining characteristics
Clinical evidence lacking in fluid volume excess
    studies
Orthopnea
S_3 heart sound
Pulmonary congestion
Change in respiratory pattern
Change in mental status
Blood pressure changes
Pulmonary artery pressure changes
Oliguria
Specific gravity changes
Azotemia
Altered electrolytes, restlessness
Anxiety

*Minimal clinical evidence present and needs further research

Gas exchange, impaired

The state in which an individual experiences an imbalance between oxygen uptake and carbon dioxide elimination at the alveolar-capillary membrane gas exchange area.

Related factors
Altered oxygen supply
Alveolar-capillary membrane changes
Altered blood flow
Altered oxygen-carrying capacity of blood

Defining characteristics
Confusion
Somnolence
Restlessness
Irritability
Inability to move secretions
Hypercapnia
Hypoxia

Grieving, anticipatory

Intellectual and emotional responses and behaviors by which individuals (families, communities) work through the process of modifying self-concept based on the perception of potential loss.

Related factors
To be developed

Defining characteristics
Potential loss of significant object
Expression of distress at potential loss
Denial of potential loss
Denial of the significance of the loss
Guilt
Anger
Sorrow
Bargaining
Alteration in: eating habits, sleep patterns, dream patterns, activity level, libido
Altered communication patterns
Difficulty taking on new or different roles
Resolution of grief prior to the reality of loss

Grieving, dysfunctional

Extended, unsuccessful use of intellectual and emotional responses by which individuals (families, communities) attempt to work through the process of modifying self-concept based on the perception of loss.

Related factors

Actual or perceived object loss (object loss is used in the broadest sense); objects may include: people, possessions, a job, status, home, ideals, parts and processes of the body.

Defining characteristics

Repetitive use of ineffectual behaviors associated with attempts to reinvest in relationships

Reliving of past experiences with little or no reduction (diminishment) of intensity of the grief

Prolonged interference with life functioning

Onset or exacerbation of somatic or psychomatic responses

Expression of distress at loss

Denial of loss

Expression of guilt

Expression of unresolved issues

Anger

Sadness

Crying

Difficulty in expressing loss

Alterations in: eating habits, sleep patterns, dream patterns, activity level, libido, concentration and/or pursuit of tasks

Idealization of lost object

Reliving of past experiences

Interference with life functioning

Developmental regression

Labile affect

Growth and development, altered

The state in which an individual demonstrates deviations in norms from his/her age-group.

Related factors

Inadequate caretaking: indifference, inconsistent responsiveness, multiple caretakers

Separation from significant others

Environmental and stimulation deficiencies

Effects of physical disability

Prescribed dependence

Defining characteristics

Delay or difficulty in performing skills (motor, social, or expressive) typical of age-group

Altered physical growth

Inability to perform self-care or self-control activities appropriate for age

Flat affect

Listlessness, decreased responses

Health maintenance, altered

Inability to identify, manage, and/or seek help to maintain health.

Related factors

Lack of or significant alteration in communication skills (written, verbal, and/or gestural)

Lack of ability to make deliberate and thoughtful judgments

Perceptual or cognitive impairment

Complete or partial lack of gross and/or fine motor skills

Ineffective individual coping; dysfunctional grieving

Lack of material resources

Unachieved developmental tasks

Ineffective family coping; disabling spiritual distress

Defining characteristics

Demonstrated lack of knowledge regarding basic health practices

Demonstrated lack of adaptive behaviors to internal or external environmental changes

Reported or observed inability to take responsibility for meeting basic health practices in any or all functional pattern areas

History of lack of health-seeking behavior

Expressed interest in improving health behaviors

Reported or observed lack of equipment, financial, and/or other resources

Reported or observed impairment of personal support system

Health-seeking behaviors (specify)

The state in which a patient in stable health is actively seeking ways to alter personal health habits and/or the environment in order to move toward optimal health. (*Stable health status* is defined as age-appropriate illness prevention measures achieved; the patient reports good or excellent health, and signs and symptoms of disease, if present, are controlled.)

Related factors

To be developed

Defining characteristics

Expressed or observed desire to seek higher level of wellness

Stated or observed unfamiliarity with wellness community resources

Demonstrated or observed lack of knowledge in health promotion behaviors

Expressed or observed desire for increased control of health practice

Expression of concern about effects of current environmental conditions on health status

Home maintenance management, impaired

Inability to independently maintain a safe growth-promoting immediate environment.

Related factors

Disease or injury of individual or family member

Insufficient family organization or planning

Insufficient finances

Unfamiliarity with neighborhood resources

Impaired cognitive or emotional functioning

Lack of knowledge
Lack of role modeling
Inadequate support systems

Defining characteristics
Subjective
Household members express difficulty in maintaining their home in a comfortable fashion

Household requests assistance with home maintenance

Household members describe outstanding debts or financial crises

Objective
Disorderly surroundings

Unwashed or unavailable cooking equipment, clothes, or linen

Accumulation of dirt, food wastes, or hygienic wastes

Offensive odors

Inappropriate household temperature

Overtaxed family members (e.g., exhausted, anxious family members)

Lack of necessary equipment or aids

Presence of vermin or rodents

Repeated hygienic disorders, infestations, or infections

Hopelessness

The subjective state in which an individual sees limited or no alternatives or personal choices available and is unable to mobilize energy on own behalf.

Related factors
Prolonged activity restriction creating isolation
Failure or deteriorating physiological condition
Long-term stress
Abandonment
Loss of belief in transcendent values/God

Defining characteristics
Passivity, decreased verbalization
Decreased affect

Verbal cues (indicating despondency, "I can't," sighing)
Lack of initiative
Decreased response to stimuli
Turning away from speaker
Closing eyes
Shrugging in response to speaker
Decreased appetite; increased/decreased sleep
Lack of involvement in care; passively allowing care

Hyperthermia

The state in which an individual's body temperature is elevated above his/her normal range.

Related factors
Exposure to hot environment
Vigorous activity
Medications/anesthesia
Inappropriate clothing
Increased metabolic rate
Illness or trauma
Dehydration
Inability or decreased ability to perspire

Defining characteristics
Increase in body temperature above normal range
Flushed skin
Warm to touch
Increased respiratory rate
Tachycardia
Seizures/convulsions

Hypothermia

The state in which an individual's body temperature is reduced below his/her normal range but not below 35.6° C (rectal)/36.4° C (rectal, newborn).

Related factors
Exposure to cool or cold environment
Illness or trauma
Inability or decreased ability to shiver
Malnutrition

Inadequate clothing
Consumption of alcohol
Medications causing vasodilation
Evaporation from skin in cool environment
Decreased metabolic rate
Inactivity
Aging

Defining characteristics
Shivering (mild)
Cool skin
Pallor (moderate)
Slow capillary refill
Tachycardia
Cyanotic nail beds
Hypertension
Piloerection

Incontinence, bowel

See Bowel incontinence.

Incontinence, functional

The state in which an individual experiences an involuntary,
unpredictable passage of urine.

Related factors
Altered environment
Sensory, cognitive, or mobility deficits

Defining characteristics
Urge to void or bladder contractions sufficiently
strong to result in loss of urine before reaching an
appropriate receptacle

Incontinence, reflex

The state in which an individual experiences an involuntary loss
of urine occurring at somewhat predictable intervals when a
specific bladder volume is reached.

Related factor
Neurological impairment (e.g., spinal cord lesion that

interferes with conduction of cerebral messages above level of reflex arc)

Defining characteristics
No awareness of bladder filling
No urge to void or feelings of bladder fullness
Uninhibited bladder contraction/spasm at regular intervals

Incontinence, stress

The state in which an individual experiences a loss of urine of less than 50 ml occurring with increased abdominal pressure.

Related factors
Degenerative changes in pelvic muscles and structural supports associated with increased age
High intraabdominal pressure (e.g., obesity, gravid uterus)
Incompetent bladder outlet
Overdistention between voidings
Weak pelvic muscles and structural supports

Defining characteristics
Reported or observed dribbling with increased abdominal pressure
Urinary urgency
Urinary frequency (more often than every 2 hours)

Incontinence, total

The state in which an individual experiences a continuous and unpredictable loss of urine.

Related factors
Neuropathy preventing transmission of reflex indicating bladder fullness
Neurological dysfunction causing triggering of micturition at unpredictable times
Independent contraction of detrusor reflex due to surgery
Trauma or disease affecting spinal cord nerves
Anatomic (fistula)

Defining characteristics

Constant flow of urine occurring at unpredictable times without distention or uninhibited bladder contractions/spasms

Unsuccessful incontinence refractory to treatments

Nocturia

Lack of perineal or bladder-filling awareness

Unawareness of incontinence

Incontinence, urge

The state in which an individual experiences involuntary passage of urine occurring soon after a strong sense of urgency to void.

Related factors

Decreased bladder capacity (e.g., history of pelvic inflammatory disease, abdominal surgeries, indwelling urinary catheter)

Irritation of bladder stretch receptors, causing spasm (e.g., bladder infection)

Alcohol

Caffeine

Increased fluids

Increased urine concentration

Overdistention of bladder

Defining characteristics

Urinary urgency

Frequency (voiding more often than every 2 hours)

Bladder contracture/spasm

Nocturia (more than 2 times per night)

Voiding in small (less than 100 ml) or in large amounts (more than 550 ml)

Inability to reach toilet in time

Infant behavior, disorganized

Alteration in integration and modulation of the physiological and behavioral systems of functioning (i.e., autonomic, motor, state, organizational, self regulatory, and attentional-interactional systems).

Related factors

Pain

Oral motor problems
Feeding intolerance
Environmental overstimulation
Lack of containment or boundaries
Prematurity
Invasive or painful procedures

Defining characteristics
  Major
   Change from baseline physiologic measures
   Tremors, startles, twitches
   Hyperextension of arms and legs
   Diffuse/unclear sleep
   Deficient self-regulatory behaviors
   Deficient response to visual/auditory stimuli
  Minor
   Yawning
   Apnea

Infant behavior, disorganized: risk for

Risk for alteration in integration and modulation of the physiological and behavioral systems of functioning (i.e., autonomic, motor, state, organizational, self-regulatory, and attentional-interactional systems).

Risk factors
Pain
Oral motor problems
Environmental overstimulation
Lack of containment or boundaries
Prematurity
Invasive or painful procedures

Infant behavior, organized: potential for enhanced

A pattern of modulation of the physiologic and behavioral systems of functioning of an infant (i.e., autonomic, motor, state, organizational, self-regulatory, and attentional-interactional systems) that is satisfactory but that can be improved, resulting in higher levels of integration in response to environmental stimuli.

Related factors
Prematurity
Pain

Defining characteristics
Stable physiologic measures
Definite sleep-wake states
Use of some self-regulatory behaviors
Response to visual or auditory stimuli

Infant feeding pattern, ineffective

A state in which an infant demonstrates an impaired ability to suck or coordinate the suck-swallow response.

Related factors
Prematurity
Neurological impairment/delay
Oral hypersensitivity
Prolonged NPO status
Anatomic abnormality

Defining characteristics
Inability to initiate or sustain an effective suck
Inability to coordinate sucking, swallowing, and
    breathing

Infection, risk for

The state in which an individual is at increased risk for being invaded by pathogenic organisms.

Risk factors
Inadequate primary defenses (broken skin, trauma-
    tized tissue, decrease in ciliary action, stasis of body
    fluids, change in pH secretions, altered peristalsis)
Inadequate secondary defenses (e.g., decreased hemo-
    globin level, leukopenia, suppressed inflammatory
    response, immunosuppression)
Inadequate acquired immunity
Tissue destruction and increased environmental
    exposure
Chronic disease

Invasive procedures
Malnutrition
Pharmaceutical agents and trauma
Rupture of amniotic membranes
Insufficient knowledge to avoid exposure to pathogens

Injury, perioperative positioning: risk for

A state in which the client is at risk for injury as a result of the environmental conditions found in the perioperative setting.

Risk factors
Disorientation
Immobilization, muscle weakness
Sensory or perceptual disturbances resulting from anesthesia
Obesity
Emaciation
Edema

Injury, risk for

The state in which an individual is at risk of injury as a result of environmental conditions interacting with the individual's adaptive and defensive resources. See also Poisoning, risk for; Suffocation, risk for; Trauma, risk for.

Risk factors
Interactive conditions between individual and environment that impose a risk to defensive and adaptive resources of individual
  Internal
  Biochemical
    Regulatory function
      Sensory dysfunction
      Integrative dysfunction
      Effector dysfunction
    Tissue hypoxia
    Malnutrition
    Immune-autoimmune
    Abnormal blood profile
      Leukocytosis or leukopenia

Altered clotting factors
Thrombocytopenia
Sickle cell
Thalassemia
Decreased hemoglobin level
Physical
Broken skin
Altered mobility
Developmental
Age
Physiological
Psychosocial
Psychological
Affective
Orientation
External
Biological
Immunization level of community
Microorganism
Chemical
Pollutants
Poisons
Drugs
Pharmaceutical agents
Alcohol
Caffeine
Nicotine
Preservatives
Cosmetics and dyes
Nutrients (vitamins, food types)
Physical
Design, structure, and arrangement of community, building, and/or equipment
Mode of transport/transportation
Nosocomial agents

People-provider
Nosocomial agents
Staffing patterns
Cognitive, affective, and psychomotor factors

Knowledge deficit (specify)

Absence or deficiency of cognitive information related to specific topic.

Related factors
Lack of exposure
Lack of recall
Information misinterpretation
Cognitive limitation
Lack of interest in learning
Unfamiliarity with information resources

Defining characteristics
Verbalization of the problem
Inaccurate follow-through of instruction
Inaccurate performance of test
Inappropriate or exaggerated behaviors (e.g., hysterical, hostile, agitated, apathetic)

Loneliness, risk for

A subjective state in which an individual is at risk of experiencing vague dysphoria.

Risk factors
Affectional deprivation
Physical isolation
Cathectic deprivation
Social isolation

Management of therapeutic regimen, community: ineffective

A pattern of regulating and integrating into community processes programs for treatment of illness and the sequelae of illness that are unsatisfactory for meeting health-related goals.

Defining characteristics
Deficits in persons and programs to be accountable for illness care of aggregates
Deficits in advocates for aggregates
Deficits in community activities for secondary and tertiary prevention

Illness symptoms above the norm expected for the number and type of population
Number of health care resources insufficient for the incidence or prevalence of illness(es)
Unavailable health care resources for illness care
Unexpected acceleration of illness

Management of therapeutic regimen, families: ineffective

A pattern of regulating and integrating into family processes a program for treatment of illness and the sequelae of illness that is unsatisfactory for meeting specific health goals.

Related factors
Complexity of health care system
Complexity of therapeutic regimen
Decisional conflicts
Economic difficulties
Excessive demands made on individual or family
Family conflict

Defining characteristics
  Major
    Inappropriate family activities for meeting the goals of a treatment or prevention program
  Minor
    Acceleration (expected or unexpected) of illness symptoms of a family member
    Lack of attention to illness and its sequelae
    Verbalized desire to manage the treatment of illness and prevention of the sequelae
    Verbalized difficulty with regulation/integration of one or more effects or prevention of complications
    Verbalizes that family did not take action to reduce risk factors for progression of illness and sequelae

Management of therapeutic regimen, individual: effective

A pattern of regulating and integrating into daily living a program for treatment of illness and its sequelae that is satisfactory for meeting specific health goals.

Defining characteristics

Appropriate choices of daily activities for meeting the goals of a treatment or prevention program

Illness symptoms within a normal range of expectation

Verbalized desire to manage the treatment of illness and prevention of sequelae

Verbalized intent to reduce risk factors for progression of illness and sequelae

Management of therapeutic regimen, individuals: ineffective

A pattern of regulating and integrating into daily living a program for treatment of illness and the sequelae of illness that is unsatisfactory for meeting specific health goals.

Related factors

Complexity of health care system
Complexity of therapeutic regimen
Decisional conflicts
Economic difficulties
Excessive demands made on individual or family
Family conflict
Family patterns of health care
Inadequate number and types of cues to action
Knowledge deficits
Mistrust of regimen and/or health care personnel
Perceived seriousness
Perceived susceptibility
    Inability to learn or retain new skills or information
    Inability to perform a previously learned skill
    Inability to recall factual information
    Inability to recall recent or past events
    Minor
    Forgets to perform a behavior at a scheduled time

Mobility, impaired physical

The state in which an individual experiences a limitation of ability for independent physical movement.

Related factors

Intolerance to activity; decreased strength and
    endurance

Pain and discomfort

Perceptual or cognitive impairment

Neuromuscular impairment

Musculoskeletal impairment

Depression; severe anxiety

Defining characteristics

Inability to purposefully move within physical envi-
    ronment, including bed mobility, transfer, and am-
    bulation

Reluctance to attempt movement

Limited range of motion

Decreased muscle strength, control, and/or mass

Imposed restrictions of movement, including me-
    chanical; medical protocol

Impaired coordination

Noncompliance (specify)

A person's informed decision not to adhere to a therapeutic
recommendation.

Related factors

Patient's value system
    Health beliefs
    Cultural influences
    Spiritual values

Client and provider relationships

Defining characteristics

Behavior indicative of failure to adhere by direct ob-
    servation or statements by patient or significant
    others

Objective tests (physiological measures, detection of
    markers)

Evidence of development of complications

Evidence of exacerbation of symptoms

Failure to keep appointments

Failure to progress

Inability to set or attain mutual goals

Nutrition, altered: less than body requirements

The state in which an individual experiences an intake of nutrients insufficient to meet metabolic needs.

Related factor

Inability to ingest or digest food or absorb nutrients because of biological, psychological, or economic factors

Defining characteristics

Loss of body weight with adequate food intake

Body weight 20% or more under ideal for height and frame

Reported inadequate food intake less than Recommended Daily Allowance

Weakness of muscles required for swallowing or mastication

Reported or evidence of lack of food

Lack of interest in food

Perceived inability to ingest food

Aversion to eating

Reported altered taste sensation

Satiety immediately after ingesting food

Abdominal pain with or without pathological conditions

Sore, inflamed buccal cavity

Nutrition, altered: more than body requirements

The state in which an individual is experiencing an intake of nutrients that exceeds metabolic needs.

Related factor

Excessive intake in relationship to metabolic need

Defining characteristics

Weight 10% to 20% over ideal for height and frame

Triceps skinfold greater than 15 mm in men and 25 mm in women

Sedentary activity level

Reported or observed dysfunctional eating patterns
   Pairing food with other activities
   Concentrating food intake at end of day
   Eating in response to external cues (e.g., time of
     day, social situation)
   Eating in response to internal cues other than
     hunger (e.g., anxiety)

Nutrition, altered: risk for more than body requirements

The state in which an individual is at risk of experiencing an intake of nutrients that exceeds metabolic needs.

Risk factors

Hereditary predisposition
Excessive energy intake during late gestational life, early infancy, and adolescence
Frequent, closely spaced pregnancies
Dysfunctional psychological conditioning in relationship to food
Membership in lower socioeconomic group
Reported or observed obesity in one or both parents
Rapid transition across growth percentiles in infants or children
Reported use of solid food as major food source before 5 months of age
Observed use of food as reward or comfort measure
Reported or observed higher baseline weight at beginning of each pregnancy
Dysfunctional eating patterns
   Pairing food with other activities
   Concentrating food intake at end of day
   Eating in response to external cues (e.g., time of
     day, social situation)
   Eating in response to internal cues other than
     hunger (e.g., anxiety)

Oral mucous membrane, altered

The state in which an individual experiences disruptions in the tissue layers of the oral cavity.

Related factors
Pathological conditions oral cavity (radiation to head
　　and/or neck)
Dehydration
Trauma
　　Chemical (e.g., acidic foods, drugs, noxious agents,
　　　　alcohol)
　　Mechanical (e.g., ill-fitting dentures; braces; tubes
　　　　endotracheal, nasogastric; surgery in oral cavity)
NPO instructions for more than 24 hours
Ineffective oral hygiene
Mouth breathing
Malnutrition
Infection
Lack of or decreased salivation
Medication

Defining characteristics
Coated tongue
Xerostomia (dry mouth)
Stomatitis
Oral lesions or ulcers
Lack of or decreased salivation
Leukoplakia
Edema
Hyperemia
Oral plaque
Oral pain or discomfort
Desquamation
Vesicles
Hemorrhagic gingivitis
Carious teeth
Halitosis
Perceived barriers
Perceived benefits
Powerlessness
Social support deficits

Defining characteristics
　Major
　　Choices of daily living ineffective for meeting the
　　　goals of a treatment or prevention program

Minor
Acceleration (expected or unexpected) of illness symptoms

Verbalized desire to manage the treatment of illness and prevention of sequelae

Verbalized difficulty with regulation/integration of one or more prescribed regimens for treatment of illness and its effects or prevention of complications

Verbalization that intimated that patient would not attempt to include treatment regimens in daily routines

Verbalization that intimated that patient would not attempt to reduce risk factors for progression of illness and sequelae

Memory, impaired

The state in which an individual experiences that inability to remember or recall bits of information or behavioral skills. Impaired memory may be attributed to pathophysiological or situational causes that are either temporary or permanent.

Related factors
Acute or chronic hypoxia
Anemia
Decreased cardiac output
Fluid and electrolyte imbalance
Neurologic disturbances
Excessive environmental disturbances

Defining characteristics
Major
Observed or reported experiences of forgetting

Inability to determine whether a behavior was performed

Pain

An unpleasant sensory and emotional experience arising from actual or potential tissue damage or described in terms of such damage (International Association for the Study of Pain);

sudden or slow onset of any intensity from mild to severe with
an anticipated or predictable end and a duration of less than 6
months.

Related factors
Injuring agents
 Biological
 Chemical
 Physical
 Psychological

Defining characteristics
 Major
 Verbal or coded report
 Observed evidence
 Antalgic position
 Protective behavior
 Guarding behavior
 Antalgic gestures
 Facial mask
 Sleep disturbance (eyes lack luster, "hecohe look,"
  fixed or scattered movement, grimace)
 Minor
 Self-focus; narrowed focus (altered time perception)
 Impaired thought process
 Reduced interaction with people and environment
 Distraction behavior (pacing, seeking out other
  people and/or activities, repetitive activities)
 Autonomic alteration in muscle tone (may span
  from listless to rigid)
 Autonomic responses (diaphoresis, blood pressure,
  respiration, pulse change, pupillary dilatation)
 Expressive behavior (restlessness, moaning, crying,
  vigilance, irritability, sighing)
 Changes in appetite and eating

Pain, chronic

An unpleasant sensory and emotional experience arising from
actual or potential tissue damage or described in terms of such
damage (International Association for the Study of Pain);
sudden or slow onset of any intensity from mild to severe,

constant or recurring without an anticipated or predictable end
and a duration of greater than 6 months.

Related factor
Chronic physical/psychosocial disability

Defining characteristics
Major
Verbal or coded report or observed evidence of:
Protective behavior
Guarding behavior
Facial mask
Irritability
Self focusing
Restlessness
Depression

Minor
Atrophy of involved muscle group
Changes in sleep pattern
Weight changes
Fatigue
Fear of reinjury
Reduced interaction with people
Altered ability to continue previous activities
Sympathetic mediated responses (temperature,
cold, changes of body position, hypersensitivity)
Anorexia

Parent/infant/child attachment, altered: risk for

Disruption of the interactive process between parent or
significant other and infant that fosters the development of a
protective and nurturing reciprocal relationship.

Risk factors
Inability of parents to meet the personal needs
Anxiety associated with the parent role
Substance abuse
Premature infant
Ill infant or child who is unable to effectively initiate
parental contact because of altered behavioral
organization

Separation
Physical barriers
Lack of privacy

Parental role conflict

The state in which a parent experiences role confusion and conflict in response to a crisis.

Related factors

Separation from child due to chronic illness
Intimidation with invasive or restrictive modalities
(e.g., isolation, intubation)
Specialized care centers, policies
Home care of a child with special needs (e.g., apnea
monitoring, postural drainage, hyperalimentation)
Change in marital status
Interruptions of family life due to home health-care
regimen (treatments, caregivers, lack of respite)

Defining characteristics

Parent(s) expresses concerns/feelings of inadequacy to
provide for child's physical and emotional needs
during hospitalization or in home
Demonstrated disruption in caretaking routines
Parent(s) expresses concerns about changes in
parental role, family functioning, family communication, and/or family health
Expresses concern about perceived loss of control over
decisions relating to child
Reluctant to participate in normal caretaking activities even with encouragement and support
Verbalizes/demonstrates feelings of guilt, anger, fear,
anxiety, and/or frustrations about effect of child's
illness on family process

Parenting, altered

The state in which a nurturing figure(s) experiences an inability
to create an environment that promotes the optimum growth
and development of another human being. (It is important to
state as a preface to this diagnosis that adjustment to parenting

in general is a normal maturational process that elicits nursing behaviors of prevention of potential problems and health promotion.)

Related factors

Lack of available role model

Ineffective role model

Physical and psychosocial abuse of nurturing figure

Lack of support between/from significant other(s)

Unmet social/emotional maturation needs of parent-ing figures

Interruption in bonding process (e.g., maternal, pater-nal, other)

Unrealistic expectation for self, infant, partner

Perceived threat to own survival, physical and emotional

Mental and/or physical illness

Presence of stress (financial, legal, recent crisis, cul-tural move)

Lack of knowledge

Limited cognitive functioning

Lack of role identity

Lack or inappropriate response of child to relationship

Multiple pregnancies

Defining characteristics

Abandonment

Runaway

Verbalization, cannot control child

Incidence of physical and psychological trauma

Lack of parental attachment behaviors

Inappropriate visual, tactile, auditory stimulation

Negative identification of infant/child's characteristics

Negative attachment of meanings to infant/child's characteristics

Constant verbalization of disappointment in gender or physical characteristics of the infant/child

Verbalization of resentment toward the infant/child

Verbalization of role inadequacy

Inattentive to infant/child needs*

Verbal disgust at body functions of infant/child

*Critical

Noncompliance with health appointments for self and/or infant/child

Inappropriate caretaking behavior (toilet training, sleep/rest, feeding)*

Inappropriate or inconsistent discipline practices

Frequent accidents

Frequent illness

Growth and development lag in the child

History of child abuse or abandonment by primary caretaker*

Verbalizes desire to have child call himself/herself by first name versus traditional cultural tendencies

Child receives care from multiple caretakers without consideration for the needs of the infant/child

Compulsively seeking role approval from others

Parenting, altered, risk for

The state in which the ability of nurturing figure(s) to create an environment that promotes the optimal growth and development of another human being is altered or at risk.

Related/risk factors
Lack of available role model

Ineffective role model

Physical and psychosocial abuse of nurturing figure

Lack of support between or from significant other(s)

Unmet social and emotional maturation needs of parenting figures

Interruption in bonding process (e.g., maternal, paternal, other)

Perceived threat to own survival: physical and emotional

Mental and/or physical illness

Presence of stress: financial or legal problems, recent crisis, cultural move

Lack of knowledge

Limited cognitive functioning

Lack of role identity

Lack of appropriate response of child to relationship

Multiple pregnancies

*Critical

Unrealistic expectation of self, infant, partner

Defining characteristics
  Actual and potential
    Lack of parental attachment behaviors
    Inappropriate visual, tactile, auditory stimulation
    Negative identification of characteristics of
      infant/child
    Negative attachment of meanings to characteristics
      of infant/child
    Constant verbalization of disappointment in
      gender or physical characteristics of infant/child
    Verbalization of resentment toward infant/child
    Verbalization of role inadequacy
    Inattention to needs of infant/child
    Verbal disgust at body functions of infant/child
    Noncompliance with health appointments for self
      and/or infant/child
    Inappropriate caretaking behaviors (toilet training,
      sleep/rest, feeding)
    Inappropriate or inconsistent discipline practices
    Frequent accidents
    Frequent illness
    Growth and development lag in child
    History of child abuse or abandonment by primary
      caretaker
    Verbalizes desire to have child call parent by first
      name despite traditional cultural tendencies
    Child receives care from multiple caretakers with-
      out consideration for the needs of a child
    Compulsive seeking of role approval from others
  Actual
    Abandonment
    Runaway
    Verbalization of inability to control child
    Evidence of physical and psychological trauma

Peripheral neurovascular dysfunction, risk for

A state in which an individual is at risk of experiencing a
disruption in circulation, sensation, or motion of an extremity.

Risk factors
Fractures
Mechanical compression (e.g., tourniquet, cast, brace,
    dressing, or restraint)
Orthopedic surgery
Trauma
Immobilization
Burns
Vascular obstruction

Personal identity disturbance

Inability to distinguish between self and nonself.

Related factors
To be developed

Defining characteristic
To be developed

Poisoning, risk for

Accentuated risk of accidental exposure to or ingestion of drugs
or dangerous products in doses sufficient to cause poisoning.

Risk factors
  Internal (individual) factors
    Reduced vision
    Verbalization of occupational setting without ade-
        quate safeguards
    Lack of safety or drug education
    Lack of proper precaution
    Cognitive or emotional difficulties
    Insufficient finances
  External (environmental) factors
    Large supplies of drugs in house
    Medicines stored in unlocked cabinets accessible to
        children or confused persons
    Dangerous products placed or stored within reach
        of children or confused persons
    Availability of illicit drugs potentially contami-
        nated by poisonous additives

Flaking, peeling paint or plaster in presence of
young children
Chemical contamination of food and water
Unprotected contact with heavy metals or
chemicals
Paint, lacquer, etc., in poorly ventilated areas or
without effective protection
Presence of poisonous vegetation
Presence of atmospheric pollutants

Post-trauma response

The state in which an individual experiences a sustained painful
response to (an) overwhelming traumatic event(s).

Related factors
Disaster
War
Epidemic
Rape
Assault
Torture
Catastrophic illness
Accident

Defining characteristics
Reexperience of traumatic event, which may be identified in cognitive, affective, and/or sensory motor
activities (flashbacks, intrusive thoughts, repetitive
dreams or nightmares, excessive verbalization of
traumatic event, verbalization of survival guilt or
guilt about behavior required for survival)
Psychic/emotional numbness (impaired interpretation
of reality, confusion, dissociation or amnesia,
vagueness about traumatic event, constricted
affect)
Altered lifestyle (self-destructiveness, e.g., substance
abuse, suicide attempt, or other acting-out behavior; difficulty with interpersonal relationships;
development of phobia regarding trauma; poor
impulse control/irritability; explosiveness)

Post-trauma response

Powerlessness

Perception that one's own action will not significantly affect an outcome; a perceived lack of control over a current situation or immediate happening.

Related factors
Health-care environment
Interpersonal interaction
Illness-related regimen
Lifestyle of helplessness

Defining characteristics
Severe
Verbal expressions of having no control or influence over situation
Verbal expressions of having no control or influence over outcome
Verbal expressions of having no control over self-care
Depression over physical deterioration that occurs despite patient compliance with regimens
Apathy
Moderate
Nonparticipation in care or decision making when opportunities are provided
Expressions of dissatisfaction and frustration over inability to perform previous tasks and/or activities
Does not monitor progress
Expression of doubt regarding role performance
Reluctance to express true feelings, fearing alienation from caregivers
Inability to seek information regarding care
Dependence on others that may result in irritability, resentment, anger, and guilt
Does not defend self-care practices when challenged
Low
Passivity
Expressions of uncertainty about fluctuating energy levels

Protection, altered

The state in which an individual experiences a decrease in the ability to guard the self from internal or external threats, such as illness or injury.

Related factors
Extremes of age
Inadequate nutrition
Alcohol abuse
Abnormal blood profiles (leukopenia, thrombocytopenia, anemia, coagulation)
Drug therapies (antineoplastic, corticosteroid, immune, anticoagulant, thrombolytic)
Treatments (surgery, radiation)
Diseases such as cancer and immune disorders

Defining characteristics
Deficient immunity
Impaired healing
Altered clotting
Maladaptive stress response
Neurosensory alterations
Chilling
Perspiring
Dyspnea
Cough
Itching
Restlessness
Insomnia
Fatigue
Anorexia
Weakness
Immobility
Disorientation
Pressure sores

Rape-trauma syndrome

Forced, violent sexual penetration against the victim's will and consent. The trauma syndrome that develops from this attack or attempted attack includes an acute phase or disorganization of the victim's lifestyle and a long-term process of reorganization of lifestyle.

Related factors
Inadequate support systems
Spouse-family blaming
Fear of reprisal, pregnancy, going out alone
Anxiety about potential health problems (e.g., AIDS, venereal disease, herpes)

Defining characteristics
  Acute phase
  Emotional reactions
      Anger
      Embarrassment
      Fear of physical violence and death
      Humiliation
      Revenge
      Self-blame
  Multiple physical symptoms
  Gastrointestinal irritability
  Genitourinary discomfort
  Muscle tension
  Sleep pattern disturbance
  Long-term phase
  Changes in lifestyle (changes in residence; dealing with repetitive nightmares and phobias; seeking family support; seeking social network support)

Rape-trauma syndrome: compound reaction

An acute stress reaction to a rape or attempted rape, experienced along with other major stressors, that can include reactivation of symptoms of a previous condition.*

Related factors
Drug or alcohol abuse
History of and/or current psychiatric illness
History of and/or current physical illness

*Definition developed by Kim, McFarland, and McLane.

Defining characteristics
All defining characteristics listed under Rape-trauma
 syndrome
Reactivated symptoms of such previous conditions
 (i.e., physical illness, psychiatric illness)
Reliance on alcohol and/or drugs

Rape-trauma syndrome: silent reaction

A complex stress reaction to a rape in which an individual is
unable to describe or discuss the rape.*

Related factors
Fear of retaliation
Intense shame
Excessive denial
Lack of support

Defining characteristics
Abrupt changes in relationships with members of the
 opposite sex
Increase in nightmares
Increasing anxiety during interview (e.g., blocking of
 associations, long periods of silence, minor stutter-
 ing, physical distress)
Marked changes in sexual behavior
No verbalization of occurrence of the rape
Sudden onset of phobic reactions

Relocation stress syndrome

Physiological and/or psychosocial disturbances as a result of
transfer from one environment to another.

Related factors
Past, concurrent, and recent losses
Losses involved with decision to move
Feeling of powerlessness
Lack of adequate support system
Little or no preparation for the impending move
Moderate to high degree of environmental change
History and types of previous transfers

*Definition developed by Kim, McFarland, and McLane.

Impaired psychosocial health status
Decreased physical health status

Defining characteristics
  Major
    Change in environment/location
    Anxiety
    Apprehension
    Increased confusion (elderly population)
    Depression
    Loneliness
  Minor
    Verbalization of unwillingness to relocate
    Sleep disturbance
    Change in eating habits
    Dependency
    Gastrointestinal disturbances
    Increased verbalization of needs
    Insecurity
    Lack of trust
    Restlessness
    Sad affect
    Unfavorable comparison of post/pre-transfer staff
    Verbalization of being concerned/upset about
      transfer
    Vigilance
    Weight change
    Withdrawal

Role performance, altered

Disruption in the way one perceives one's role performance

Related factors
To be developed

Defining characteristics
Change in self-perception of role
Denial of role
Change in others' perception of role
Conflict in roles
Change in physical capacity to resume role
Lack of knowledge of role
Change in usual patterns or responsibility

70

Self-care deficit, bathing/hygiene

The state in which one experiences an impaired ability to perform or complete bathing/hygiene activities for oneself.

Related factors
To be developed

Defining characteristics
Inability to wash body or body parts
Inability to obtain or get to water source
Inability to regulate temperature or flow

Self-care deficit, dressing/grooming

The state in which one experiences an impaired ability to perform or complete dressing and grooming activities for oneself.

Related factors
To be developed

Defining characteristics
Impaired ability to put on or take off necessary items of clothing
Impaired ability to obtain or replace articles of clothing
Impaired ability to fasten clothing
Inability to maintain appearance at satisfactory level

Self-care deficit, feeding

The state in which one experiences an impaired ability to perform or complete feeding activites for oneself.

Related factors
To be developed

Defining characteristic
Inability to bring food from receptacle to mouth

Self-care deficit, toileting

The state in which one experiences an impaired ability to perform or complete toileting activities for oneself.

Related factors
Impaired transfer ability
Impaired mobility status
Intolerance to activity; decreased strength and
    endurance
Pain, discomfort
Perceptual or cognitive impairment
Neuromuscular impairment
Musculoskeletal impairment
Depression, severe anxiety

Defining characteristics
Inability to get to toilet or commode
Inability to sit on or rise from toilet or commode
Inability to manipulate clothing for toileting
Inability to carry out proper toilet hygiene
Inability to flush toilet or empty commode

Self-concept, disturbance in

See Body image disturbance; Personal identity disturbance; Self-esteem disturbance.

Self-esteem disturbance

Negative self-evaluation/feelings about self or self-capabilities, which may be directly or indirectly expressed.

Related factors
To be developed

Defining characteristics
Self-negating verbalization
Expressions of shame/guilt
Evaluation of self as unable to deal with events
Rationalization/rejection of positive feedback and ex-
    aggeration of negative feedback about self
Hesitancy to try new things/situations
Denial of problems obvious to others
Projection of blame /responsibility for problems
Rationalization of personal failures
Hypersensitivity to criticism
Grandiosity

Self-esteem, chronic low

Long-standing negative self-evaluation/feelings about self or self-capabilities.

Related factors
To be developed

Defining characteristics
  Major
  Long-standing or chronic: self-negating verbalization
  Expressions of shame/guilt
  Evaluates self as unable to deal with events
  Rationalizes away/rejects positive feedback and exaggerates negative feedback about self
  Hesitant to try new things/situations
  Minor
  Frequent lack of success in work or other life events
  Overly conforming, dependent on others' opinions
  Lack of eye contact
  Nonassertive/passive
  Indecisive
  Excessively seeks reassurance

Self-esteem, situational low

Negative self-evaluation/feelings about self that develop in response to a loss or change in an individual who previously had a positive self-evaluation.

Related factors
To be developed

Defining characteristics
  Major
  Episodic occurrence of negative self-appraisal in reponse to life events in a person with a previous positive self evaluation
  Verbalization of negative feelings about the self (helplessness, uselessness)
  Minor
  Self-negating verbalizations
  Expressions of shame/guilt

Evaluates self as unable to handle situations/events
Difficulty making decisions

Self-mutilation, risk for

A state in which an individual is at high risk to perform an act on the self to injure, not kill, that produces tissue damage and tension relief.

Risk factors
Groups at risk:

Clients with borderline personality disorder, especially females 16 to 25 years of age

Clients in psychotic state—frequently males in young adulthood

Emotionally disturbed and/or battered children

Mentally retarded and autistic children

Clients with a history of self-injury

History of physical, emotional, or sexual abuse
Inability to cope with increased psychological/physiological tension in a healthy manner

Feelings of depression, rejection, self-hatred, separation anxiety, guilt, and depersonalization

Fluctuating emotions

Command hallucinations

Need for sensory stimuli

Parental emotional deprivation

Dysfunctional family

Sensory/perceptual alterations (specify) (visual, auditory, kinesthetic, gustatory, tactile, olfactory)

The state in which an individual experiences a change in the amount or patterning of incoming stimuli accompanied by a diminished, exaggerated, distorted, or impaired response to such stimuli.

Related factors
Environmental factors
Therapeutically restricted environments (isolation,

intensive care, bed rest, traction, confining illnesses, incubator)

Socially restricted environment (institutionalization, homebound, aging, chronic illness, dying,
   infant deprivation); stigmatized (mentally ill,
   mentally retarded, mentally handicapped);
   bereaved

Altered sensory reception, transmission, and/or
   integration:
   Neurological disease, trauma, or deficit
   Altered status of sense organs
   Inability to communicate, understand, speak, or
      respond
   Sleep deprivation
   Pain

Chemical alteration

Endogenous (electrolyte imbalance, elevated blood
   urea nitrogen (BUN) level, elevated ammonia,
   hypoxia)

Exogenous (central nervous system stimulants or
   depressants, mind-altering drugs)

Psychological stress (narrowed perceptual fields
   caused by anxiety)

Defining characteristics

Disoriented in time, place, or with persons
Altered abstraction
Altered conceptualization
Change in problem-solving abilities
Reported or measured change in sensory acuity
Change in behavior pattern
Anxiety
Apathy
Change in usual response to stimuli
Indication of body image alteration
Restlessness
Irritability
Altered communication patterns
Disorientation
Lack of concentration
Daydreaming
Hallucinations

Sensory/perceptual alterations (specify) (visual, auditory, kinesthetic, gustatory, tactile, olfactory)—cont'd

Noncompliance
Fear
Depression
Rapid mood swings
Anger
Exaggerated emotional responses
Poor concentration
Disordered thought sequencing
Bizarre thinking
Visual and auditory distortions
Motor incoordination

Other possible defining characteristics
Complaints of fatigue
Alteration in posture
Change in muscular tension
Inappropriate responses
Hallucinations

Sexual dysfunction

The state in which an individual experiences a change in sexual function that is viewed as unsatisfying, unrewarding, or inadequate

Related factors
Biopsychosocial alteration of sexuality
   Ineffectual or absent role models
   Physical abuse
   Psychosocial abuse (e.g., harmful relationships)
   Vulnerability
   Misinformation or lack of knowledge
   Values conflict
   Lack of privacy
   Lack of significant other
   Altered body structure or function: pregnancy, recent childbirth, drugs, surgery, anomalies, disease process, trauma, radiation

Defining characteristics
Verbalization of problem
Alterations in achieving perceived sex role
Actual or perceived limitation imposed by disease and/or therapy

Conflicts involving values
Alterations in achieving sexual satisfaction
Inability to achieve desired satisfaction
Seeking of confirmation of desirability
Alteration in relationship with significant other
Change in interest in self and others

Sexuality patterns, altered

The state in which an individual expresses concern regarding his/her sexuality.

Related factors
Knowledge/skill deficit about alternative responses to health-related transitions, altered body function or structure, illness, or medical treatment
Lack of privacy
Lack of significant other
Ineffective or absent role models
Conflicts with sexual orientation or variant preferences
Fear of pregnancy or of acquiring sexually transmitted disease
Impaired relationship with significant other

Defining characteristics
Reported difficulties, limitations, or changes in sexual behaviors or activities

Skin integrity, impaired

The state in which an individual's skin is adversely altered.

Related factors
External (environmental)
Hyperthermia or hypothermia
Chemical substance
Mechanical factors
   Shearing forces
   Pressure
   Restraint
   Radiation
   Physical immobilization

Skin integrity, impaired

Humidity
Internal (somatic)
Medication
Altered nutritional state: obesity, emaciation
Altered metabolic state
Altered circulation
Altered sensation
Altered pigmentation
Skeletal prominence
Developmental factors
Immunological deficit
Alterations in turgor (change in elasticity)
Excretions/secretions
Psychogenic
Edema

Defining characteristics
Disruption of skin surface
Destruction of skin layers
Invasion of body structures

Skin integrity, impaired, risk for

The state in which an individual's skin is at risk of being adversely altered.

Risk factors
External (environmental)
Hypothermia or hyperthermia
Chemical substance
Mechanical factors
Shearing forces
Pressure
Restraint
Radiation
Physical immobilization
Excretions and secretions
Humidity
Internal (somatic)
Medication
Altered nutritional state: obesity, emaciation
Altered metabolic state

Altered circulation
Altered sensation
Altered pigmentation
Skeletal prominence
Developmental factors
Alterations in skin turgor (change in elasticity)
Psychogenic
Immunological

Sleep pattern disturbance

Disruption of sleep time causes discomfort or interferes with desired lifestyle.

Related factors
Sensory alterations
    Internal factors
        Illness
        Psychological stress
    External factors
        Environmental changes
        Social cues

Defining characteristics
Verbal complaints of difficulty in falling asleep
Awakening earlier or later than desired
Interrupted sleep
Verbal complaints of not feeling well-rested
Changes in behavior and performance
    Increasing irritability
    Restlessness
    Disorientation
    Lethargy
    Listlessness
Physical signs
    Mild, fleeting nystagmus
    Slight hand tremor
    Ptosis of eyelid
    Expressionless face
Thick speech with mispronunciation and incorrect words
Dark circles under eyes
Frequent yawning

Changes in posture
Not feeling well-rested

Social interaction, impaired

The state in which an individual participates in an insufficient or excessive quantity or ineffective quality of social exchange.

Related factors
Knowledge/skill deficit about ways to enhance mutuality
Communication barriers
Self-concept disturbance
Absence of available significant others or peers
Limited physical mobility
Therapeutic isolation
Sociocultural dissonance
Environmental barriers
Altered thought processes

Defining characteristics
Verbalized or observed discomfort in social situations
Verbalized or observed inability to receive or communicate a satisfying sense of belonging, caring, interest, or shared history
Observed use of unsuccessful social interaction behaviors
Dysfunctional interaction with peers, family, and/or others
Family report of change in style or pattern of interaction

Social isolation

Aloneness experienced by an individual and perceived as imposed by others and as a negative or threatened state.

Related factors
Factors contributing to the absence of satisfying personal relationships, such as the following:
   Delay in accomplishing developmental tasks
   Immature interests
   Alterations in physical appearance
   Alterations in mental status

Unaccepted social behavior
Unaccepted social values
Altered state of wellness
Inadequate personal resources
Inability to engage in satisfying personal relationships

Defining characteristics
Objective
Absence of supportive significant other(s)—family, friends, group
Sad, dull affect
Inappropriate or immature interests and activities for developmental age or stage
Uncommunicative, withdrawn; no eye contact
Preoccupation with own thoughts; repetitive, meaningless actions
Projects hostility in voice, behavior
Seeks to be alone or exists in subculture
Evidence of physical and/or mental handicap or altered state of wellness
Shows behavior unaccepted by dominant cultural group

Subjective
Expresses feeling of aloneness imposed by others
Expresses feelings of rejection
Experiences feelings of indifference of others
Expresses values acceptable to subculture but is unable to accept values of dominant culture
Inadequacy in or absence of significant purpose in life
Inability to meet expectations of others
Insecurity in public
Expresses interests inappropriate to developmental age or stage

Spiritual distress (distress of the human spirit)

Disruption in the life principle that pervades a person's entire being and that integrates and transcends one's biological and psychosocial nature.

Related factors

Separation from religious and cultural ties

Challenged belief and value system (e.g., result of moral or ethical implications of therapy or result of intense suffering)

Defining characteristics

Expresses concern with meaning of life and death and/or belief systems

Anger toward God (as defined by the person)

Questions meaning of suffering

Verbalizes inner conflict about beliefs

Verbalizes concern about relationship with deity

Questions meaning of own existence

Inability to choose or chooses not to participate in usual religious practices

Seeks spiritual assistance

Questions moral and ethical implications of therapeutic regimen

Displacement of anger toward religious representatives

Description of nightmares or sleep disturbances

Alteration in behavior or mood evidenced by anger, crying, withdrawal, preoccupation, anxiety, hostility, apathy, etc.

Regards illness as punishment

Does not experience that God is forgiving

Inability to accept self

Engages in self-blame

Denies responsibilities for problems

Description of somatic complaints

Spiritual well-being, potential for enhanced

Spiritual well-being is the process of an individual's developing or unfolding of mystery through harmonious interconnectedness that springs from inner strengths.

Defining characteristics

Inner strengths

A sense of awareness, self consciousness, sacred source, unifying force, inner core, and transcendence

Unfolding mystery

One's experience about life's purpose and meaning, mystery, uncertainty, and struggles

Harmonious interconnectedness

Relatedness, connectedness, harmony with self, others, higher power or God, and the environment

Suffocation, risk for

Accentuated risk of accidental suffocation (inadequate air available for inhalation).

Risk factors
Internal (individual) factors
  Reduced olfactory sensation
  Reduced motor abilities
  Lack of safety education
  Lack of safety precautions
  Cognitive or emotional difficulties
  Disease or injury process
External (environmental) factors
  Pillow placed in infant's crib
  Vehicle warming in closed garage
  Children playing with plastic bags or inserting small objects into their mouths or noses
  Discarded or unused refrigerators or freezers without doors removed
  Children left unattended in bathtubs or pools
  Household gas leaks
  Smoking in bed
  Use of fuel-burning heaters not vented to outside
  Low-strung clothesline
  Pacifier hung around infant's head
  Eating large mouthfuls of food
  Propped bottle placed in infant's crib

Swallowing, impaired

The state in which an individual has decreased ability to voluntarily pass fluids and/or solids from the mouth to the stomach.

Related factors
Neuromuscular impairment (e.g., decreased or absent

gag reflex, decreased strength or excursion of muscles involved in mastication, perceptual impairment, facial paralysis)
Mechanical obstruction (e.g., edema, tracheotomy tube, tumor)
Fatigue
Limited awareness
Reddened, irritated oropharyngeal cavity

Defining characteristics
Observed evidence of difficulty in swallowing (e.g., stasis of food in oral cavity, cough/choking)
Evidence of aspiration

Thermoregulation, ineffective

The state in which an individual's temperature fluctuates between hypothermia and hyperthermia.

Related factors
Trauma or illness
Immaturity
Aging
Fluctuating environmental temperature

Defining characteristics
Fluctuations in body temperature above or below normal range
See also defining characteristics of hypothermia and hyperthermia

Thought processes, altered

The state in which an individual experiences a disruption in cognitive operations or activities.

Related factors
To be developed

Defining characteristics
Inaccurate interpretation of environment
Cognitive dissonance
Distractibility
Memory deficit or problems

Egocentricity
Hypervigilance/hypovigilance

Other possible defining characteristics
Inappropriate/nonreality-based thinking

Tissue integrity, impaired

The state in which an individual experiences damage to mucous membrane or corneal, integumentary, or subcutaneous tissue. See also Oral mucous membrane, altered.

Related factors
Altered circulation
Nutritional deficit/excess
Fluid deficit/excess
Knowledge deficit
Impaired physical mobility
  Irritants
  Chemical (including body excretions, secretions, medications)
  Thermal (temperature extremes)
  Mechanical (pressure, shear, friction)
  Radiation (including therapeutic radiation)

Defining characteristic
Damaged or destroyed tissue (cornea, mucous membrane, integumentary, or subcutaneous)

Tissue perfusion, altered (specify type) (renal, cerebral, cardiopulmonary, gastrointestinal, peripheral)

The state in which an individual experiences a decrease in nutrition and oxygenation at the cellular level due to a deficit in capillary blood supply.

Related factors
Interruption of flow, arterial
Interruption of flow, venous
Exchange problems
Hypervolemia
Hypovolemia

Defining characteristics
Skin temperature: cold extremities
Skin color
    Dependent, blue or purple
    Pale on elevation, and color does not return on
        lowering leg
    Diminished arterial pulsations
Skin quality: shining
Lack of lanugo
Round scars covered with atrophied skin
Gangrene
Slow-growing, dry, thick, brittle nails
Claudication
Blood pressure changes in extremities
Bruits
Slow healing of lesions

Trauma, risk for

Accentuated risk of accidental tissue injury (e.g., wound, burn, fracture).

Risk factors
  Internal (individual) factors
    Weakness
    Poor vision
    Balancing difficulties
    Reduced temperature and/or tactile sensation
    Reduced large—or small—muscle coordination
    Reduced hand-eye coordination
    Lack of safety education
    Lack of safety precautions
    Insufficient finances to purchase safety equipment
        or effect repairs
    Cognitive or emotional difficulties
    History of previous trauma
  External (environmental) factors
    Slippery floors (e.g., wet or highly waxed)
    Snow or ice on stairs, walkways
    Unanchored rugs
    Bathtub without hand grip or antislip equipment
    Use of unsteady ladder or chairs

Entering unlighted rooms
Unsturdy or absent stair rails
Unanchored electric wires
Litter or liquid spills on floors or stairways
High beds
Children playing without gates at tops of stairs
Obstructed passageways
Unsafe window protection in homes with young children
Inappropriate call-for-aid mechanisms for bed-resting client
Pot handles facing toward front of stove
Bathing in very hot water (e.g., unsupervised bathing of young children)
Potential igniting of gas leaks
Delayed lighting of gas burner or oven
Experimenting with chemicals or gasoline
Unscreened fires or heaters
Wearing of plastic aprons or flowing clothing around open flame
Children playing with matches, candles, cigarettes
Inadequately stored combustibles or corrosives (e.g., matches, oily rags, lye)
Highly flammable children's toys or clothing
Overloaded fuse boxes
Contact with rapidly moving machinery, industrial belts, or pulleys
Sliding on coarse bed linen or struggling within bed restraints
Faulty electrical plugs, frayed wires, or defective appliances
Contact with acids or alkalis
Playing with fireworks or gunpowder
Contact with intense cold
Overexposure to sun, sun lamps, radiotherapy
Use of cracked dishware or glasses
Knives stored uncovered
Guns or ammunition stored unlocked
Large icicles hanging from roof
Exposure to dangerous machinery
Children playing with sharp-edged toys
High-crime neighborhood and vulnerable patient

Driving a mechanically unsafe vehicle
Driving after partaking of alcoholic beverages or
    drugs
Driving at excessive speeds
Driving without necessary visual aids
Children riding in front seat of car
Smoking in bed or near oxygen
Overloaded electrical outlets
Grease waste collected on stoves
Use of thin or worn pot holders or mitts
Unrestrained babies riding in car
Nonuse or misuse of seat restraints
Nonuse or misuse of necessary headgear for motor-
    ized cyclists or young children carried on adult
    bicycles
Unsafe road or road-crossing conditions
Play or work near vehicle pathways (e.g., drive-
    ways, lanes, railroad tracks)

Unilateral neglect

The state in which an individual is perceptually unaware of and
inattentive to one side of the body.

Related factors
Effects of disturbed perceptual abilities (e.g., hemi-
    anopsia)
One-sided blindness
Neurological illness or trauma

Defining characteristics
Consistent inattention to stimuli on affected side
Inadequate self-care
Positioning and/or safety precautions in regard to
    affected side
Does not look toward affected side
Leaves food on plate on affected side

Urinary elimination, altered

The state in which an individual experiences a disturbance in
urine elimination. See also Incontinence (functional, reflex,
stress, total, urge).

Related factors
Sensory motor impairment
Neuromuscular impairment
Mechanical trauma

Defining characteristics
Dysuria
Frequency
Hesitancy
Incontinence
Nocturia
Retention
Urgency

Urinary retention

The state in which an individual experiences incomplete emptying of the bladder.

Related factors
High urethral pressure caused by weak detrusor
Inhibition of reflex arc
Strong sphincter
Blockage

Defining characteristics
Bladder distention
Small, frequent voiding or absence of urine output
Sensation of bladder fullness
Dribbling
Residual urine
Dysuria
Overflow incontinence

Ventilation, inability to sustain spontaneous

A state in which the response pattern of decreased energy reserves results in an individual's inability to maintain breathing adequate to support life.

Related factors
Metabolic factors
Respiratory muscle fatigue

Defining characteristics
  Major
    Dyspnea
    Increased metabolic rate
  Minor
    Increased restlessness
    Apprehension
    Increased use of accessory muscles
    Decreased tidal volume
    Increased heart rate
    Decreased pO_2 level
    Increased pCO_2 level
    Decreased cooperation
    Decreased SaO_2 level

Ventilatory weaning response, dysfunction (DVWR)

A state in which an individual cannot adjust to lowered levels of mechanical ventilator support, which interrupts and prolongs the weaning process.

Related factors
  Physical
    Ineffective airway clearance
    Sleep pattern disturbance
    Inadequate nutrition
    Uncontrolled pain or discomfort
  Psychological
    Knowledge deficit of the weaning process/patient role
    Patient-perceived inefficacy about the ability to wean
    Decreased motivation
    Decreased self-esteem
    Anxiety: moderate, severe
    Fear
    Hopelessness
    Powerlessness
    Insufficient trust in the nurse
  Situational
    Uncontrolled episodic energy demands or problems

Inappropriate pacing of diminished ventilator
support
Inadequate social support
Adverse environment (noisy, active environment;
negative events in the room; low nurse-patient
ratio; extended nurse absence from bedside; unfamiliar nursing staff)
History of ventilator dependence > 1 week
History of multiple unsuccessful weaning attempts

Defining characteristics
Mild DVWR
Major
Responds to lowered levels of mechanical ventila-
tor support with the following:
Restlessness
Slight increased respiratory rate from baseline
Minor
Responds to lowered levels of mechanical ventila-
tor support with the following:
Expressed feelings of increased need for oxygen;
breathing discomfort; fatigue, warmth
Queries about possible machine malfunction
Increased concentration on breathing
Moderate DVWR
Major
Responds to lowered levels of mechanical ventila-
tor support with the following:
Slight increase from baseline blood pressure
<20 mm Hg
Slight increase from baseline heart rate <20
beats/minute
Baseline increase in respiratory rate <5
breaths/minute
Minor
Hypervigilance to activities
Inability to respond to coaching
Inability to cooperate
Apprehension
Diaphoresis
Eye widening
Decreased air entry on auscultation

Color changes; pale; slight cyanosis
Slight respiratory accessory muscle use
Severe DVWR
Major
Responds to lowered levels of mechanical ventilator support with the following:
Agitation
Deterioration in arterial blood gas levels from current baseline
Increase from baseline blood pressure >20 mm Hg
Increase from baseline heart rate >20 beats/minute
Respiratory rate increases significantly from baseline
Minor
Profuse diaphoresis
Full respiratory accessory muscle use
Shallow, gasping breaths
Paradoxical abdominal breathing
Discoordinated breathing with the ventilator
Decreased level of consciousness
Adventitious breath sounds, audible airway secretions
Cyanosis

Violence, risk for: directed at others*

Behaviors in which an individual demonstrates that he/she can be physically, emotionally, and/or sexually harmful to others.

Risk factors
History of violence:
Against others (hitting someone, kicking someone, spitting at someone, scratching someone, throwing objects at someone, biting someone, attempted rape, rape, sexual molestation, urinating/defecating on a person
Threats (verbal threats against property, verbal threats against person, social threats, cursing, threatening notes/letters, threatening gestures, sexual threats)

Against self (suicidal threats or attempts, hitting or injuring self, banging head against wall)

Social (stealing, insistent borrowing, insistent demands for privileges, insistent interruption of meetings, refusal to eat, refusal to take medication, ignoring instructions)

Indirect (tearing off clothes, ripping objects off walls, writing on walls, urinating on floor, defecating on floor, stamping feet, temper tantrum, running in corridors, yelling, throwing objects, breaking a window, slamming doors, sexual advances)

Other factors

Neurological impairment (positive electroencephalogram, computerized axial tomography (CAT) or magnetic resonance image, head trauma, positive neurological findings, seizure disorders)

Cognitive impairment (learning disabilities, attention deficit disorder, decreased intellectual functioning)

History of childhood abuse

History of witnessing family violence

Cruelty to animals

Firesetting

Prenatal and perinatal complications/abnormalities

History of drug/alcohol abuse

Pathological intoxication

Psychotic symptomatology (auditory, visual, command hallucinations)

Paranoid delusions

Loose, rambling or illogical thought processes

Motor vehicle offenses (frequent traffic violations, use of motor vehicle to release anger)

Suicidal behavior

Impulsivity

Availability and/or possession of weapon(s)

Body language: rigid posture, clenching of fists and jaw, hyperactivity, pacing, breathlessness, and threatening stances

Related factors

Antisocial character

Battered women

Catatonic excitement
Child abuse
Manic excitement
Organic brain syndrome
Panic states
Rage reactions
Suicidal behavior
Temporal lobe epilepsy
Toxic reactions to medication

*In 1996 NANDA split the diagnosis "Violence, risk for: self-directed or directed at others" into two diagnoses, "Violence, risk for: self-directed:" and "Violence, risk for: directed at others"

NURSING DIAGNOSES

Prototype Care Plans

Key to the Care Plan Format

Patient goals
Expected outcomes
  Associated nursing/collaborative interventions *and
    scientific rationale*

LINDA K. YOUNG, MARIE MAGUIRE, MARILYN HARTER, AND AUDREY M. MCLANE

Activity intolerance

CLINICAL CONDITION/ MEDICAL DIAGNOSIS	RISK FACTORS
Myocardial infarction; nearing discharge from acute care hospital	Imbalance between oxygen supply and demand; ineffective pain management

---

Patient goals
Expected outcomes
  Associated nursing/collaborative interventions *and scientific rationale*

Develop activity/rest pattern consistent with physiological limitations as evidenced by the following:

Monitors physiological response to activity
Manages pain effectively
Engages in regular exercise of 4 METS or less
Tolerates job-related activities without pain or fatigue

  Teach patient to monitor physiological responses to activity, e.g., pulse rate, shortness of breath. *Self-monitoring facilitates determination/evaluation of activity level consistent with physical status.*

  Develop individualized activity/exercise program including home exercises. *Patients are more likely to follow individualized programs of activity/exercise to obtain the beneficial effects on cardiac performance.*

  Collaborate with patient to tailor medication taking to demands of activities. *Taking medications as prescribed can enhance activity tolerance and reduce pain.*

  Assist patient to identify factors that decrease/increase activity tolerance. *Accurate determination of factors that decrease/increase activity tolerance provides a foundation for effective problem solving.*

  Teach patient to eliminate/reduce activities that cause pain or fatigue.

  Discuss necessity to pace activities. *Pacing activity levels lessens cardiac workload.*

Activity intolerance

97

Teach patient use of exercise log to record exercise
activities and responses (pulse, shortness of
breath, anxiety). *Keeping a log may increase compliance.*

Teach patient warning signs of cardiac decompensation, e.g., difficulty breathing, dependent
edema.

**Recognize influences of emotional responses on
exercise tolerance as evidenced by the following:**

Discusses emotional responses with significant other
Learns/practices relaxation techniques
**Significant other understands reasons for use
of cognitive coping strategies**

Teach patient/significant other influence of
fears/anxiety on exercise tolerance. *Fear and
anxiety may decrease activity tolerance.*

Teach/monitor use of cognitive coping strategies,
e.g., imagery relaxation, controlled breathing.
*Emotional responses to activity may be managed
through the use of cognitive coping strategies.*

Encourage significant other to learn coping strategies and/or assist patient in use of the strategies.

**Use social support network to maintain desired
lifestyle as evidenced by the following:**

**Significant other assists with activities of daily living
to prevent activity level from exceeding 4 METs**
Friends/family/neighbors help with home maintenance activities

Collaborate with patient/significant other to establish a plan of daily activities consistent with desired lifestyle and exercise prescription of <4
METs.

Teach significant other to help patient pace
activities.

Encourage patient/significant other to seek assistance with home maintenance activities from
friends, family, neighbors. *Social support enhances
compliance and recovery.*

Determine interest of patient/significant other in sexual counseling. *Sexual activity is often a great concern to patients and their sexual partners.*

REFERENCES

Buchannan L and others: Measurement of recovery from myocardial infarction using heart rate variability and psychological outcomes, *Nurs Res* 42(2):74, 1993.

Davis M, Eshel E: *The relaxation and stress reduction workbook*, Oakland, Calif, 1988, Hew Herbinger.

Froelicheres and others: Return to work, sexual activity and other activities after acute myocardial Infarction. *Heart Lung: Crit Care* 23(5):423-435, 1994.

Holm K, Penckofer SM: Women's cardiovascular health. In *Annual review of women's health,* New York, 1993, National League for Nursing Press, pp 289-310.

Johnson JC, Mouse JM, Regaining control: the process of adjustment after myocardial infarction, *Heart Lung* 19(2):126, 1990.

Low KG: Recovery from myocardial infarction and coronary artery bypass surgery in women: psychosocial factors, *Women's Health* 2(2):133-139, 1993.

McCaffery M, Beebe A: *Pain: clinical manual for nursing*, St Louis, 1989 Mosby.

Miller P and others: Influence of a nursing intervention on regimen adherence and societal adjustment post myocardial infarction, *Nurs Res* 37(5):297, 1988.

Activity intolerance, risk for

CLINICAL CONDITION/ MEDICAL DIAGNOSIS	RISK FACTORS
Myocardial infarction	Fatigue, >15%

> **Patient goals**
> **Expected outcomes**
> > Associated nursing/collaborative interventions *and scientific rationale*

Participate in cardiac rehabilitation program as evidenced by the following:

Enrolls in cardiac rehabilitation program

Negotiate with patient to participate in cardiac rehabilitation program. *Cardiac rehabilitation programs can facilitate the patient's ability to achieve and maintain a vital and productive life while remaining within the heart's ability to respond to increases in activity and stress.*

Encourage spouse to accompany patient on walks. *Social support may enhance participation in the activity.*

Clarifies values with nurse's assistance

Assist patient and significant other with clarification of values. *Becoming aware of one's own values may enhance compliance with prescribed regimen.*

Teach patient long-term value of increased activity. *Highlighting positive long-term effects may increase compliance.*

Verbalizes fears about increasing level of activity

Assist patient in verbalizing anxiety/fear/concerns about engaging in exercise. *Recognizing fears and anxiety is the first step to managing them.*

Integrate exercise prescription into daily living by the following:

Experiences less fatigue after exercise regimen over a period of time

Teach patient/significant other benefits of exercise regimen in decreasing fatigue/weakness.

Activity intolerance, risk for

Uses written list of activities with MET levels to guide activities

Teach patient/significant other the importance of using MET levels to guide and prioritize activities.

Provide written specifications for duration, intensity, frequency, and METs levels of activities of daily living (ADLs) and recreational activities. Knowledge of METs of ADLs and recreational activities promotes safe functioning.

Uses exercise log to record distance walked and symptoms experienced

Teach patient/significant other use of exercise log to record activities, time, duration, intensity, and physiologic responses (e.g., pulse rate, shortness of breath, lightheadedness). *Use of log may increase compliance.*

Teach self-monitoring of heart rate during exercise. *Self-monitoring promotes self-care.*

Teach self-evaluation of response to activity, including actions for specific signs and symptoms.

Gradually reduce body weight as evidenced by the following:

Consults with dietician to begin weight reduction program

Negotiate with patient to make decision to lose weight. *Client input and motivation are factors affecting patient participation in weight reduction.*

Refer to dietician for diet instruction and for recommending caloric requirements.

Encourage spouse to participate in weight reduction instructions.

Assist patient/significant other in preparing shopping list for low-caloric meals. *Predetermined low-caloric meals and snacks help increase the likelihood of limited caloric intake.*

Discuss low-caloric food preparation (e.g., broiling, baking, and poaching).

Achieves desired body weight

Set realistic weekly weight-loss goal.

Monitor weight twice a week *to help patient realize*

weight loss and gain, which can reinforce changed behavior.

Encourage spouse to support patient effort in weight loss.

REFERENCES

Buchannan L and others: Measurement of recovery from myocardial infarction using heart rate variability and psychological outcomes, *Nurs Res* 42(2):74, 1993.

Christ J: Weight management. In Bulechek GM, McCloskey JC, eds: *Nursing interventions: essential nursing treatments*, ed 2, Philadelphia, 1992, WB Saunders.

Conn VS, Taylor SG, Casey B: Cardiac rehabilitation program participation and outcomes after myocardial infarction, *Rehab Nurs* 17(2):58-63, 1992.

Froelicheres, K and others: Return to work, sexual activity and other activities after acute myocardial infarction. *Heart Lung: Crit Care* 23(5):423-435, 1994.

Johnson JC, Mouse JM: Regaining control: the process of adjustment after myocardial infarction, *Heart Lung* 19(2):126, 1990.

Magnan MA: A Bayesian methodological approach to validation of a nursing diagnosis: activity intolerance. In Rantz MJ, Lemone P: *Classification of nursing diagnosis: proceedings of the eleventh conference*, pp 97-111. Glendale, Calif, 1995, CINAHL Information Systems.

Miller P and others: Influence of a nursing intervention on regimen adherence and societal adjustment post myocardial infarction, *Nurs Res* 37(5):297, 1988.

Activity intolerance, risk for—cont'd

Adaptive capacity, decreased: intracranial

CLINICAL CONDITION/ MEDICAL DIAGNOSIS	RELATED FACTORS
Traumatic, closed head injury	Sustained increase in intracranial pressure (ICP) of ≥15 mm Hg and decreased cerebral perfusion pressure (CPP) of ≤50-60 mm Hg.

Patient goals
Expected outcomes
  Associated nursing/collaborative interventions *and*
    scientific rationale

Experience reduced ICP as evidenced by the following:

Decreased or no evidence of deleterious effects of increased ICP

  Perform neuralgic assessment every hour or as needed in order to detect progressive signs of increased ICP.

  Observe for decreasing levels of consciousness, including restlessness, irritability, drowsiness, lethargy, confusion, obtundation, stupor, lower Glasgow Coma Score (GCS), and ability to follow commands.

  Assess pupillary responses: ovoid pupil, hippus, sluggish reactivity progressing to fixed, unilateral change in pupil size (midposition of gradual dilation).

  Assess for visual deficits: decreased visual acuity, blurred vision, papilledema, field cuts, diplopia, nystagmus, and ptosis.

  Assess motor function: progressive paresis, hemiplegia, Babinski sign, or decorticate or decerebrate posturing.

  Observe for headache, vomiting, and seizures.

  Monitor vital signs every hour or as needed: watch for elevation in blood pressure with widening pulse pressure and bradycardia. Signs of decompensation include a decrease in blood pressure,

Adaptive capacity, decreased: intracranial

tachycardia, and irregular respirations (Cheyne-Stokes respiration progressing to neurogenic hyperventilation to irregular brainstem patterns). *Cushing reflex is seen when ICP approaches systemic arterial pressure (SAP), producing pressure and ischemia on the vasomotor center. This triggers a sympathetic response, causing a rise in systolic blood pressure, widening pulse pressure, pulse slowing, and irregular repirations.*

Monitor for cardiac arrhythmias. *Cardiac dysrhythmias are often associated with intracranial pathologic conditions and result in decreased cerebral blood flow (CBF) and ischemia, contributing further to cerebral edema and increased ICP.*

Observe for loss of brainstem reflexes: corneal, gas and swallow, oculocephalic, and oculovestibular reflexes.

Report to physician any evidence of deterioration in neurologic status and initiate interventions to reverse process immediately. *Changes in neurologic status indicate increasing ICP. Early intervention to increase intracranial adaptive capacity and decrease demands prevents deleterious effects of ICP.*

Experience reduced or no elevations in ICP and maintain CCP as evidenced by the following:

ICP within normal limit of 10 to 15 mm Hg
Repeated or sustained elevations in ICP are prevented or minimized
CPP within normal limit of 60 to 100 mm Hg
Patent airway and adequate gas exchange maintained (e.g., PaO_2 80 to 100 mm Hg, $PaCO_2$ 25 to 30 mm Hg, and ability to manage secretions)
Maintain in slightly hypovolemic state
Normothermia to hypothermia maintained

Accurately measure ICP and monitor trends continuously.

Regulate CSF drainage through ventricular catheter.

Calculate CPP every hour and as needed.

Maintain blood pressure within accepted patent parameters. *Hypotension causes ischemia, whereas hypertension causes edema leading to increased ICP and tissue damage.*

Monitor ABGs and regulate ventilator to keep $PaCO_2$ 25 to 30 mm Hg.

Synchronize manual hyperventilation with inspiration. *Hyperventilation lowers $PaCO_2$ levels, leading to vasoconstriction and a decreased ICP. Synchronization of manual hyperventilation prevents increases in intrathoracic pressure and ICP.*

Closely monitor physiologic parameters when using positive end-expiratory pressure *(PEEP). PEEP reduces arterial BP, thereby reducing CPP. PEEP decreases cerebral venous outflow, increasing ICP.*

Suction patient to maintain patent airway only as needed, adhering to the following guidelines: Preoxygenate patient with 100% FiO_2 prior to suctioning. *Hyperoxygenation prevents hypoxemia during suctioning.*

Limit suction duration to 10 seconds and suction passes to 1 or 2. *Limiting suction time and number of suction passes avoids or minimizes cerebral hypertension.*

Allow 2 minutes of undisturbed rest between catheter passes. *Two minutes of undisturbed rest is needed to allow mean SAP, mean ICP, CPP and heart rate to reach baseline levels. MICP increases in a step-wise fashion from baseline to first suctioning episode and from first to second suctioning episode.*

Do not rotate head from side to side. *Passive rotation of head to the right and left is known to increase ICP, with return to baseline levels taking more than 10 minutes.*

Keep negative suction pressure < 120 mm Hg. *Negative suction pressure of < 120 mm Hg is sufficient to remove secretion without reducing residual capacity or contributing to excessive tracheal mucosal damage.*

Use suction catheters with outer to inner diameter ratios < 0.50. *Suction catheters with an OD/ID ration of < 0.50 allows for passive influx of air into the endotracheal tube.*

Minimize or prevent seizure activity

Administer anticonvulsants to maintain therapeutic levels. *Seizure activity increases demand for ATP approximately 250%.*

Maintain neutral body alignment at all times with head of bed elevated 30 degrees unless contraindicated. *Neutral head position maintains CSF flow and prevents obstruction of the jugular veins, increasing venous return and lowering ICP.*

Avoid securing endotracheal tube to neck area. *Prevents obstruction of the jugular veins, increasing venous return and lowering ICP.*

Avoid procedures that increase thoracic and abdominal pressure (e.g., turning and positioning, hip flexion, coughing, restraints, isometric exercises, noxious stimuli, and Valsalva maneuver). Log roll and instruct patient to exhale during activity. Use narcotics sedating or paralyzing agents, hyperventilation, or local anesthetics to blunt response to stimuli. Assess ICP waves during activity and avoid stimulation when elevation of P_2 component occurs. *Increases in thoracic pressure decrease venous return, increase CSF pressure, decrease cardiac output and increase blood pressure, causing additional rise in ICP. Elevation of P_2 occurs with rise in ICP. Analysis of waveforms allows individualization of care.*

Minimize patient activity levels: provide nonstimulating environment, avoid clustering patient care activities, and prevent shivering. Individualize care on the basis of physiologic responses—ICP, CPP, SAP, and cerebral blood flow. *Continued stimulation may lead to undesirable increases in physiologic parameters and deleterious effects on brain function.*

Administer oxygen to maintain PaO_2 above 80 to 100 mm Hg. Monitor arterial blood gasses (ABGs), O_2 saturations, and jugular bulb O_2 extraction. *Hypoxia and hypercapnia produce synergistic effects and increase CBF more than either factor alone.*

Adaptive capacity, decreased: intracranial—cont'd

Use hyperventilation combined with hyperoxygenation *with caution* in head-injured patients with low PaCO$_2$. *Reduction of PaCO$_2$ to below 25 mm Hg significantly decreases CBF further and may actually cause cerebral ischemia.*

Use hyperosmotics, corticosteroids, and diuretics as directed.

Limit fluid intake to a slightly dehydrated level (1500 to 2000 ml). Monitor fluid balance every hour, and electrolytes, CVP or pulmonary artery catheter, urine or serum osmolality, specific gravity, and blood count as needed. Observe for diabetes insipidus or syndrome of inappropriate diuretic hormone. Replace fluids with isotonic fluids, crystalloids, or colloids. *Decrease in intracellular volume decreases cerebral edema and ICP. Hypotonic fluids increase cerebral edema.*

Maintain temperature at normothermic levels or lower by using cooling blanket, antipyretics, antibiotics, aseptic technique. *Each degree centigrade rise in body temperature raises the metabolic demand of the brain by 10%.*

REFERENCES

Barker E: *Neuroscience nursing,* St Louis, 1994, Mosby.

Keller C, Williams A: Cardiac dysrhythmias associated with central nervous system dysfunction, *J Neurosci Nurs* 25(6):349, 1993.

Kerr ME, Lovasik O, Darby J: Evaluating cerebral oxygenation using jugular venous oximetry in head injuries, *AACN Clin Issues* 6(1):11-20, 1995.

Kerr ME and others: Head-injured adults: Recommendations for endotracheal suctioning, *J Neurosci Nurs* 25(2):86, 1993.

March K and others: Effect of backrest position on inracranial and cerebral perfusion pressures. *J Neurosci Nurs* 22(6):375, 1990.

McClelland M and others: Continuous midazolam/atracurium infusions for the management of increased intracranial pressure, *J Neurosci Nurs* 27(2):96-101, 1995.

Prendergast V: Current trends in research and treatment of intracranial hypertension, *Crit Care Nurs Q* 17(1):1, 1994.

Adaptive capacity, decreased: intracranial—cont'd

Adjustment, impaired

CLINICAL CONDITION/ MEDICAL DIAGNOSIS	RISK FACTORS
Myocardial infarction	Disability requiring change in lifestyle or behavior

Patient goals
Expected outcomes
> Associated nursing/collaborative interventions *and scientific rationale*

Modify lifestyle to reduce risk of disease recurrence, decrease impact of disability and increase independence within limits imposed by change of health status as recognized by the following:

Recognized that choice of self-care practices can influence adjustment to disability

> Assist patient in working through emotional responses to MI (e.g., denial, anxiety, or depression) by using communication techniques that help patient to maintain appropriate control over own care and health.

> Provide opportunity for expression of fears related to MI and potential physical limitations; *the patient's perception of disability associated with the MI influences the patient's adaptation to the change in health status.*

> Teach patient and family to differentiate between denial of the presence of change in health status due to MI and denial of possible limitations *to maximize physiological and psychosocial adaptation.*

> Consistently convey value of self-directive behavior on patient's part.

> Assist patient in identifying and understanding how choice of health care practices can influence adjustment from MI.

> Encourage use of problem-focused coping strategies (e.g., discussing own health problems with oth-

ers in a similar situation, pacing changes in health care and lifestyle by setting monthly goals with related daily activities). *Patients who use problem-focused coping strategies experience increased perception of self-control, and appear to have less psychosocial difficulty with post-MI adjustment.*

Demonstrates self-care practices that are within prescribed treatment regimen

Provide information about MI and what to expect during and after hospitalization, based on assessment of learning readiness, *to reduce fear and anxiety associated with hospitalization and to reinforce positive psychological and social outcomes.*

Promote patient's making decisions related to specific aspects of care, sharing observations of physical status and progress with caregivers, and assuming responsibility for selected aspects of care *to maximize patient's achieving and maintaining a sense of control (within physical limitations).*

Assist patient to select self-care practices that enhance risk factor modification, adjustment to disability (e.g., maintaining balanced exercise/rest regimen) including need for modification of activities of daily living during convalescence.

Uses strengths and potential to engage in maximally independent and constructive lifestyle

Convey hope that patient is able to overcome difficulties in current situation.

Use the patient's family as a resource to promote discussion of topics that are not related to disability (e.g., current events, family activities, hobbies, recreation interests).

Encourage identification of personal strengths and intact roles *to maximize sense of ability for regaining control and minimizing perception of disability as a handicap.*

Have patient identify previous coping behaviors and support systems used for past problem solving *to help patient mobilize previous coping strengths and skills that can be used in current situation.*

Makes future plans that are congruent with changed health status

Assess for possible correlation between extent of family's willingness to support patient's changed lifestyle and patient's ability to adapt to changes in health status.

Actively include family and significant others in entire cardiac rehabilitation process. *The perceived beliefs of significant others are important for patient's adherence to medical regimen.*

Collaborate with patient and other staff *to assist in determining factors that will promote control and management of patient's health status change.*

Facilitate compromise when patient's identified goals differ from goals developed by health-care providers or from family expectations.

Uses available health-care system and community resources

Assess for presence of closed networks (e.g., closed family system or closed cultural system). *Social support plays a significant role in coping with disability and lifestyle management. Closed family or closed cultural systems may influence appropriate help-seeking by patient and/or family.*

Encourage patient and family to explore such resources as Medicare, Social Security, and disability insurance.

Refer patient and significant other to community resources such as cardiac support groups or the American Heart Association for assistance with ongoing informational needs, advocacy issues, and current developments in treatment and research.

REFERENCES

Hilbert GA: Cardiac patients and spouses: family functioning and emotions, *Clin Nurs Res* 3(3):243, 1994.

Johnson JI, Morse JM: Regaining control: the process of adjustment after myocardial infarction, *Heart Lung* 19(2):126, 1990.

Malan SS: Psychosocial adjustment following MI: Current view and nursing implications, *J Cardiovasc Nurs* 6(4):57, 1992.

McCauley, KM: Assessing social support in patients with cardiac disease, *J Cardiovasc Nurs* 10(1):73, 1995.

Moser DK, Dracup KA: Psychosocial recovery from a cardiac event: the influence of perceived control, *Heart Lung* 23(4):273, 1995.

Adjustment, impaired—cont'd

Riegel BJ, Dracup KA: Does overprotection cause cardiac invalidism after acute myocardial infarction? *Heart Lung* 21(6):529, 1992.

Rose SK and others: Anxiety and self-care following myocardial infarction, *Issues Ment Health Nurs* 15(4):433, 1994.

Webb M and Riggin O: A comparison of anxiety levels of female and male patients with myocardial infarction, *Crit Care Nurs* 14(1):118, 1994.

Airway clearance, ineffective

CLINICAL CONDITION/ MEDICAL DIAGNOSIS	RISK FACTORS
Tracheostomy with tracheal intubation	Ineffective coughing; excessive secretions with intubated trachea

Patient goals
Expected outcomes
    Associated nursing/collaborative interventions *and scientific rationale*

Manage secretions more effectively as evidenced by the following:

Secretions are easily expectorated or suctioned
Breath sound are clear following treatments

Assist patient to cough after several deep breaths.

Help patient to assume a comfortable cough position (e.g., high Fowler's with knees bent and a light weight pillow over abdomen) *to augment expiratory pressures and minimize discomfort. Effective cough requires a deep breath and contraction of expiratory muscles especially the abdominal muscles to increase the intrathoracic pressure and expel secretions.*

Remove expectorated secretions from opening of tracheostomy tube using aseptic technique. Use clean technique in home. Note volume, viscosity, and color of secretions.

Avoid deep suctioning; if patient can cough secretions to tracheal tube, suction the tube only.

Perform chest physical therapy maneuvers to drain remote areas of lung by gravity (add percussion, if not contraindicated). *Chest physical therapy consists of vibration, percussion, and postural drainage of selected lung units (e.g., segments). Vibration applied to chest wall, together with gravity and slow exhalation after deep breathing, dislodges retained secretions from the underlying airways and facilitates mucous clearance.*

Airway clearance, ineffective

Vibrate affected area during exhalation; be prepared to collect expectorated secretions or suction as described later.

Initiate cough assists (as described previously) or provide a fast manual resuscitative bag breath to stimulate cough receptors. Quickly release hand pressure on bag and again be ready to collect secretions.

Adjust frequency of therapy according to achievement of expected outcomes, target times, and patient comfort.

Tracheal tube is free of plugs

Provide systemic hydration which is calculated from patient's intake, output, and body weight. *The usual water loss from expired gas is 300 ml per day, depending on respiratory rate and route of inspiration. Systemic dehydration or fluid excess adversely affects the mucociliary escalator (i.e., relationship of cilia, sol, and gel layers) and impairs mucociliary clearance.*

Provide humidified gas at 37° C and 100% saturation via ventilator, T-piece connector attached to wide-bore tubing or tracheostomy mask. *Normally inspired gas is filtered, warmed, and humidified by the upper airway, primarily the nose. By the time the inspired gas reaches the trachea it is 37° C and 100% humidified. When the normal host defenses are bypassed, dryer and cooler air dehydrates the respiratory mucous membranes and impairs mucociliary clearance and causes inspissated tracheobronchial secretions.*

Remove condensed vapor from inspiratory line as needed and change humidifier, connectors, and tubing every day.

Protect opening of tracheal tube from unfiltered ambient air and avoid introduction of foreign objects and blind instillation of fluids (e.g., saline).

Perform intratracheal suctioning only when secretions are reachable by catheter and patient cannot cough effectively.

Prepare patient for this uncomfortable and potentially traumatic procedure and explain purpose and sequence of maneuvers.

Use aseptic technique during suctioning; clean technique is appropriate in home.

Preoxygenate with 100% oxygen before suctioning.

If patient is spontaneously breathing and has a dominant hypoxic drive to breathe, adjust FiO_2 accordingly.

After preoxygenation and hyperinflations, use a sterile catheter which is one half the diameter of the tracheal tube and apply intermittent negative pressure for less than 15 seconds per pass; reoxygenate and remain with patient until return to baseline vital signs. *Suctioning removes air as well as secretions from the airways and induces hypoxemia.*

Use minimal cuff inflation. If patient is spontaneously breathing and can swallow oropharyngeal secretions and oral feedings without aspiration, the cuff can be left deflated to minimize tracheal damage.

Consult physician for adjunctive therapies and further assessment, mucolytics, bronchodilators, antibiotics, fiberoptic bronchoscopy, diagnostic tests (e.g., sputum for culture, sensitivity and Gram stain, or chest x-ray).

Patient or significant other is able to perform airway clearance procedures

Provide patient with cues/devices to motivate independent deep breathing exercises (e.g., visual or tactile feedback).

Teach patient to cough after several deep breaths.

Teach patient alternate cough techniques (e.g., huff or quad) if patient is having difficulty.

Teach patient or significant other airway clearance procedure and administration of medical adunctive therapies as appropriate.

REFERENCES

Bach JR: Mechanical insufflation-exsufflation. Comparison of peak expiratory flows with manually assisted and unassisted coughing techniques, *Chest*, 104(5):1553-1562, 1993.

Copnell B, Ferguson D: Endotracheal suctioning: time worn ritual or timely intervention? *Am J Crit Care* 4(2):100-105, 1995.

Hagler DA, Traver GA: Endotracheal saline and suction catheters sources of lower airway contamination, *Am J Crit Care* 3(6):444-447, 1994.

Hanley MV, Rudd T, Butler J: What happens to intratracheal saline instillations? *Am Rev Respir Dis* 117(part 2 suppl):124, 1978.

Hanley MV, Tyler ML: Ineffective airway clearance related to airway infection, *Nurs Clin North Am* 22(1):135-150, 1987.

Johnson KL and others: Closed versus open endotracheal suctioning: costs and physiologic consequences, *Crit Care Med* 22(4):658-666, 1994.

Kerr ME and others: Head injured adults: Recommendations for endotracheal suctioning, *J Neuroscience Nurs* 25(2):86-91, 1993.

Raymond SJ: Normal saline instillation before suctioning: Helpful or harmful? A review of literature, *Am J Crit Care* 4(4):267, 1995.

Stone KS and others: The effect of lung hyperinflation and endotracheal suctioning on cardiopulmonary hemodynamics, *Nurs Res* 40(2):76-80, 1991.

Swartz MS and others: A national survey of endotracheal suctioning techniques in the pediatric population, *Heart Lung* 25(1):52-61, 1996.

Anxiety

CLINICAL CONDITION/ MEDICAL DIAGNOSIS	RELATED FACTORS
Major depression, single episode	Maturational Crisis (mid-life aging process)
	Situational crisis (increasing job uncertainties)

Patient goals
Expected outcomes
  Associated nursing/collaborative interventions *and*
    scientific rationale

Experience reduced anxiety levels of at least one level as evidenced by the following:

Experiences a decrease in symptoms; e.g., decreased tension, apprehension, insomnia, tremors, irritability, isolation, fatigue, restlessness, perceptual distortions, physical reactions to anxiety

Assess level of anxiety (e.g., ability to comprehend, problem-solving ability, narrowing perceptual field, level of functioning, ability to perform activities of daily living, appropriateness of response to situation).

Maintain calm and safe environment.

Decrease stimuli.

Talk to and reassure patient.

Encourage involvement in activities, depending on level of anxiety.

Guide participation in self-care.

Redirect as necessary.

Assist patient in identifying possible sources of stress.

Introduce the use of humor in reducing anxiety.

Provide health teaching about anxiety in the following areas:

- Impact of anxiety on the body
- Levels of anxiety
- Impact of chemicals on the body

Assess use of alcohol, caffeine, nicotine, and other drugs.

Anxiety

116

*It is important to reduce level of anxiety to none, low or
moderate levels so that patient can begin to concentrate on participating in developing plan of care and
achieving behavioral change.*

**Recognize own anxiety and participate in
developing plan of care to effect change as
evidenced by the following:**

Discusses and monitors own behavior every shift
Identifies stressors
Actively participates in unit activities
Initiates interactions with peers
Develops realistic goals
**Connects behavior with feelings (i.e., loss of job,
changes on job)**

Help patient to connect behavior with feelings.
Encourage patient to discuss feelings about anxiety.
Obtain patient's perception of the anxiety experi-
enced.
Focus on the "here and now."
Develop room plan with patient (e.g., remain out
of room for 50 minutes each hour).
Help patient to identify how anxiety is manifested
through behavior.
Explore with patient ways of anticipating anxiety.
Provide health teaching in the following areas:
• Stress management
• Goal setting

**Accept physical and emotional changes of the
aging process as evidenced by the following:**

Acknowledges limitations
Verbalizes fears of aging process
Functions at optimal level
**Uses strengths to develop ways of coping with the
aging process**

Provide health teaching about the aging process including grief reaction.
Encourage patient to function as independently as
possible.
Encourage patient to discuss feelings/fears.

Anxiety—cont'd

Assist patient in identifying effective coping strategies.

Assist patient in identifying support systems.

Explore with patient effective use of support systems.

The aging process can be anxiety provoking to some persons.

Demonstrate effective coping strategies in relation to situational and maturational crisis as evidenced by the following:

Develops a personal plan to decrease anxiety using problem-solving process

Identifies community resources/support

Demonstrates relaxation techniques

Meets self-care needs

Forms interpersonal relationships

Participates in discharge planning

Explore coping mechanisms with patient; help patient to identify those coping mechanisms that were successful in decreasing anxiety.

Help patient to identify adaptive coping mechanisms within patient's own cultural expectations.

Discuss importance of regular exercise program.

Provide health teaching in the problem-solving process (e.g., organize, prioritize, implement, evaluate)

Uses relaxation techniques including deep breathing

Instruct patient to take slow, deep breaths (eyes may be opened or closed); repeat and demonstrate as necessary; use progressive relaxation.

Tell patient to sit or lie in a comfortable position in a quiet area (patient should close eyes unless that makes him or her uncomfortable).

At periods throughout exercise ask patient to focus on breathing (slow and deep).

To begin exercise, instruct patient to get in a comfortable position and imagine being in a quiet, comfortable place (e.g., on a beach, listening to a gentle rain). Then instruct patient to gently tense (for 5 seconds) (without injury) and then relax each muscle group (10 to 15 seconds).

Begin with toes and feet and move progressively upward—calf of leg, thigh, buttock, lower back, hands (make fist), lower arm, upper arm, shoulders, neck, and ending with face (grimace). After relaxing face, patient should remain quiet for 15 minutes (or as patient can tolerate), concentrating on peace, quiet, and breathing.

Instruct patient to use entire exercise or just for areas of tension when time allows.

Instruct patient to use the deep breaths portion when time is limited.

REFERENCES

Coplan J, Tiffon L, Gorman J: Therapeutic strategies for the patient with treatment resistant anxiety, *J Clin Psychiatry*, 54:5 (suppl.): 69, 1993.

Davis M, Eshelman ER, McKay M: *The relaxation and stress reduction workbook*, Oakland, Calif, 1982, New Harbinger.

Flannery, Jr RB: *Becoming stress resistant: through the project smart program*, New York, 1990, Continuum.

Gaberson K: The effect of humorous and musical distraction on preoperative anxiety, *AORN* 6d:(5):784, 1995.

Peplau H: *Interpersonal relationships in nursing*, New York, 1952, GP Putnam's Sons.

Shuldham CM and others: Assessment of anxiety in hospital patients, *J Adv Nurs* 22:87, 1995.

Stinemetz J and others: *Rx for stress: a nurses' guide*, Palo Alto, Calif, 1984, Bull Publishing.

Whitley GG: Anxiety: defining the diagnosis, *J Psychosoc Nurs Ment Health Serv* 27(10):7, 1989.

Aspiration, risk for

CLINICAL CONDITION/ MEDICAL DIAGNOSIS	RISK FACTORS
Decreased level of consciousness as a result of severe trauma	Enteral feeding via nasoenteric tubes

Patient goals
Expected outcomes
> Associated nursing/collaborative interventions *and scientific rationale*

Tolerate nasoenteric feedings without complication, as evidenced by the following:

No signs of symptoms of aspiration related to nasoenteric feedings

Orient patient and teach significant other about procedure for enteral feeding via nasoenteric tube. Emphasize the use of frequent hand washing and clean techniques when handling enteral feeding and related equipment *to decrease formula contamination.*

Confirm tube placement after insertion and at regular intervals at least every 4 to 8 hours with continuous feeding or before each intermittent feeding.

Confirm initial tube placement by chest x-ray examination in collaboration with physician.

Aspirate stomach contents. If needed, check aspirate for pH level to confirm initial tube placement. An acidic pH indicates that the nasogastric tube is in the stomach (pH 0 to ≤ 6.0). Acid inhibitors cause pH ≥ 6.0. Alkaline reaction suggests duodenal/jejunal placement ($\geq$ pH 6.0). If the tube becomes dislodged after feedings are initiated, check the respiratory secretions for presence of glucose. *Glucose is not usually present in tracheal or pulmonary secretions. Diabetics may exhibit glucose in respiratory secretions due to high serum levels. False positives for glucose can occur if blood is visible in the pulmonary secretions and the presence of complex carbohydrates may cause erroneous results.*

Inject 10 cc of air using at least a 30 cc to 60 cc syringe before aspiration, if aspiration of stomach contents is difficult. *This will prevent the small-bore tube from collapsing during aspiration.* Position patient on the right side to help pool secretions, *making it easier to obtain gastric contents when aspirating through a small-bore feeding tube.*

Monitor potential risk factors such as decreased levels of consciousness, sedated state, decreased cough/gas reflex, and incompetent lower esophageal sphincter.

To avoid dislodging tube:
- Monitor coughing, vomiting and suctioning.
- Tape feeding tube securely and monitor external tube markings for possible tube migration every 4 hours and before each feeding.

Assess for gastric retention every 4 hours through the following procedures:
- Check gastric residuals.
- If residuals are two times the infusion rate or >100 mL and there are clinical signs and symptoms such as nausea, vomiting, and abdominal distention, hold tube feeding and recheck residual in 1 hour.
- Notify physician if this occurs for two consecutive measurements of residuals (tube feedings may need to be discontinued or a prokinetic agent may need to be ordered).

Evaluate gastric motility at least every 4 hours through the following procedures:
- Auscultate bowel sounds
- Percuss abdomen for air
- Assess for nausea/vomiting
- Assess for diarrhea/constipation
- Assess for gastric distention by checking abdominal girths serially. Measure from one anterior iliac crest to the other. An increase of 8 to 10 cm above baseline should be considered

significant, and tube feeding should be stopped and physician notified.

Hold the tube feedings and notify the physician if bowel sounds are absent, distention is present, or there is nausea/vomiting. *The absence of bowel sounds with abdominal distention and nausea and/or vomiting may indicate a paralytic ileus and thus contraindicate tube feedings. Jejunal feedings can be administered in the absence of bowel sounds.*

Maintain proper patient positioning during tube feeding administration through the following procedures:

- Elevate head of bed 30 to 45 degrees during feeding *to minimize amount of feeding in stomach and reduce the chance of aspirating.*
- Turn patient to right side to facilitate passage of stomach contents through pylorus, if unable to elevate head of bed. *The side lying position also allows emesis to drain from the mouth rather than be aspirated into the lungs. (When side lying is not possible, consider an alternate feeding method.)*
- Stop tube feeding 30 to 60 minutes before physical activity and procedures that require lowering of patient's head.

Monitor patient for signs of aspiration (cyanosis, dyspnea, cough, wheezing, tachycardia, fever, massive atelectasis with pulmonary edema, hyposemia, temperature greater than 38° C for 24 hours).

Check vital signs, temperature every 4 to 8 hours.

Auscultate breath sounds every 4 to 8 hours.

Observe and record color and character of sputum every 8 hours. Add blue food coloring to tube feedings. *The presence of blue food coloring in the pulmonary secretions indicates that tube feeding has been aspirated. Blue food coloring may cause false-positive hemocult readings for stool.*

Check pulmonary-tracheal secretions for glucose with reagent strip every 4 to 8 hours in high-risk patients. *Positive glucose indicates presence of for-*

mula in pulmonary secretions (false-positive may occur with presence of blood in pulmonary secretions, or an increase in glucose in the blood).

Consider use of combination gastirc-jejunal tubes to decompress the stomach while feeding into the jejunum *to prevent gastric secretion aspiration.*

REFERENCES

Ibanez J and others: Gastroesophageal reflux in intubated patients receiving enteral nutrition: effect of supine and semi-recumbent positions, *JPEN* 16:419-422, 1992.

Kinsey GC and others: Tracheal glucose as a detector of enteral feeding aspiration, *JPEN* 16 (Suppl)35S (From 16th Clinical Congress Program Summary & Abstracts, Abstract No. 105), 1992.

McClave S and others: Use of residual volume as a marker for enteral feeding intolerance: prospective blinded comparison with physical examination and radiographic findings, *JPEN* 16(2):99, 1992.

Metheny, N: Minimizing respiratory complications of nasoenteric tube feedings. State of the science, *Heart Lung* 22(3):213-223, 1993.

Metheny NA and others: Effectiveness of pH measurements in predicting feeding tube placement, *Nurs Res* 38(5):280-285, 1989.

Metheny, N and others: pH testing of feeding-tube aspirates to determine placement, *NCP* 9:185-190, 1994.

Montecalvo MA and others: Nutritional outcome and pneumonia in critical care patients randomized to gastic versus jejunal tube feedings, *Crit Care Med* 20(10):1377-1387, 1992.

Mullan H and others: Risks of pulmonary aspiration among patients receiving enteral nutrition support, *JPEN* 16(2):160, 1992.

Potts RG and others: Comparison of blue dye visualization and glucose oxidase test strip methods for detecting pulmonary aspiration of enteral feedings in intubated adults, *Chest* 103(1):117-121, 1993.

Strong RM and others: Equal aspiration rates from postpylorus and intragastric-placed small-bore nasoenteric feeding tubes: a randomized prospective study, *JPEN* 16:59-63, 1992.

Aspiration, risk for—cont'd

Body image disturbance

CLINICAL CONDITION/ MEDICAL DIAGNOSIS	RELATED FACTORS
Mastectomy for breast cancer	Difficulty accepting postoperative body image

Patient goals
Expected outcomes
    Associated nursing/collaborative interventions *and scientific rationale*

Accept body image change and incorporate into self-concept as evidenced by the following:

Verbalizes feelings related to disfigurement and loss of body part

    Acknowledge feelings expressed by patient and communicate acceptance to *support normal grieving and adjustment.*

    Encourage patient to verbalize feelings about perceived changes and meaning of altered body image.

    Assess patient's perception of impact of mastectomy on relationship with present or future partner *to determine patient's fears and possible distortions.*

    Respect patient's need for privacy, emotional withdrawal, or denial (e.g., concealing or minimizing change). *These behaviors are consistent with normal grieving and intrusiveness may increase vulnerability of the patient.*

Personalizes loss of body part and acknowledges changes

    Encourage patient to view and touch altered body part and participate in self-care activities.

    Provide information about cosmetic aids and use of clothing styles *to improve self-image of patient.*

    Acknowledge patient's problem-solving efforts to enhance own appearance *to reinforce adaptive behaviors.*

Body image disturbance

124

Uses available resources for information and support

Provide information about support services and self-help groups in the community and encourage participation *to connect with peers for information and validation.*

Include partners and family members when providing support and education to patient, and make referrals for additional follow-up, if indicated.

REFERENCES

Cronan L: Management of the patient with altered body image, *Brit J Nurs* 2:257, 1993.

Helman C: The body image in health and disease: exploring patients' maps of body and self, *Patient Ed Coun* 26:169, 1995.

McCloskey JC, Bulechek GM, editors: *Nursing interventions classification (NIC)*, ed 2, St Louis, Mosby, 1996.

Newell B: Body image disturbance: cognitive behavioral formulation and intervention, *J Adv Nurs* 16:1400, 1991.

Northouse LL, Cracciolo-Caraway A, Appel CP: Psychological consequences of breast cancer on partner and family, *Semin Oncol Nurs* 7(3):216, 1991.

Price B: A model for body-image care, *J Adv Nurs* 15:585, 1990.

Price B: *Body image, nursing concepts and care*, London, 1990, Prentice Hall.

Royak-Schaler R: Psychological processes in breast cancer: a review of selected research, *J Psychosoc Oncol* 9(4):71, 1991.

Wainstock JM: Breast cancer: psychosocial consequences for the patient, *Semin Oncol Nurs* 7(3):207, 1991.

Wong CA, Bramwell L: Uncertainty and anxiety after mastectomy for breast cancer, *Cancer Nurs* 15(5):363, 1992.

Body image disturbance—cont'd

Body temperature, altered, risk for

CLINICAL CONDITION/ MEDICAL DIAGNOSIS	RISK FACTORS
Head injury	Trauma affecting hypothalamus

Patient goals
Expected outcomes
  Associated nursing/collaborative interventions *and scientific rationale*

Maintain normothermia as evidenced by the following:

Temperature remains within normal range

Monitor temperature every 4 hours; if elevated, monitor more frequently, or use continuous rectal or pulmonary artery temperatures.

Administer steroids as ordered *to decrease edema around the area of hypothalamus.*

Administer antipyretic agents as ordered; *antipyretics reduce fever by affecting hypothalamic response to pyrogens.*

Apply external cooling measures: cooling blankets should be kept at a temperature of 23.9° C. *This temperature causes less shivering and is effective in reducing febrile temperatures.*

Apply ice packs in axillae and groin. *Axillae and groin are close to large blood vessels that will lose heat readily by conduction.*

Wrap hands and feet in terry-cloth toweling to prevent shivering: *hands and feet have many nerve endings sensitive to heat loss; shivering should be avoided as it causes increases in metabolic rate, CO_2 production, oxygen consumption and myocardial work and decreases in O_2 saturation and glycogen stores.*

Administer intravenous fluids at room temperature.

Consider other causes of fever, including drug fever (check liver function studies) and infectious process (check complete blood count cultures).

REFERENCES

Bruce J, Grove S: Fever: pathology and treatment, *Crit Care Nurs* 12(1):40, 1992.

Caruso C and others: Cooling effects and comfort of four cooling blanket temperatures in humans with fever, *Nurs Res* 41(2):68, 1992.

Cunha B, Tu R: Fever in the neurosurgical patient, *Heart Lung* 17(6):608, 1988.

Holtzclaw B: Shivering, *Nurs Clin North Am* 25(4):977, 1990.

Holtzclaw B: The febrile response in critical care: state of the science, *Heart Lung* 21(5):482, 1992.

Sherman DW: Managing an acute head injury, *Nursing* 20(4):47, 1990.

Body temperature, altered, risk for—cont'd

Bowel incontinence

CLINICAL CONDITION/ MEDICAL DIAGNOSIS	RELATED FACTORS
Pelvic floor trauma	Defecation pain; excessive use of laxatives

---

Patient goals
Expected outcomes
   Associated nursing/collaborative interventions *and*
      scientific rationale

Take an active role in pain management as evidenced by the following:

Records pain experienced during defecation, measures used to control pain, and pain relief

   Use lubricated gloved finger to examine rectum for presence of stool, areas of pain/tenderness, and impairment of external and sphincter; use local anesthetic cream if necessary. Place lubricated index finger approximately 7 cm into the rectum and hook posteriorly. Instruct patient to tighten the muscles to avoid defecation. The puborectalis muscle will move anteriorly and narrow the anal canal constricting the finger.

   Teach/monitor patient's ability to rate pain on a scale of 1 to 10, and to use pain log and measures to obtain pain relief. *Participation in pain management increases patient's perception of control.*

   Elicit from patient measures used to increase comfort prior to seeking assistance (e.g., warm soaks).

   Refer to physician to evaluate resolution of pelvic trauma.

Establish a regular pattern of bowel elimination as evidenced by the following:

Gradually decreases reliance on laxatives to control stool consistency

   Provide written information about use of bulk

forming agents and a high-fiber diet *to achieve desired stool consistency.*

Teach/monitor use of food diary *to gain awareness of pattern of food intake.*

Collaborate with patient to develop/monitor a plan for increasing fluid intake to six to eight glasses of water a day.

Practices pelvic floor exercises three times a day

Discuss with physician patient's readiness to begin pelvic floor exercises (PFEs).

Teach PFEs and coach practice sessions. *PFEs strengthen the external and sphincter and help prevent incontinence.*

Instruct patient to maintain contractions for 3 to 4 seconds and then repeat without tensing muscles of legs, buttocks, or abdomen. If *contractions are maintained for 1 minute, sphincters tend to fatigue and go into a refractory stage.*

Reports easy passage of soft formed stool and decrease in episodes of bowel incontinence

Collaborate with patient to plan and implement a toileting routine.

Teach patient to respond immediately to urge to defecate. *Stool will harden in rectum when evacuation is delayed.*

Alert patient to avoid fatty acids in triggering meal (usually breakfast). *Fatty acids delay stimulation of the gastrocolic and duodenocolic reflexes.*

REFERENCES

Gattuso JM, Kamm MA: Adverse effects of drugs used in the management of constipation and diarrhea, *Drug Safety* 10(1):47-65, 1994.

Keck JO and others: Biofeedback training is useful in fecal incontinence but disappointing in constipation, *Dis Colon Rectum,* 37(12):1271-1276, 1994.

Maas M, Specht J: Bowel incontinence. In Maas M, Buckwalter KC, Hardy M, eds: *Nursing diagnosis and interventions for the elderly,* ed 2, Redwood City, Calif, 1991, Addison-Wesley.

McCloskey JC, Bulechek GM, editors: Bowel incontinence care. In *Nursing interventions classification (NIC),* ed 2, St Louis, 1996, Mosby, p 149.

McCormick KA, Burgio KL: Incontinence: update on nursing care measures, *J Gerontol Nurs* 10:16, 1984.

McLane AM, McShane RE: Bowel management. In Bulechek GM, McCloskey JC, eds: *Nursing interventions: essential nursing treatments,* Philadelphia, 1992, WB Saunders.

McLane AM, McShane RE: Bowel incontinence. In Thompson JM and others: *Mosby's Clinical Nursing,* ed 3, St Louis, 1993, Mosby.

Breastfeeding, effective

CLINICAL CONDITION/ MEDICAL DIAGNOSIS	RELATED FACTORS
Adequate lactation and transfer	Appropriate knowledge; support sources

Patient goals
Expected outcomes
> Associated nursing/collaborative interventions *and scientific rationale*

Adequate lactation is maintained as evidenced by the following:

Infant demonstrates adequate weight gain appropriate to age.

Mother meets her intended breastfeeding goal

> Review present pattern of breastfeeding. *Knowledge of physiology of milk production is crucial in the management of lactation.*

> Discuss nutritious diet from all four major food groups.

> Instruct to avoid intentional weight loss. *Proper nutrition is necessary to maintain health of mother and infant and maintain adequate lactation.*

> Encourage to maintain adequate fluid intake and drink to satisfy thirst; discourage taking excessive fluids. *Forcing fluids negatively affects milk production.*

> Encourage frequent rest or nap while the baby is asleep. *Fatigue may inhibit the milk ejection reflex and diminish milk supply.*

> Encourage mother to avoid use of cigarettes, caffeine, alcohol, and illegal drugs. *These substances may enter breastmilk and be harmful to the infant. Nicotine may decrease prolactin levels and inhibit milk ejection reflex.*

> Provide anticipatory guidance for infant developmental changes that affect lactation (growth spurts at 2 to 3 weeks, 6 weeks, and 3 months). *Mother may misperceive an inadequate milk supply due to increased infant feedings.*

Breastfeeding, effective

Avoid introducing solids until infant is 5 to 6 months of age. *Current recommendations stress delaying the addition of solids; solids may diminish milk supply.*

Demonstrate how to express/pump breastmilk and store properly. *Adequate stimulation of the breasts is necessary to maintain lactation when mother and infant are separated.*

Discuss with mother her feelings about breastfeeding outside the home.

Prevent breast complications as evidenced by the following:

Mother develops no breast or nipple complications

Encourage use of supportive bra 24 hours a day.

Advise how to choose correct bra and bra size. Bra should give support and not bind.

Avoid underwires and elastic around the cups, *which may prevent sufficient drainage by pressing on milk ducts.*

Advise to wash the breast and nipples with warm water daily. Avoid soaps and other drying agents *that may irritate the nipple and remove natural oils.*

Stress importance of preventing engorgement through unrestricted feeding. *Breast engorgement can be painful, may predispose to the development of nipple fissures and breast abscesses, and is associated with lactation failure.*

Encourage mother to use both breasts at a feeding. *Inadequate drainage of milk sinuses can lead to a diminished milk production.*

Encourage mother to nurse at least 10 minutes per breast before switching. Allow adequate time for the milk ejection reflex to occur *to ensure that the infant receives the hindmilk and not only the low-calorie foremilk.*

Demonstrate how to massage breasts during feeding. *Breast massage causes the hindmilk to move from the alveoli to the lactiferous sinuses, thus facilitating the milk ejection reflex and emptying of the breasts.*

Encourage mother to alternate infant's feeding positions. *Changing positions will help alleviate stress on the nipples and minimize irritation.*

Stress importance of the infant getting as much of the areola as possible in his/her mouth *to compress the lactiferous sinuses, not just the nipple.*

Instruct mother to avoid external pressure on the breasts (e.g., positions that put pressure on one spot for long periods).

Demonstrate how to empty breast manually or with pump if baby does not drain breast adequately. *Ducts may become plugged and mastitis develop if inadequate emptying occurs.*

Maintain family adaptation to breastfeeding process as evidenced by the following:

Family members verbalize support of the breastfeeding mother

Provide age-appropriate literature about breastfeeding to family members. *Support and encouragement from the partner and family significantly influence breastfeeding duration and the maintenance of lactation.*

Encourage mother to answer questions from her other children.

Role play with mother possible situations related to questions of her child(ren).

Family sleep patterns are maintained with minimal disruption

Discuss sleep pattern disruptions that may occur.

Encourage significant others to demonstrate their support by assisting with household duties.

Provide praise and positive reinforcement to family members.

Family activities are not curtailed

Discuss how to plan family activities, including trips, conducive to breastfeeding.

Discuss selection of clothing that allows for discreet breastfeeding such as loose-knit pullovers, button-fronted blouses, and shawl.

REFERENCES

Buchko BL and others: Comfort measures in breastfeeding primiparous women, *J Obstet Gynecol Neonatal Nurs* 23:46-52, 1994.

Humenick SS, Hill PD, Anderson MA: Breast engorgement: patterns and selected outcomes, *J Hum Lact* 10:87-93, 1994.

Hill PD, Humenick SS: Nipple pain during breastfeeding: the first two weeks and beyond, *J Hum Lact* 2:21-35, 1993.

Hill PD: The enigma of insufficient milk supply, *Am J Matern Child Nurs* 16(6):313, 1991.

Hill PD, Humenick SS: Nipple pain during breastfeeding: the first two weeks and beyond, *J Hum Lact* 2(2):21, 1993.

Matich JR, Sims LS: A comparison of social support variables between women who intend to breast or bottle feed, *Soc Sci Med* 34(8):919, 1992.

Newton N: The quantitative effect of oxytocin (pitocin) on human milk yield, *Ann N Y Acad Sci* 652:597, 1992.

Newton N: The relation of the milk-ejection reflex to the ability to breast feed, *Ann N Y Acad Sci* 652:597-610, 1992.

Perez-Escamilla R and others: Determinants of lactation performance across time in an urban population from Mexico, *Soc Sci Med* 37:1069-1078, 1993.

Rajan L: The contribution of professional support, information and consistent correct advice to successful breast feeding, *Midwifery* 9:197-209, 1993.

Breastfeeding, ineffective

CLINICAL CONDITION/ MEDICAL DIAGNOSIS	RELATED FACTORS
Insufficient milk supply syndrome	Previous history of breastfeeding failure; poor infant suck reflex

Patient goals
Expected outcomes
>   Associated nursing/collaborative interventions *and scientific rationale*

Establish optimal lactation as evidenced by:

Verbalizes accurate information related to breast-feeding

> Interview patient to assess patient's level of knowledge.

> Initiate teaching to reduce patient's inadequate knowledge about breastfeeding. *Patients who are knowledgeable about breastfeeding tend to be more successful at breastfeeding.*

> Include patient's significant other in teaching.

Identifies personal and family support for breast-feeding

> Identify cultural barriers to breastfeeding. *The acceptance/success of breastfeeding may be negatively influenced in certain cultures.*

> Encourage patient/significant others to verbalize emotional attitudes about breastfeeding. *The acceptance/success of breastfeeding can positively influence successful breastfeeding.*

Feeds infant with minimal assistance

> Use nipple shells if nipples are flat or inverted. *The nipple protrudes through a hole in the center and constant gentle pressure around the nipple causes it to evert.*

> Demonstrate colostrum expression to entice infant.

> Promote appropriate positioning for feeding; side lying, football hold, sitting, or across abdomen.

> Provide suggestions for waking a sleepy baby.

Demonstrate techniques to help infant "latch on" correctly. *Incorrect position of the infant's mouth abrades the nipple, causes soreness, and contributes to early weaning.*

Observe infant during feeding for faulty sucking mechanism.

Do not restrict sucking time.

Offer both breasts at each feeding.

Provide for frequent feedings on demand every 2 to 3 hours.

Has fewer breast complications as evidenced by:

No evidence of breast/nipple trauma

Observe breast for engorgement, warmth, redness of nipple, cracks or fissures in nipple, or anomaly of breast.

Monitor for frequency of analgesia use.

Patient demonstrates breast care techniques used to decrease breast complications

Encourage frequent feedings with proper positioning.

Encourage patient to apply warm, moist packs 10 to 15 minutes before feeding or encourage patient to take warm showers before feeding.

Assist patient with hand expression or by pumping breast to soften areola and make nipple protrude.

Encourage use of varying positions of baby's mouth on breast by changing holding position with each feeding.

Teach proper technique to break suction of nursing infant.

Encourage air drying nipples after feeding and use of a supportive bra.

Discourage use of soaps or lotions containing alcohol; use ointments as prescribed.

Maintains the breastfeeding process as evidenced by:

Expresses confidence in ability to handle future situations

Encourage appropriate changes in nutrition and rest.

Breastfeeding, ineffective—cont'd

Discuss implications for using medications while breastfeeding. *Passive diffusion, carrier mediated diffusion, or active transport allow passage of a drug from plasma to milk.*

Discourage delaying or skipping feedings.

Discuss observing for signs of adequate letdown reflex.

Teach patient how to evaluate if infant is getting enough. *Perceived insufficient milk supply leads to supplementing and early discontinuation of breast-feeding.*

Discourage supplements. *Substitute bottles may confuse infant. Supplementation can negatively affect milk production.*

Identifies resources for problems and/or support

Provide consistent information, support and positive reinforcement. *Patients who have support in their network tend to be more successful in breast-feeding.*

Provide anticipatory guidance for developmental changes that affect breastfeeding (i.e., growth spurts).

Provide written information about resources/support groups for breastfeeding.

Demonstrate use of assistive devices for infants with problems.

Discuss strategies to continue breastfeeding after returning to work. *Knowledge about methods to facilitate breastfeeding can delay discontinuation of breastfeeding after returning to work.*

Discuss role of father/significant other while breast-feeding.

Discuss effects of breastfeeding on sexuality.

REFERENCES

Duckett L, Henly SJ, Garvis M: Predicting breastfeeding duration during the postpartum hospitalization, *West J Nurs Res* 15(2):177-198, 1993.

Hill PD, Aldag JC: Insufficient milk supply among black and white breastfeeding mothers, *Res Nurs Health* 16(3):203-11, 1993.

Isabella PH, Isabella RA: Correlates of successful breastfeeding: A study of social and personal factors, *Human Lactation* 10(4):257-264, 1994.

Kessler LA and others: The effect of a woman's significant other on her breastfeeding decision, *Human Lactation* 11(2):103-109, 1995.

Breastfeeding, ineffective—cont'd

Lawrence RA: *Breastfeeding: a guide for the medical profession*, ed 4, St Louis, 1994, Mosby.

Leff EW, Gagne MP, Jeffries SC: Maternal perceptions of successful breastfeeding, *Human Lactation* 10(2):99-104, 1994.

Lothian JA: It takes two to breastfeed: the baby's role in successful breastfeeding, *J Nurse-Midwifery* 40(4):328-334, 1995.

Quarles A and others: Mothers' intention, age, education and the duration and management of breastfeeding, *Maternal-Child Nurs* 22(3):102-108, 1994.

Rodriquez-Garcia R, Frazier L: Cultural paradoxes relating to sexuality and breastfeeding, *Human Lactation* 11(2):111-115, 1995.

Breastfeeding, interrupted

CLINICAL CONDITION/ MEDICAL DIAGNOSIS	RELATED FACTORS
Prematurity	Uncoordinated sucking, swallowing, and breathing mechanisms

Patient goals
Expected outcomes
    Associated nursing/collaborative interventions *and*
        scientific rationale

Demonstrate a commitment to provide adequate and bacteriologically safe breast milk to the preterm infant for gavage feeding as evidenced by the following:

Participates in initial consultation with nurse with expertise in breastfeeding premature infants

Encourage mother to consult (NICU) breastfeeding specialist. *NICU breastfeeding specialist has expertise in both lactation and in the clinical care of high-risk infants.*

Provide privacy during consultation.

Recognizes the immunological, nutritional, and emotional benefits of breastfeeding as they relate to the infant's special condition

Reinforce the mother's knowledge about the immunological and nutritional benefits of breastfeeding. *Milk produced by mothers who deliver preterm infants differs in composition from milk produced by mothers who deliver at term. It has higher concentration of protein, sodium, calcium, lipids, and selected antiinfective properties, which is consistent with the unique nutritional needs of preterm infants. Evidence indicates that breastfeeding affords protection against illness such as respiratory and gastrointestinal infections, specifically during infancy.*

Discuss the emotional benefits of breastfeeding. *Mothers of preterm infants have stated repeatedly that breastfeeding is the one thing they can do for their preterm infants when professionals have assumed other caregiving activities.*

Recognizes that the expressed milk will be given to the infant by artificial feeding method such as gavage

Provide information to the mother that most small, preterm infants cannot be breastfed directly. Therefore preterm infants receive expressed mother's milk (EMM) by artificial feeding such as gavage infusion until they have demonstrated the ability to feed orally. *Preterm infant's ability to coordinate sucking, swallowing, and breathing varies from 32 to 36 weeks of gestation depending on feeding method.*

Discuss two major problems that may occur during gavage feeding, such as significant nutrient loss and bacterial growth of already colonized milk, *to understand the risks in gavage feeding.*

Maintains adequate milk supply by pumping breast correctly 8 to 12 times daily in the early postpartum period

Develop a workable plan that incorporates physiological principles of early and frequent milk expression in the postpartum period. *Stimulating lactation is easier in the early postpartum period than it is several days later. Milk produced in early lactation, especially colostrum, contains antiinfective properties that are more beneficial to the infant. Frequent pumping contributes to adequate milk supply.*

Uses recommended pump and collecting equipment for optimal production of milk

Encourage the patient to rent an electric breast pump with a double pump collecting kit for home use, *to optimize prolactin levels and decrease pumping times.*

Help with breast pump rentals and purchases from referral agencies, *to relieve mother of the burden of phone calls at a stressful time. Nurse's assistance ensures services from the agencies that benefit the mother, such as (1) delivery of appropriate pump and collecting equipment, (2) directs billing of third-party payers, if the mother so desires, and (3) picking up pump from the home, when no longer needed.*

Teach mother the correct use of pump, proper cleaning, and the assembly and disassembly of the equipment.

Inform mother that with few exceptions, pumping will continue for at least 2 weeks after the infant has been discharged from NICU, *to empty breasts completely and increase prolactin levels.*

Recognizes importance of adequate nutrition and implications of drugs for safe milk supply

Reinforce the importance of adequate nutrition, fluids, and rest, *to ensure adequate milk supply.*

Discuss on individual basis concerns related to medications, smoking, or alcohol ingestion while mother is expressing milk for her preterm infant. *Depending on maternal dosage and clinical condition of the infant, a drug that is considered "safe" if present in EMM for full-term healthy infants may not be equally safe for a 750-gm, 26-week infant.*

Produces expressed mother's milk (EMM) with "abnormally" low bacteriological contamination (e.g., an absence of all bacteria except skin flora in minimal concentrations (10^2 to 10^4 colony-forming units per mL)

Develop protocol for maternal breast care and bacteriologic surveillance of EMM. *EMM is never sterile and contains Staphylococcus epidermidis that may be pathogenic to preterm infants.*

Explain the milk expression techniques and the reasons for special precautions. *Assure mother that her hygiene is not being questioned but that precautions are needed to reduce the bacteria to "abnormally" low levels.*

Complies with the established protocol for milk expression

Teach mothers about bacteria-reducing techniques for milk expression as recommended by Meier and Wilks. *The smaller, sicker preterm infant has a compromised immune system and may be more susceptible to bacteria in EMM.*

Send mother's EMM for culture per protocol to *en-*

sure that mother is exercising appropriate expression techniques.

Uses recommended containers for storage of EMM to minimize the bacteriologic contamination except skin flora concentration at 10^2 to 10^4 colony-forming units per ml

Instruct mothers to collect EMM in sterile, graduated plastic feeders with twist-on, air-tight caps. This EMM can be refrigerated or frozen for later use, by the nurses who will prepare the milk for gavage or bottle feeding. *Such feeders are ideal for EMM storage and easier to defrost and handle without contaminating the contents.*

Label each bottle with baby's name, date, time milk was pumped, and any medication the mother is taking.

Uses EMM within 24 hours after refrigeration

Advise mothers to use fresh and/or previously frozen EMM for feeding within 24 hours after refrigeration. *No definitive guidelines are available for the length of time EMM can remain refrigerated until it is fed to the infant, except for conservative policy based on American Academy of Pediatrics Committee on Nutrition.*

Encourage mother to express milk just before each feeding. *This approach is optimal in minimizing bacterial growth and maximizing antiinfective properties of the milk received by the infant.*

Take an active role in the management of in-hospital breastfeeding sessions as evidenced by:

Recognizes that the intended outcomes of early breastfeeding sessions are positioning the infant correctly at breast and physiologic stability during feeding

Determine the readiness to breastfeed by assessing whether the infant can coordinate the suck-swallow-breathe mechanisms *rather than currently used criteria such as infant weight, ability to bottle-feed, type of thermal support an infant requires, and gestational age.*

Initiate breastfeeding according to the criteria currently being used for initiating bottle-feeding, *until the time a research based tool is available to enable the nurse and the physician to make decisions about readiness to feed. Specific NICU policy, such as bottle-feeding at 34 weeks of gestation when an infant weighs a minimum of 1500 gm, can be used for breastfeeding.*

Delay bottle-feeding for at least 1 week while the infant learns to breastfeed, *to introduce the preterm infant to breastfeeding before bottle-feeding.*

Assess prefeeding vital signs of the preterm infant *to provide baseline data.*

Explain rationale for test-weighing to the mothers. *Mothers should understand that test-weighing is not being used as a determinant of a "successful" breastfeeding session and that adequate infant intake is not the goal of early breastfeeding.*

Perform test-weighing by using electronic scales *to determine the volume of milk the preterm infant consumes during breastfeeding so that other fluids (e.g., supplemental gavage feeding or parenteral fluids) can be adjusted accordingly.*

Prepare the breast for feeding by cleansing it with sterile water and gauze pads.

Assist in positioning the infant (cross-chest position) at breast *to facilitate "latch-on."*

Consider skin-to-skin contact by positioning the infant chest-to-chest with the mother. *Preterm infants held skin-to-skin (kangaroo care) are warm enough and have regular heart rate and respiration. Breastfeeding may be enhanced by skin-to-skin contact where lactation becomes more productive and lasts longer. Parents may become attached to their infants and feel confident about caring for them.*

Monitor physiologic variables during breastfeeding *to determine infant's responses.*

Provide gavage supplementation during or after the feeding as needed.

Recognizes that the intended outcome of *later breastfeeding* sessions is the infant's consumption of ade-

quate volumes of milk in order to prepare for discharge

Implement the same nursing interventions as in early breastfeeding.

Conduct and evaluate serial test weighing by using electronic scales. *Ideally, volume of intake during breastfeeding should approximate that consumed by the infant during gavage or bottle feeding and should demonstrate a trend of increasing volume over time. If mothers are concerned that their infants do not consume volumes comparable to those they receive by gavage or bottle, they should be reassured that small volumes of intake are normal, especially until milk ejection and mature infant sucking patterns are synchronized.*

Implement cue-based feeding during the last 1 to 2 weeks of the infant's hospitalization. *Mothers will experience what "demand" feeding is and will have an opportunity to observe their infants awaken in response to hunger.*

Use postdischarge consultation services to support breastfeeding at home as evidenced by:

Recognizes that postdischarge consultation can influence successful adjustment in breastfeeding at home

Provide an individualized written plan for breastfeeding management at home.

Allow for liberal complementation/supplementation of breastfeeding in the individualized plan.

Develop a schedule for telephone consultation and an occasional home visit.

REFERENCES

Bell E, Geyer J, Jones, L: A structured intervention improves breastfeeding success for ill or preterm infants, *MCN Am J Matern Child Nurs,* 20:309-314, 1995.

Meier PP and others: Breastfeeding support services in the neonatal intensive care, *J Obstet Gynecol Neonatal Nurs* 22(4):338, 1993.

Meier PP, Mangurten HH: Breastfeeding the preterm infant. In Riordan J, Auerbach KG, eds: *Breastfeeding and human lactation,* Boston, 1993, Jones and Bartlett.

Meier PP, Wilks SO: The bacteria in expressed mothers milk, *MCN Am J Matern Child Nurs* 12:420-423, 1987.

Orlando, Susan: The immunologic significance of breast milk, *J Obstet Gynecol Neonatal Nurs* 24(7):678, 1995.

Breastfeeding, interrupted—cont'd

Breathing pattern, ineffective

CLINICAL CONDITION/ MEDICAL DIAGNOSIS	RELATED FACTORS
Stable chronic obstructive pulmonary disease	Respiratory muscle fatigue, impaired respiratory mechanics

Patient goals
Expected outcomes
   Associated nursing/collaborative interventions *and scientific rationale*

Minimize energy expenditure of respiratory muscles as evidenced by the following:

Respiratory rate and tidal volume within normal limits, minimal dyspnea

Teach pursed-lip breathing, abdominal stabilization, and controlled coughing techniques; provide optimal care for mechanical assistance (e.g., ventilatory) if necessary. *Pursed-lip breathing forces patients to breathe more slowly and deeply and reduces dyspnea during exertion. Coughing can be fatiguing, hence abdominal stabilization and controlled coughing techniques are used to provide support to the expiratory muscles and assist in removing airway secretions while minimizing energy expenditure. These techniques will be beneficial only to patients who are producing excessive mucus.*

Increase inspiratory muscle strength and endurance as evidenced by the following:

Increases maximal inspiratory pressure and reports decreased exertional dyspnea.

Evaluate status of inspiratory muscle for training and, if appropriate, initiate inspiratory muscle training. *Inspiratory muscle training improves conscious control of respiratory muscles and decreases anxiety associated with increased inspiratory effort. Increased strength of the inspiratory muscles may allow some patients to tolerate submaximal levels of activity for longer periods with less dyspnea.*

Breathing pattern, ineffective

144

Assess the nutritional status of the patient. If lean body mass is depleted, plan to add nutritional support to build muscle mass in the diaphragm and intercostal muscles. *Repletion of lean body mass will rebuild muscles, including the diaphragm and intercostal muscles. This will promote increases in inspiratory muscle strength and endurance, as well as enhance the effects of inspiratory muscle training.*

Monitor oxygen saturation with pulse oximeter during training session to verify that patient does not desaturate. Encourage patient to breathe as deeply as possible during inspiratory muscle training. *Use of very small tidal volumes during inspiratory muscle training could decrease alveolar ventilation and cause some patients to experience oxyhemoglobin desaturation.*

Limit work of breathing as evidenced by the following:

Reports taking as-needed antibiotics when sputum color changes (yellow or green)

Teach patient to monitor color, consistency, and volume of sputum *because respiratory infections increase work of breathing. Early treatment of bacterial infection of the lungs may speed recovery and thereby reduce the work of breathing.*

Reports taking bronchodilator medications as prescribed

Teach patient name, dosage, method of administration, schedule, and appropriate behavior if side effects occur, and teach consequences of improper use of medications. *Anticholinergics (ipratropium bromide), beta agonists, and methylxanthines are commonly prescribed bronchodilators that can be beneficial in decreasing airway resistance and work of breathing.*

Evaluate patient's technique for taking inhaled medications. Recommend a spacer device for patients who have difficulty with timing during the procedure. *Under optimal conditions, no more than 10% of the drug from each puff is deposited into the lungs; with a spacer device, as much as 15% of the drug will be deposited.*

Demonstrates ability to pace ADLs in line with ventilatory function

Teach patient to modify ADLs within ventilatory limits.

Induce periodic hyperinflation of lungs with a series of slow, deep breaths. *Hyperinflation works like a deep sigh, expanding alveoli that are partially closed, mobilizing airway secretions, and increasing lung tissue compliance.*

REFERENCES

Anthonisen M and others: Antibiotic therapy in exacerbations of chronic obstructive pulmonary disease, *Ann Intern Med* 106:196-203, 1987.

Ferguson GT, Cherniack RM: Management of chronic obstructive pulmonary disease, *N Engl J Med* 328:1017-1022, 1993.

Fishman, AP: Pulmonary Rehabilitation Research: NIH Workshop Summary, *Am Respir Crit Care Med* 149:825-833, 1994.

Harris RS, Lawson TV: The relative mechanical effectiveness and efficiency of successive voluntary coughs in healthy young adults, *Clin Sci* 34:569-577, 1968.

Kim MJ and others: Inspiratory muscle training in patients with chronic obstructive pulmonary disease, *Nurs Res* 42:356-362, 1993.

Larson JL and others: Maximal inspiratory pressure: Learning effect and test-retest reliability in patients with chronic obstructive pulmonary disease, *Chest* 104:448-453, 1993.

Larson JL and others: Inspiratory muscle training with a pressure threshold breathing device in patients with chronic obstructive pulmonary disease, *Am Rev Respir Dis* 138:689-696, 1988.

Schols AMW, and others: Prevalence and characteristics of nutritional depletion in patients with stable COPD eligible for pulmonary rehabilitation. *Am Rev Respir Dis,* 147:1151-1156, 1993.

Sharp JT and others: Postural relief of dyspnea in severe chronic obstructive pulmonary disease, *Am Rev Respir Dis* 122:201-211, 1980.

Sutton PP and others: Assessment of forced expiration technique, postural drainage and directed coughing in chest physiotherapy, *Eur J Respir Dis* 64:62-68, 1983.

Cardiac output, decreased

CLINICAL CONDITION/ MEDICAL DIAGNOSIS	RELATED FACTORS
Myocardial infarction (MI)	Electrophysiologic rhythm disturbances: tachyarrhythmias (heart rate ≥ 160/minute)
Heart failure	

> **Patient goals**
> **Expected outcomes**
> > Associated nursing/collaborative interventions *and scientific rationale*

Regain normal range of cardiac output (CO) as evidenced by the following:

Has normal blood pressure (BP)

Review history of patient's BP to determine normal range.

Monitor BP at regular intervals and when there is a significant heart rate/rhythm change.

Assess for change in sensorium in presence of hypotension because a decrease in cardiac output will reduce cerebral blood flow.

Consult with physician in presence of significant heart rate/rhythm changes or BP changes for indicated drug therapy or treatment (e.g., cardiac pacing).

Has cardiac rate/rhythm within normal range, free of tachyarrhythmias without intravenous (IV) medication; with or without maintenance oral medications; with or without support of implantable cardioverter defibrillator (ICD)

Monitor the patient's physiologic responses to the tachyarrhythmias (e.g., altered mentation, hypotension, pallor, diaphoresis, abnormal breath sounds or heart sounds, hypoxia, change in the quality of pulse, and loss of consciousness).

Set alarm limits on electrocardiogram (ECG) monitor (rate, rhythm, S-T trending).

Monitor for ECG changes that increase the risk for development of arrhythmias (e.g., prolonged

Cardiac output, decreased

147

QRS, or Q-T interval; frequent premature atrial or ventricular beats; or R on T phenomenon).

Determine the need for continuous monitoring in collaboration with the physician.

In the presence of a tachycardia, analyze the rhythm for regularity and the morphology of the complexes. Determine the site of origin of the tachyarrhythmia in the conduction system (sinus, atrial, junctional, or ventricular). *In general, the treatment for sinus tachycardia is to determine and treat the cause. However, in the presence of a myocardial infarction (MI) a beta blocker may be used. Heart rates >160 that originate above the ventricles, atrial or junctional, referred to as supraventricular tachycardia (SVT), are not imminently life-threatening but may seriously compromise CO. The diastolic filling time is shortened, diminishing preload, stroke volume, and ultimately decreasing CO (CO = SV × HR).*

In the presence of an SVT, assess the following: (1) Assess the rate and quality of peripheral pulses and detect pulse deficits. *In atrial fibrillation (and other atrial rhythms that are extremely fast and/or uncoordinated) the atrial contribution to CO (the "atrial kick") is lost by as much as 30%.* (2) Monitor blood pressure for hypotension and signs of decreased perfusion and auscultate for extra heart sounds, specifically S_3. *When the left ventricle is failing and noncompliant, the sudden deceleration of the filling wave produces an audible third sound.* (3) Monitor and evaluate the 12-lead ECG for precipitous changes and signs of myocardial ischemia (e.g., depressed ST segments and significant T-wave changes). (4) Determine the presence of and evaluate chest pain/discomfort. *With sustained tachycardia, there is the potential for decreased cardiac perfusion (related to the shortened diastolic filling time), decreased oxygen to the myocardium, and increased myocardial workload.* (5) Monitor pulmonary status, respiratory rate and effort, and adverse behavioral changes, *all of which indicate a serious decrease in oxygen deliv-*

ery to the tissues. If pulse oximetry is available, monitor oxygen saturation. (6) If the patient is being anticoagulated *(disorganized atrial activity may result in thrombus formation and emboli),* monitor partial thromboplastin and prothrombin times and, if not, discuss with the physician the feasibility of anticoagulation. *Heart rates ≥ 160 that originate above the ventricles (atrial or junctional), referred to as SVT, are not imminently life-threatening but may seriously compromise CO. The diastolic filling time is shortened, diminishing preload, stroke volume, and ultimately decreasing CO (CO = SV × HR). In general, the treatment for sinus tachycardia is to determine and treat the cause. However, in the presence of an MI, a beta blocker may be used.*

Initiate oxygen therapy, an IV, and hemodynamic monitoring as indicated and ordered.

Notify the physician of significant changes and discuss therapeutic options.

Monitor the patient's response to Valsalva maneuver or carotid sinus stimulation as indicated. *These actions increase parasympathetic (vagal) responses, producing a block in the atrioventricular (AV) node and reducing the ventricular rate.*

Administer medication as ordered (e.g., adenosine IV *which interrupts the re-entrant circuit;* verapamil or diltiazem IV *which interrupt the re-entrant circuit and increase the delay in the AV node;* digoxin, *to slow AV conduction, increasing degrees of heart block and slowing the ventricular rate;* and/or metoprolol, esmolol, or propranolol IV *to decrease automaticity and conduction velocity slowing the heart rate).* Monitor response to drug therapy and report untoward reactions to the physician.

Prepare the patient for electrical cardioversion if indicated and ordered. *Cardioversion delivers a synchronized direct current charge to the myocardium causing all the cells to depolarize simultaneously and allowing the sinus node to gain control.* Assist as indicated with synchronizing the charge with the patient's QRS to avoid the vulnerable period of the cardiac cycle and potential ventricular fibrillation. Initial charge is 100 joules (j), followed by 200 j, 300 j, and 360 j.

Explain the procedure in accurate but nonthreatening terms, secure a written consent, and reassure the patient that he/she will receive a medication before the treatment to avoid pain and discomfort.

Monitor blood pressure, heart rate, rhythm, and level of consciousness until stable, after cardioversion.

If overdrive pacing is ordered, explain the treatment to the patient, secure a consent, and assist as indicated. *Overdrive pacing is usually effective in controlling the fast rate and may convert some SVTs to normal sinus rhythm.*

In the presence of ventricular tachycardia (VT), assess level of consciousness and presence of carotid pulse. *VT not only causes a decrease in CO as described with SVTs, but may also rapidly progress to ventricular fibrillation (VF) and death.* In the monitored patient who is unresponsive, not breathing, and pulseless, initiate cardiopulmonary resuscitation (CPR), administer chest thump, and alert the CPR team. Thump chest only if a defibrillator is not available, *because doing so could precipitate ventricular fibrillation.* If a defibrillator is available, immediately deliver unsynchronized countershock stat at 200 j, followed by 300 j and 360 j, and proceed with CPR/ACLS as outlined in hospital policy.

If the patient is conscious and hemodynamically stable, initiate drug regimen according to hospital policy (e.g., a lidocaine bolus 1.5 mg/kg, followed by an IV infusion with lidocaine).
Lidocaine reduces ventricular automaticity and may terminate VT.

Administer procainamide 20 to 30 mg/min IV and, if no response, bretylium IV 5 to 10 mg/kg IV, as ordered, if VT persists. *Procainamide reduces automaticity and slows AV conduction and may terminate VT. Bretylium raises the VF threshold.*

Monitor response to drug therapy and report untoward reactions to the physician.

Prepare the patient for synchronized cardioversion if indicated. Talk with the patient throughout the procedure, calmly and reassuringly explaining the treatment.

Monitor serum potassium and magnesium levels and replace as indicated. *Hypokalemia may cause AV blocks, ventricular arrhythmias, and asystole. Hypomagnesemia may cause ventricular arrhythmias.*

If electrophysiology study (EPS) is indicated, explain the treatment to the patient, secure a consent, and assist as indicated. *EPS is an invasive, diagnostic procedure in which four or five catheters are placed inside the heart to determine the sites of origin and mechanism of tachyarrhythmias.*

If radiofrequency ablation (RFA) is indicated, explain the treatment to the patient, secure a consent, and assist as indicated. *RFA is an invasive, therapeutic procedure in which radiofrequency energy is delivered to a small portion of the heart, causing necrosis of the tissue that is responsible for the tachyarrhythmia.*

If an implantable cardioverter defibrillator (ICD) is implanted, a detailed teaching plan with the patient and family should include purpose, restrictions, how it works, what to do when it does not, how a shock feels, how to perform CPR, and follow-up care. *An ICD is a programmable device designed to deliver burst or ramp overdrive pacing, synchronized cardioversion shocks, or defibrillation shocks for VT or defibrillation shocks for VF episodes.*

Review appropriate precautions (e.g., electrical safety precautions, avoidance of contact sports); reassure patient about cosmetic appearance and self-image in general; introduce concept regular clinic visits. *Simplify the regimen to meet patient's level of understanding and interest.* Counsel the patient when fears and concerns persist. *The foregoing will maximize patient adherence to therapy and potentially improve patient outcomes.*

Cardiac output, decreased—cont'd

Expresses freedom from chest pain/discomfort, dyspnea, dizziness, lightheadedness, palpitations, and syncope

Assess/document/evaluate the patient's perceptions related to the tachyarrhythmias (e.g., dizziness or lightheadedness, dyspnea, feelings of anxiety or alarm, fatigue, palpitations, chest pain).

Experience less stress as evidenced by the following:

Verbalizes understanding of and acceptance of therapy, drugs, and treatment

Explain, if indicated, the purpose of ICU or surveillance unit to patient/significant others and reassuringly discuss the advantages of "having your heartbeat watched continuously."

Assess emotional response to tachyarrhythmias and the environment.

Individualize patient teaching appropriate to age, reading level, and ethnic background.

Review all antiarrhythmic medications, that is, purpose, side effects, diet, and activity restrictions, if indicated, and promote positive "upbeat" attitude/behavior.

Explain the procedural and describe the sensory aspects of therapies (e.g., how the instrument is placed and how it will feel). *Preparation for stressful events, particularly description of the sensory aspects, can reduce stress and facilitate coping.*

Relates positive social interaction

Encourage family/significant others to visit at optimal times for the patient.

Monitor the patient's physiological/emotional response to interactions between the patient, visitors, and staff.

REFERENCES

American Heart Association, *Textbook of advanced cardiac life support,* 1994.

Bremner SM, McCauley KM, Axtrell, KA: A follow-up of patients with implantable cardioverter defibrillators, *J Cardiovasc Nurs* 7(3):40, 1993.

Craney J: Radiofrequency catheter ablation of supraventricular tachycardias: clinical consideration and nursing care, *J Cardiovasc Nurs* 7(3):26, 1993.

Cardiac output, decreased—cont'd

Garvin BJ, Huston GP, Baker CF: Information used by nurses to pre-
pare patients for a stressful event, *Appl Nurs Res* 5(4):158, 1992.
Lupker RV: Patient adherence: a 'risk factor' for cardiovascular disease,
Cardiovasc Dis 2(5):418, 1993.
McCloskey JC, Bulechek GM, eds: Dysrhythmia management. In
Nursing interventions classification (NIC), St Louis, 1992, Mosby.
Witherell CL: Cardiac rhythm control devices, *Crit Care Clin North Am*
6(1):85-101, 1994.

Caregiver role strain

CLINICAL CONDITION/ MEDICAL DIAGNOSIS	RELATED FACTORS
Wife caring for husband with cognitive impairment	Physical/emotional demands of caregiving; perceived isolation of caregiver

> **Patient goals**
> **Expected outcomes**
>   Associated nursing/collaborative interventions *and scientific rationale*

Obtain assistance with meeting demands of caregiving role as evidenced by the following:

Increases skill in the management of patient behaviors

Guide use of daily log to record patient's behaviors and caregiver's management strategies.

Assist caregiver with analysis of recordings to identify disruptive behaviors that add to caregiving burden. *Caregiver involvement in the identification of problems and potential solutions will increase likelihood of successful resolution.*

Provide practical advice in the management of specific behaviors. *Practical advice reduces perceived burden by enhancing a sense of control.*

Verbalizes caregiving tasks that could be delegated

Review/discuss requirements for care with patient and caregiver.

Assist caregiver with identification of caregiving resources (e.g., family member, friends, community agencies).

Develop options for delegation of specific tasks.

Obtains information about costs of home health care services and respite care

Provide/discuss information about respite care.
    Provide caregiver with list of caregiving resources within budgetary limits.

Contracts with health care providers for specific services

Help caregiver develop a daily schedule that includes pacing direct care activities. *Delegation of specific tasks to formal caregivers may enable patient to remain in home setting despite an expected negative trajectory.*

Explore use of a computer link to supplement in-home services.

Develop support system with friends/neighbors as evidenced by the following:

Identifies social resources that could by mobilized
Requests that neighbors sit/visit with patient while caregiver attends to personal needs
Socializes with a friend on a regular basis

Help caregiver/patient to identify type/source of support that would be most helpful.

Help caregiver negotiate with patient to resume preferred leisure time activity.

Improve caregiver's health status as evidenced by the following:

Develops and implements a plan for daily exercise
Makes and keeps appointments for annual physical/pelvic examinations and mammography

Develop a plan for monitoring caregiver's health status.

Teach and monitor use of daily log for recording caregiver's activities, rest/exercise periods, and hours of sleep.

Help patient/caregiver to develop an alternate plan for patient's care in the event of caregiver's illness. *Demands/stress of caregiving increase vulnerability by depleting energizer reserves.*

REFERENCES

Archbold P and others: The PREP system of nursing interventions: a pilot test with families caring for older members, *Res Nurs Health* 18(1):3-16, 1995.

Brennan PF, Moore SM, Smyth KA: ComputerLink: Electronic support for the home caregiver, *Adv Nurs Sci* 13(4):14-27, 1991.

Brennan PF, Moore SM, Smythe KA: The effects of a special computer network on caregivers of persons with Alzheimer's disease, *Nurs Res* 44(3):166-172, 1995.

Bull MJ: Managing the transition from hospital to home, *Qual Health Res* 2(1):27-41, 1992.

Burns C, and others: New diagnosis: caregiver role strain, *Nurs Diagn* 4(2):70-76, 1993.

Caregiver role strain—cont'd

Carruth AK. Development and testing of the caregiver reciprocity scale. *Nurs Res* 45(2):92-97, 1996.

Given BA, Given CW: Family caregiving for the elderly, *Ann Rev Nurs Res* 9:77, 1991.

Given CW and others: The caregiver reaction assessment (CRA) for caregivers to persons with chronic physical and mental impairments, *Res Nurs Health* 15(4):271-283, 1992.

Kuhlman GJ and others: Alzheimer's disease and family caregiving: critical synthesis of the literature and research agenda, *Nurs Res* 40(6):331-337, 1991.

Langner SR: Ways of managing the experience of caregiving to elderly relatives, *West I Nurs Res* 15(5):582-594, 1993.

Lindgren CL: The caregiver career, *Image: J Nurs Schol* 25(3):214, 1993.

Reinhard SC: Living with mental illness: effects of professional support and personal control on caregiver burden, *Res Nursing Health* 17(2):79-88, 1994.

Stetz KM: Response to caregiving demands: their difficulty and effects on well-being of elderly caregivers, *Schol Inq Nurs Pract* 6(2):129-133, 1992.

Willhagen I: Caregiving demands: their difficulty and effects on well-being of elderly caregivers, *Schol Inq Nurs Pract* 6(2):111-127, 1992.

Caregiver role strain—cont'd

Caregiver role strain, risk for

CLINICAL CONDITION/ MEDICAL DIAGNOSIS	RISK FACTORS
Diabetic wife, primary wage earner, caring for husband with cardiopulmonary disease (COPD) following hospital discharge	Competing role demands: severity of care recipient's illness

Patient goals
Expected outcomes
   Associated nursing/collaborative interventions *and scientific rationale*

Establish a pattern of caregiving that is compatible with role demands as evidenced by the following:

Negotiates with employer for temporary reduction in work hours without loss of benefits

Contracts with health care provider for specific services

Requests alternating weekend assistance from daughter and son who live within driving distance

   Formulate with caregiver alternatives for decreasing role demands (e.g., temporary reduction in work hours; use of formal health care services).

   Plan and facilitate a family conference to negotiate care commitments with caregiver's son and daughter.

   Provide caregiver with a list of home health care providers and other community resources. *Early recognition of "at risk" status of caregiver will facilitate realistic planning.*

Provide competent care for spouse as evidenced by the following:

Requests assistance with complex care activities

Keeps appointments to participate in patient care activities before discharge

Verbalizes confidence in ability to provide care

Caregiver role strain, risk for

Contracts with health care providers for specific services

Help caregiver and patient to develop a written plan of care.

Determine caregiver's competence to carry out required care.

Provide instruction of patient care activities.

Discuss with caregiver the importance of spending time with patient when no care is being provided. *Patient needs to feel the nurturing aspects of the relationship in contrast to "burden" of care.*

Establish a self-care pattern consistent with role demands and caregiver's health impairment as evidenced by the following:

Makes appropriate sleeping arrangements
Equips husband's bedroom with electronic communication device to respond to his needs during night
Continues to follow diabetic regimen

Negotiate with patient/caregiver for appropriate sleeping arrangements with some form of electronic communication.

Teach caregiver/recipient to recognize signs/symptoms of fatigue.

Teach importance of keeping lights at low level during night to prevent difficulty in falling asleep after responding to husband's request for assistance.

Teach caregiver to use a daily log to monitor own health status (e.g., hours of sleep, feelings, loss of weight).

REFERENCES

Archbold P and others: The PREP system of nursing interventions: a pilot test with families caring for older members, *Res Nurs Health* 18(1):3-16, 1995.

Brennan PF, Moore SM, Smyth KA: ComputerLink: electronic support for the home caregiver, *Adv Nurs Sci* 13(4):14-27, 1991.

Bull MJ, Maruyama G, Luo D: Testing a model for posthospital transition of family caregivers for elderly persons, *Nurs Res* 44(3):132-138, 1995.

Bull MJ: Managing the transition from hospital to home, *Qual Health Res* 2(1):27-41, 1992.

Burns C and others: New diagnosis: caregiver role strain, *Nurs Diagn* 4(2):70-76, 1993.

Caregiver role strain, risk for—cont'd

Carruth AK. Development and testing of the caregiver reciprocity scale, *Nurs Res* 45(2):92-97, 1996.

Cossette S, Levesque L: Caregiving tasks as predictors of mental health of wife caregiver of men with chronic obstructive pulmonary disease, *Res Nurs Health* 16:251-263, 1993.

Fink SV: The influence of family resources and family demands on the strains and well-being of caregiving families, *Nurs Res* 44(3):139-146, 1995.

Given BA, Given CW: Family caregiving for the elderly, *Ann Rev Nurs Res* 9:77, 1991.

Given CW and others: The caregiver reaction assessment (CRA) for caregivers to persons with chronic physical and mental impairments, *Res Nurs Health* 15:271-283, 1992.

Langner SR: Ways of managing the experience of caregiving to elderly relatives, *West J Nurs Res* 15(5):582-594, 1993.

Lindgren CL: The caregiver career, *Image J Nurs Schol* 5(3):214, 1993.

Stetz KM: Response to caregiving demands: their difficulty and effects on the well-being of elderly caregivers, *Schol Inq Nurs Pract* 6(2):129-133, 1992.

Willhagen MI: Caregiving demands: their difficulty and effects on the well-being of elderly caregivers, *Schol Inq Nurs Pract* 6(2):111-127, 1992.

Communication, impaired verbal

CLINICAL CONDITION/ MEDICAL DIAGNOSIS	RELATED FACTORS
Schizophrenia	Psychological barriers

> **Patient goals**
> **Expected outcomes**
> Associated nursing/collaborative interventions *and scientific rationale*

Overcome psychological barriers to increase ability to use or understand language in human interaction as evidenced by the following:

Transmits clear, concise, and understandable messages

Use facilitative communication techniques while interacting with patient.

Teach and support use of effective communication techniques. *Use of effective communication techniques, such as reflection, validation, and clarification, results in transmission of understandable messages.*

Encourage initiation of conversations.

Encourage expression of feelings.

Attends to appropriate stimuli

Reduce stimuli to assist patient in attending to pertinent stimuli or increase stimuli to motivate patient.

Assist in correction of faulty perception.

Give clear, simple messages using language patient can understand.

Teach patient to identify and focus on relevant stimuli. *Through manipulation of the environment, teaching, and role modeling, the nurse facilitates the patient's accurate perception of and response to stimuli.*

Uses congruent verbal and nonverbal communication

Match verbal and nonverbal communication during nurse-patient interactions.

Validate meaning of nonverbal communication.

Point out discrepancies in verbal and nonverbal communication. *The message component of communication depends on translation of ideas, purpose, and intent into congruent verbal and nonverbal communication.*

Teach and encourage use of stress reduction techniques.

Sends and receives feedback

Increase patient's awareness of strengths and limitations in communication with others.

Describe, demonstrate, and encourage use of active listening skills.

Provide feedback to patient.

Teach patient to accept, request, and send both positive and negative feedback. *Communication is modified or corrected through the regulatory process of feedback.*

Support efforts to use feedback.

Experience gratification from communication

Model, teach, and support use of confirming responses when communicating with others.

Teach patient evaluation of own and others' communication.

Demonstrate and support responsibility for communication. *Motivation to communicate is related to the gratification experienced from communication.*

REFERENCES

Bulechek G, McCloskey J: *Nursing interventions: essential nursing treatments,* Philadelphia, 1992, WB Saunders.

Lekander B, Lehman S, Lindquist R: Therapeutic listening: key intervention for several nursing diagnosis, *Dimens Crit Care Nurs* (US) 12(1):24, 1993.

McFarland G, Naschinski C: Communication. In Thompson JM, McFarland GK, Hirsh JE and Tucker SM: *Mosby's clinical nursing,* ed 4, St Louis, 1997, Mosby.

Naschinski CE, McFarland GK: Impaired verbal communication. In McFarland GK, McFarlane EA: *Nursing diagnosis and intervention: planning for patient care,* ed 3, St Louis, 1997, Mosby.

Stewart J, Creed J: Aphasia: a care study, *Br J Nurs* 3(5):226-229, 1994.

VanCura B, Dawson S: A program to assist sensory-impaired patients, *Medsurg Nurs* 2(2):131-135, 1993.

Communication, impaired verbal—cont'd

Community coping, potential for enhanced

CLINICAL CONDITION/
MEDICAL DIAGNOSIS

Health care services not available to meet emerging patient needs related to the increasing incidence of human immunodeficiency virus (HIV) positive cases in a community that provides county public health services through not-for-profit agencies. The nurse, who is the director of the Sexually Transmitted Disease Clinic, initiates and coordinates the planning and intervention.

RELATED FACTORS

Lacks a plan for coordinating services between agencies to meet the emerging needs of HIV-positive clients.

Patient goals
Expected outcomes
Associated nursing/collaborative interventions *and
scientific rationale*

The community will experience enhanced coping by providing and maintaining the necessary health care services for HIV-positive clients as evidenced by the following:

Develops a comprehensive plan in conjunction with the not-for-profit agencies in the county to monitor persons with HIV from the time of screening

Consult with an infectious disease specialist to identify necessary screening and interventions for persons with HIV. *The time span from primary HIV infection through the asymptomatic HIV seropositive phase to the symptomatic seropositivity phase and AIDS diagnosis can be more than 10 years.*

Consult with persons with HIV to identify needs.

Successful programs include consumers during the planning stages.

Identify agencies that have the potential for providing necessary services. *Monitoring of persons with HIV requires numerous services, such as sophisticated laboratory test, substance abuse counseling and treatment, and home care.*

Identify sources for financing the expansion of existing programs and the development of new ones to meet the emerging needs of persons with HIV. *Funds are available from public and private sources; not-for-profit agencies generally have limited resources.*

Keep state and county health officers apprised of the ongoing efforts to provide services for persons with HIV. *When not-for-profit health care facilities are contractors that provide care for the county or state, it is mandatory that they communicate changing health care delivery needs and potential changes in a timely manner.*

Provide a designated place and time for routine monitoring and screening specific to HIV-positive clients. *Limiting the clinic to persons with HIV provides an atmosphere where needs specific to these clients (such as social support, education, substance abuse intervention, and grief counseling) can be met.*

Provides resources for continuous and timely monitoring of persons with HIV

Facilitate timely referral to the HIV-positive clinic. *Baseline physical findings are required. Providing emotional support is requisite for coping with the diagnosis.*

Facilitate timely referral of persons with HIV once AIDS is diagnosed. *Care is generally available for patients once AIDS has been diagnosed.*

The community will experience enhanced coping by the coordination of multiagency provision of services to persons with HIV as evidenced by the following:

Identifies strategies for providing care across agencies

Facilitate an ongoing committee composed of community advocates for persons with HIV and a representative from each agency with the potential to provide care to persons with HIV. *Caregivers and advocates can work together to develop and implement a plan that delivers care efficiently.*

Provide a case manager for each person with HIV. *Case managers visit clients in their homes to identify individual needs that may not be recognized in a clinic setting. They monitor changes in health status and arrange for needed care expeditiously.*

Encourage on-site HIV screening of all patients receiving substance abuse treatment. *Intravenous (IV) drug users are at increased risk for HIV infection. Making assessment available on site will facilitate early diagnosis and monitoring of HIV-positive cases.*

Provide a substance abuse counselor at all HIV-positive clinics. *Alcohol and drugs are often used by persons with HIV to cope with their diagnosis; these can interfere with immune status.*

Provide education across agencies to keep providers of health care updated with current HIV knowledge. *Research is ongoing that can impact care of HIV-positive clients. For example, screening at-risk pregnant patients is important, because recent studies have shown that treating the mother with zidovudine (AZT) will decrease chances of the baby developing AIDS.*

REFERENCES

Anderson E, McFarlene J: *Community as partner: theory and practice in nursing*, ed 2, Philadelphia, 1996, JB Lippincott.

Boswell S: Approach to the patient with HIV infection. In Groll A, editor: *Primary care medicine: office evaluation and management of the adult patient*, ed 3, Philadelphia, 1995, JB Lippincott.

Flynn B, Wiles D, Rider M: Empowering communities: action research through healthy cities, *Health Educ* Q 21(3):395, 1994.

Israel B, Checkoway B, Schulz A, Zimmerman M: Health education and community empowerment: Conceptualizing and measuring perceptions of individual, organizational and community control, *Health Educ* Q 21(2):149, 1994.

Jemmott JB III, Jemmott LS: Alcohol and drug use during sexual activity: predicting the HIV-risk-related behaviors of inner-city black male adolescents, *J Adolesc Res* 8(1):41, 1993.

US Department of Health and Human Services: *Evaluation and management of early HIV infection: clinical practice guideline number 7* (AHCPR Publication No. 94-0572) Washington, DC, 1994, U.S. Government Printing Office.

Zidovudine for the prevention of HIV transmission from mother to infant, *MMWR* 43(16):285, 1994.

Community coping, potential for enhanced—cont'd

Community coping, ineffective

CLINICAL CONDITION/ MEDICAL DIAGNOSIS	RELATED FACTORS
Inadequate immunization status of many children from a metropolitan school district's poorest school, delaying school entry which in turn affects the school budget.	Isolation of families related to fear of gang violence
The school nurse does the community assessment and intervention.	

Patient/Community goals
Expected outcomes
> Associated nursing/collaborative interventions *and scientific rationale*

The community will develop a pattern of coping for meeting threats to its health status as evidenced by the following:

Meets the immunization crisis by immunizing all children immediately so they can attend school

Mobilize the resources of the health department to provide immunizations at the school. *This is resource management to deal with the crisis and is not a method to meet the ongoing needs of the community.*

Notify parents of the availability of immunizations at the school, with both the mass media and flyers/posters in the community. *Disenfranchised citizens are difficult to reach, so interventions need to be at several levels.*

Monitor the immunization status of students so that referrals are made in a timely manner. *Families that do not take advantage of available immunizations may be dysfunctional, with a potential for child abuse.*

Community coping, ineffective

Meets the well-child needs of all community children in a timely manner rather than in response to a crisis.

Collaborate with health department clinic staff to identify issues associated with delivery of well-child services to children from the area with deficits in immunization coverage. *Immunization status is often inadequate for poor, preschool children. One fourth of preschool children and one third of poor children lack recommended immunizations. Organizational readiness is associated with success of programs.*

Identify a cohort of key informants (parents of children whose well-child needs have not been met). *Knowledge of individual perceptions of community problems is requisite to solving deficits in health care. Underuse is often a result of inadequate community involvement during the planning stage.*

Facilitate communication between health care providers of well-child care and community members disenfranchised from care. *Providers and consumers may have different perceptions of the problems associated with nonuse of services by the neediest community members.*

Empower community members to negotiate for needed well-child services. *Transferring power to the community enables members to begin sharing responsibility for their health.*

Mobilize available resources to immunize children in a timely manner. *This will ultimately save the system money by preventing childhood illnesses.*

The community will experience competence for dealing with threats to it as evidenced by the following:

Identifies strategies for reversing the trend toward gang anarchy and violence.

Facilitate formation of a community organizing group. *Community health nurses can be effective in using the social action model to help bring about change for areas with limited resources.*

Arrange for a meeting between area police and the community to develop a plan for better police coverage in this high-crime area. *The school nurse can act as an advocate for the community. There may be fear and resentment of the police, and arranging for them to communicate with community members is necessary for improving neighborhood safety.*

Enhance community competence by indicating community strengths. *Identifying community strengths is one method of capacity building in a community.*

Identify a safe place for children to receive health care. *Services will not be used if they are located in opposing gang territory.*

REFERENCES

Flynn B, Wiles D, Rider M: Empowering communities: action research through healthy cities, *Health Educ Q* 21(3):395, 1994.

Hahn M: What's new in immunizations? *Nurse Pract* 4(2):35, 1996.

Huesman LR, Eron LD, Lekowitz NM, Walder LO: Stability of aggression over time and generations, *Dev Psychol* 20(6):1120, 1984.

Israel B, Checkoway B, Schulz A, Zimmerman M: Health education and community empowerment: conceptualizing and measuring perceptions of individual, organizational and community control, *Health Educ Q* 21(2):149, 1994.

Martaus TM, Bell ML, Kenyon V, Snow L, Hefty LV: Realities of developing community health orientation programs, *Pub Health Nurs* 10(3):173, 1993.

Plaut T, Landis S, Trevor J: Focus group and community mobilization. In Morgan D, ed: *Successful focus group,* Newbury Park, Calif, 1993, Sage.

Report of the Committee on Infectious Diseases of the American Academy of Pediatrics. *Red Book,* ed 3, Elk Grove Village, Illinois, 1994, American Academy of Pediatrics.

Rosenberg ML: *Violence in America,* New York, 1993, Oxford University Press.

Community coping, ineffective—cont'd

Confusion, acute

CLINICAL CONDITION/ MEDICAL DIAGNOSIS	RELATED FACTORS
Patient, age 67, with history of chronic obstructive pulmonary disease and peripheral vascular disease recovering from abdominal aortic aneurysm surgery and embolectomy for lower extremity emboli and arterial occlusion.	Delirium

> **Patient goals**
> **Expected outcomes**
> Associated nursing/collaborative interventions *and scientific rationale*

Resolution of transient cerebral dysfunction as evidenced by the following:

No injury to self or others

Monitor for presence of signs and symptoms of acute confusion (e.g., fluctuation in levels of consciousness, attention, concentration; orientation; psychomotor activity; perceptual disturbances; sleep-wake disturbance that may include daytime somnolence and increased wakefulness at night; disorganization of thoughts and speech). *Patients with acute confusion are at increased risk to impulsively attempt to harm themselves (e.g., pulling out tubes of intravenous (IV) lines, getting out of bed) or others (by striking out).*

Collaborate with patient's physician and other members of multidisciplinary treatment team *to determine underlying causes for delirium (e.g., metabolic disturbances, systemic disease, infection, drug reactions) because delirium can become life-threatening if untreated and inappropriately managed.*

Explain safety mechanisms in patient's immediate environment, such as call light, side rails, equipment alarm systems, surveillance by nurse. *Repeating the information, using short simple sentences, until patient's acute confusion subsides, will assist the patient in understanding the explanations.*

Provide ongoing close surveillance by staff, such as one-to-one around the clock if patient exhibits behaviors that are indicative of self-injury or self-harm.

Ensure close observation by nursing staff if patient becomes highly agitated to *minimize use of soft or leather restraints. Restraints can increase paranoia and agitation, and contribute to additional complications, including pulmonary embolism, deep vein thrombosis, atelectasis, pneumonia, and decubitus ulcers.*

Have a calm family member or friend remain with patient if he/she becomes extremely frightened or agitated *to provide reassurance from a familiar person while minimizing risk for self-harm.*

Achieves satisfactory sleep pattern

Avoid or minimize the use of benzodiazepines and drugs with anticholinergic properties such as diphenhydramine (Benadryl) to promote sleep *because of the propensity of these drugs to potentiate existing acute confusion.*

Collaborate with members of the health team to adhere to patient's scheduled periods of undisturbed rest *to minimize exacerbation of confusion because of sleep deprivation.*

Incorporate patient's usual technique for achieving rest and sleep (e.g., soothing music, back rub, routine hygiene activities) *to promote satisfactory sleep pattern.*

Eliminate unnecessary environmental stimulation (e.g., staff interactions, excessive television or radio, monitoring equipment) *to facilitate improved sleep-wake cycle.*

Differentiates between reality and unreality

Ensure that all staff members introduce self by

name and call patient by preferred name *to reinforce patient's perception of reality.*

Ensure adequate non-glare lighting in patient's immediate environment, including night light, *to facilitate patient's reorientation to sensory cues and to reduce likelihood of visual distortions, misperceptions.*

Have patient's eyeglasses and hearing aids available (check to be sure that they are in working order) *to maximize accuracy of sensory input and to reduce potential for distortion of reality.*

Place appropriate visual cues within easy viewing of patient (e.g., calendar, clock, familiar photographs).

Do not argue with patient about his/her misinterpretations, and distortions of reality; acknowledge recognition that the experience is real and distressing for the patient.

Meets self-care needs to extent possible

Encourage patient to participate as much as possible in self-care activities such as hygiene, bathing, grooming.

Provide a reasonable length of time for patient to complete self-care activities *based on assessment of patient's compromised mentation.*

Defer patient's participation in treatment team expectations such as patient education, specific aspects of discharge planning, and major decision-making until there is tangible evidence of improved mentation *because cognitive impairments compromise the patient's ability to participate in these activities.*

Reduction in patient and family distress associated with mental status changes as evidenced by:

Family experiences reduced distress

Convey assurance to patient and family that the patient is safe in the present environment.

Encourage family and friends to maintain ongoing contact with patient; keep the patient informed of family activitities and plans.

Provide assurance to patient and family that total

clearing from the acute confusion may take from several days to several weeks. *This will reduce anxiety associated with recognition of cognitive disturbance and uncertainty about its outcome.*

Conduct an assessment to determine need for debriefing both patient and family after acute confusion has been resolved. *This will reduce undue fear and anxiety about what actually happened and clarify patient's possible distortions of events that transpired during the period of acute confusion.*

REFERENCES

American Psychiatric Association: *Diagnostic and statistical manual of mental disorders,* ed 4, Washington, DC, 1994, American Psychiatric Association.

Clark S: Psychiatric and mental health concerns in the patient with sepsis, *Crit Care Clin North Am* 6(2):389, 1994.

Evans CA, Kenny PJ, Rizzuto: Caring for the confused geriatric surgical patient, *Geriatric Nurs* 14(5):237, 1993.

Foreman MD: Complexities of acute confusion, *Geriatric Nurs* 11(3):136, 1990.

Foreman MD: Confusion in the hospitalized elderly: incidence, onset, and associated factors, *Res Nurs Health,* 12:21, 1989.

Inaba-Roland K, Maricle RA: Assessing delirium in the acute care setting, *Heart Lung* 21(1):48, 1992.

Lipowski ZJ: *Delirium: acute confusional states,* New York, 1990, Oxford University Press.

McFarland GK, Wasli EL, Gerety EK: *Nursing diagnosis and process in psychiatric mental health nursing,* ed 7, Philadelphia, 1997, JB Lippincott.

St Pierre J: Delirium in hospitalized elderly patients: off track, *Crit Care Nurs Clin North Am* 8(1):53, 1996.

Sullivan-Marx EM: Delirium and physical restraint in the hospitalized elderly, *Image J Nurs Schol* 26(4):295, 1994.

Confusion, chronic

CLINICAL CONDITION/ MEDICAL DIAGNOSIS	RELATED FACTORS
Elderly male diagnosed with dementia of the Alzheimer's type (early onset) currently living in a residential care home.	Displays a behavioral inconsistency with the environment; response to environmental stimuli, problem-solving ability, and capacity to follow complex instruction is compromised.

Patient goals
Expected outcomes
>   Associated nursing/collaborative interventions *and*
>   *scientific rationale*

Maintain ability to function in a structured environment as evidenced by the following:

Establishing a consistent daily routine and environment that will enable the patient to compensate for inability to plan activities.

>   Post a written daily routine for patient to follow. *Provide written directions or additional cues to the chronically confused individual who retains the ability to read.*

>   Provide a consistent caregiver(s). *Patients will experience increased security when cared for by people they recognize.*

>   Provide a daily time for small group activity that is valued by patient (i.e., music, art, reminiscence group, selected television program, bible therapy). *Planned activities are beneficial if they are pleasurable and incorporate the patient's culture, habits, values, manners, preferences and occupation.*

>   Place meaningful possessions in the patient's environment, such as photographs, mementos, favorite furniture. *Familiar belongings promote a sense of security.*

>   Avoid change in room environment (i.e., reassignment of patient's room, rearrangement of furniture or items, holiday decorations). *Frequent*

environment change may produce conflicting cues.

Ensuring that the patient has optimal sensory input to enable him to participate within the environment.

Make provision for optimal sensory input (e.g., eyeglasses are clean, hearing aid is functional, absence of cerumen impaction). *The cognitively impaired individual is at risk for misinterpretation of environment when sensory input is not accurate.*

Provide adequate nonglare lighting. *Visual perceptions may be altered by glare or shadows.*

Eliminate unnecessary environmental stimuli such as excessive noise level, multiple conversation/activity, violent/aggressive movies or television programs. *Disturbing visual images or loud noise can precipate a catastrophic reaction.*

Providing opportunities for meaningful communication and socialization.

Provide opportunity for one-on-one conversation with caregiver(s). *Providing sufficient time for interacting with patient reinforces socialization skill and a sense of self-worth.*

Maintain eye contact, smile and present a pleasant affect when interacting with the patient. *Verbal and nonverbal communications are important in establishing a relationship with a cognitively impaired person.*

Encourage continued interaction with a pet, that is, allow the pet to remain with patient or provide access to animal-assisted therapy. *Pets provide links to the past, encourage conversation and provide a pleasurable activity option.*

REFERENCES

Abraham IL and others: Multidisciplinary assessment of patients with Alzheimer's disease, *Nurs Clin North Am* 29(1):13-128, 1994.

Armstrong-Esther CA, Browne KD, McAfee JG: Elderly patients: still clean and sitting quietly, *J Adv Nurs* 19:264-271, 1994.

Barry PP: Medical evaluation of the demented patient, *Med Clin North Am* 78(4):779-784, 1994.

Beck CK, Shue VM: Interventions for treating disruptive behavior in demented elderly people, *Nurs Clin North Am* 29(1):143-155, 1994.

Bowie P, Mountain: Using direct observation to record the behavior of long-stay patients with dementia, *Int J Geriatric Psychiatry* 8:857-864, 1993.

Daly JM, Maas M, Buckwalter K: Use of standardized nursing diagnosis and interventions in long-term care, *J Gerontol Nurs* 21(8):29-36, 1995.

Confusion, chronic—cont'd

Fisher JE, Fink CM, Loomis CC: Frequency and management difficulty of behavioral problems among dementia patients in long-
term care facilities, *Clin Gerontol* 13(1):3-12, 1993.

Forges EJ: Spirituality, aging and the community-dwelling caregiver
and care recipient, *Geriatric Nurs* 15(6):296-301, 1994.

Hall GR: Caring for people with Alzheimer's disease using the conceptual model of progressively lowered stress threshold in the clinical
setting, *Nurs Clin North Am* 29(1):129-141, 1994.

Harvath TA and others: Dementia related behaviors in Alzheimer's
disease and AIDS, *J Psychosocial Nurs* 33(1):35-39, 1995.

Khovzam HR: Bible study: a treatment in elderly patients with
Alzheimer's disease, *Clin Gerontol* 15(2):71-74, 1994.

Loewenstein DA: Neuropsychological assessment in Alzheimer's disease, *Med Clin North Am* 78(4):789-793, 1994.

Rantz MJ, McShane RE: Nursing interventions for chronically confused nursing home residents, *Geriatric Nurs* 16(1):22-27, 1995.

Stolley JM and others: Managing the care of patients with irreversible
dementia during hospitalization for comorbidities, *Nurs Clin North
Am* 28(4):767-782, 1993.

Ugarriza DN, Gray T: Alzheimer's disease: nursing interventions for
clients and caretakers, *J Psychosocial Nurs* 31(10):7-10, 1993.

Constipation

CLINICAL CONDITION/ MEDICAL DIAGNOSIS	RELATED FACTORS
Chronic depression	Inadequate fluid and fiber in diet; daily ingestion of constipating medications

Patient goals
Expected outcomes
> Associated nursing/collaborative interventions *and scientific rationale*

Experience fewer incidences of constipation as evidenced by the following:

Obtains immediate relief

> Insert bisacodyl (Dulcolax) suppository within 1 hour of breakfast *to increase stimulation of gastro-colic reflex*; or use lubricated, gloved finger to break up large masses of hard stool. Follow with tap-water enema.

> Teach patient to exclude fatty acids from breakfast or triggering meal. *Fatty acids delay reflex stimulation and slow digestion.*

Takes fiber supplement once a day
Reports return to usual pattern of elimination: every 2 to 3 days
Verbalizes understanding of constipating effects of selected medications

> Recommended use of fiber supplement such as psyllium (Metamucil) once a day while on constipating medications with increase to twice a day if needed.

> Teach patient about constipating effects of medications.

Increase ingestion of fluids and fiber-rich foods as evidenced by the following:

Eats bran muffin or high-fiber bread daily
Eats one high-fiber vegetable daily and gradually increases to two or more

Constipation

Increase fluid intake to eight glasses daily

Teach patient to record all intake for 48 hours. Analyze eating pattern with patient. Recommend diet changes to increase bulk in diet. *Gradual addition of fiber helps to avoid cramping and flatus.* Recommend intake of eight glasses of water daily.

REFERENCES

Gattuso JM, Kamm MA: Adverse effects of drugs used in the management of constipation and diarrhea, *Drug Safety* 10(1):47-65, 1994.

Georges JM, Heitkemper MM: Dietary fiber and distressing gastrointestinal symptoms in midlife women, *Nurs Res* 43(6):357-361, 1994.

Hall GR and others: Managing constipation using a research-based protocol, *Medsurg Nurs* 4(1):11-20, 1995.

McCloskey JC, Bulechek GM: Constipation/impaction management. In *Nursing interventions classification (NIC)*, ed 2, St Louis, 1996, Mosby.

McLane AM, McShane RE: Constipation. In Mass M, Buckwalter KC, Hardy M, eds: *Nursing diagnosis and intervention for the elderly*, Redwood City, Calif, 1991, Addison-Wesley.

McLane AM, McShane RE: Constipation. In Thompson JM and others: *Mosby's clinical nursing*, ed 3, St Louis, 1993, Mosby.

Neal LJ: Power pudding: natural laxative therapy for the elderly who are homebound, *Home Health Nurse,* 13(3):88-71, 1995.

Rodriques-Fisher L, Bourguignon C, Good B: Dietary fiber nursing intervention: prevention of constipation in older adults, *Clin Nurs Res* 2(4):464-477, 1993.

Wolfsen CR, Barker JC, Mittenss LS: Constipation in the daily lives of frail elderly people, *Arch Fam Med* 2(8):853-858, 1993.

Constipation, colonic

CLINICAL CONDITION/ MEDICAL DIAGNOSIS	RELATED FACTORS
Elderly widower, six weeks after knee replacement	Preference for nonfibrous foods; restricted mobility (uses a walker)

Patient goals
Expected outcomes
　　Associated nursing/collaborative interventions *and*
　　　　scientific rationale

Establish a regular pattern of bowel movements as evidenced by the following:

Has a bowel movement at least every 3 days
Stool passes easily
Experiences sensation of complete passage of stool
Responds immediately to urge to defecate
　　Suggest trial of bisacodyl (Dulcolax) suppository instead of oral laxatives within 1 hour of breakfast or triggering meal, *which will elicit gastrocolic reflexes. Reflexes are strongest when stomach is empty.*
　　Establish toileting routine without use of suppositories or oral laxative.
　　Teach patient importance of immediate response to urge to defecate. *Stool will harden in rectum in the presence of chronic distention.*

Modify dietary intake to increase ratio of high-fiber foods as evidenced by the following:

Eats bran in some form daily
Eats one high-fiber vegetable daily
Substitutes whole grain for white bread
Eats prunes, banana, or preferred fresh fruit daily
　　Teach patient to record all intake for 48 hours.
　　Analyze eating pattern with patient.
　　Recommend diet changes to increase bulk in diet, consistent with financial limitations; substitute whole grain for white bread.
　　Recommend gradual addition of dietary fiber; 6 to

Constipation, colonic

10 gm of fiber each day. *Slow addition of fiber help to avoid cramping and flatus.*

Increase activity level as evidenced by the following:

Increases length of walks 10 ft per week
Engages in active range of motion twice daily
Exercises abdominal muscles daily
Substitutes 3-point cane for walker as increase in strength permits

Encourage outdoor walking (weather permitting). Increase ambulation distance from 20 ft to 40 ft and then to tolerance level.

Teach active range of motion and abdominal strengthening exercises. *Inadequate exercise is a major contributor to change in stool consistency.*

REFERENCES

Gattuso JM, Kamm MA: Adverse effects of drugs used in the management of constipation and diarrhea, *Drug Safety* 10(1):47-65, 1994.

Hall GR, et al: Managing constipation using a research-based protocol, *Medsurg Nurs* 4(1):11-20, 1995.

McLane AM, McShane RE: Bowel management. In Bulechek GM, McCloskey JC, eds: Nursing interventions: essential treatments, Philadelphia, 1993, JB Lippincott.

McLane AM, McShane RE: Constipation. In Mass M, Buckwalter KC, Hardy M, eds: *Nuring diagnosis and intervention for the elderly,* Redwood City, Calif, 1991, Addison-Wesley.

McLane AM, McShane RE: Colonic constipation. In Thompson JM, and others: *Mosby's clinical nursing,* ed 3, St Louis, 1993, Mosby.

Neal LJ: Power pudding: natural laxative therapy for the elderly who are homebound, *Home Health Nurse* 13(3):88-71, 1995.

Rodriques-Fisher L, Bourguignon C, Good B: Dietary fiber nursing intervention: Prevention of constipation in older adults, *Clin Nurs Res* 2(4):464-477, 1993.

Constipation, colonic—cont'd

Constipation, perceived

CLINICAL CONDITION/ MEDICAL DIAGNOSIS	RELATED FACTORS
Cholecystectomy, day surgery	Cultural health beliefs (expects to have a daily bowel movement; overuse of laxatives)

Patient goals
Expected outcomes
   Associated nursing/collaborative interventions *and scientific rationale*

Modify cultural health beliefs of family with respect for perceived need for having bowel movement as evidenced by the following:

Verbalizes receptivity to suggestion to have a bowel movement every 2 to 3 days

   Explore and acknowledge health beliefs and convictions.

   Confront health beliefs that maintain dysfunctional behavior. *Out-of-date information leads to faulty appraisal of pattern of elimination and need for laxatives.*

Modify toileting routines as evidenced by the following:

Drinks hot liquid before breakfast
Reports use of rectal suppository less than once a week

   Prescribe lemon juice and hot water every morning for 1-week trial.

   Teach patient to recognize and attend to stimulus behaviors (i.e., actions/behaviors that stimulate urge to defecate). *Gastrocolic reflexes are strongest when stomach is empty.*

   Teach patient to use a suppository to stimulate evacuation instead of using laxatives if bowel movements are less frequent than every 2 to 3 days.

Decrease use of laxatives as evidenced by the following:

Substitutes fresh fruit and vegetable sticks for desserts

Gradually increases walking to 1 mile three times per week

Provide instructions about increasing use of bulk and fiber in brown-bag lunches if patient carries a lunch.

Discuss temporary use of psyllium (Metamucil) to supplement gradual increase of natural fiber in diet. *Gradual addition of fiber to diet helps to avoid cramping and flatus.*

Teach patient role of exercise in developing and maintaining acceptable pattern of bowel elimination.

REFERENCES

Hall GR and others: Managing constipation using a research-based protocol. *Medsurg Nurs* 4(1):11-20, 1995.

Gattuso JM, Kamm MA: Adverse effects of drugs used in the management of constipation and diarrhea. *Drug Safety* 10(1):47-65, 1994.

McLane AM, McShane RE: Perceived constipation. In Thompson JM, McFarland GK, Hirsch JE and Tucker SM and others: *Mosby's clinical nursing,* ed. 3, St Louis, 1993, Mosby.

McLane AM, McShane RE: Constipation. In Maas M, Buckwalter KC, Hardy M, eds: *Nursing diagnosis and intervention for the elderly,* Redwood City, Calif, 1991, Addison-Wesley.

McShane RE, McLane AM: Constipation: impact of etiological factors, *J Gerontol Nurs* 14(4):31, 1988.

Constipation, perceived—cont'd

Coping, defensive

CLINICAL CONDITION/ MEDICAL DIAGNOSIS	RELATED FACTORS
Cancer	Stressful events, threat to self-esteem

> **Patient goals**
> **Expected outcomes**
>   Associated nursing/collaborative interventions *and*
>   *scientific rationale*

Experience defenses that are protective against stressful event and threat to self-esteem as evidenced by the following:

No further insult to self-esteem

Support patient's personhood, uniqueness, and right to be involved in decision making.

Seek to understand patient's perspective of situation and what is stressful or threatening. Seek to understand patient's sense of self and role expectations of self. *Enhancing an individual's self-esteem involves, as a first step, exploring the discrepancies within his/her self-concept.*

Gently clarify misconceptions.

Reduce stressful aspects of life (e.g., encourage expression of emotions).

Encourage maintenance of social support, including support from family, neighbors, and clergy.

Assist patient in becoming aware of behaviors that are harmful to others, such as ridiculing others, but do not try to pressure patient from defensive stance.

Demonstrates reduction in use of maladaptive defensive behaviors as evidenced by the following:

Verbalizes a realistic appraisal of the event, its demands, and coping resources available.

Verbalizes comfort with ideal and perceived roles and competencies to manage situation.

Communicates a sense of personal integrity.

Coping, defensive

181

Assist patient in exploring nature and characteristics of demands of cancer and coping resources required: identify where discrepancies exist between ideal and perceived roles in the situation. *Pace intervention to patient's readiness for assistance because a period of denial may be present.*

Help patient to identify desired goals in adjusting to cancer.

Where possible, reduce stressful aspects of the event and enhance patient's coping abilities through setting realistic, concrete goals with individual; identifying specific strategies for achieving goals; setting realistic time frames for reaching goals, reviewing capabilities and learning from past experiences; exploring patterns of thinking (especially negative thoughts); learning necessary knowledge and skills; acknowledging accomplishments toward desired goals; maintaining social networks; and encouraging expression of fears and concerns. *Pacing interventions with the patient's progression helps the patient adapt to the situation.*

REFERENCES

Aguilera D, Messick L: *Crisis intervention,* ed 7, St Louis, 1994, Mosby.

Curbow B and others: Self concept and cancer in adults, *Sci Med* 31(2):115-129, 1990.

Gammon J: Which way out of the crisis? Coping strategies for dealing with cancer, *Profes Nurse* 8(8):488-490, 1993.

Hagopian GA. Cognitive strategies used in adapting to a cancer diagnosis, *Oncol Nurs Forum* 20(5):759-763, 1993.

Katz MR, Rodin G, Devins GM: Self-esteem and cancer: theory and research, *Can J Psychiatry* 40(10):608-615, 1995.

Lazarus RS, Folkman S: *Stress, appraisal and coping,* New York, 1986, Springer.

Norris J: Nursing interventions for self-esteem disturbance, *Nurs Diagn* 3(30):48-53, 1992.

Ritz-Thomas D: Repression, self-concealment and rationality/emotional defensiveness: correspondence between three questionnaire measures of defensive coping, *Personal Indiv Diff* 20(1):95-102, 1996.

Ward S, Leventhal H, Easterling D: Social support, self esteem and communication in persons receiving chemotherapy, *J Psychosoc Oncol* 9:98-116, 1991.

Coping, defensive—cont'd

Coping, family: potential for growth

CLINICAL CONDITION/ MEDICAL DIAGNOSIS	RELATED FACTORS
Birth of second child	Adaptive tasks effectively addressed; progress toward self-actualization

---

Patient goals
Expected outcomes
 Associated nursing/collaborative interventions *and*
   scientific rationale

Actualize growth potential of family as evidenced by:

Verbalizes changes in family roles/relationships

Assist family to identify changes in family dynamics resulting from birth of second child.

Assist family to identify effects of changes on family process.

Verbalizes changes in individual attitudes, values and goals

Assist family to identify changes in individual family members resulting from birth of second child.

Assist family to identify strengths in coping with changes.

Assist family to transfer learning achieved with first child to parenting second child

Chooses goals and experiences that foster growth of child

Discuss goals and experiences that maximize growth potential for all family members.

Provide information as needed to enable individuals/family to develop new goals that relate to individuals and total family system.

Facilitate development of new methods of goal attainment.

Collaborate with family members in planning and implementing lifestyle changes. *Most families may be viewed as healthy but in need of temporary support. Intervention should be aimed at promoting family competence.*

Coping, family: potential for growth

Develop broader base of support as evidenced by:

Verbalizes interest in contacting others experiencing a similar situation

Identify family readiness to accept support from additional sources.

Assist family members to identify types of support needed.

Develops additional relationships that provide support during crisis

Inform family members of appropriate health care and community resources.

Refer family to appropriate resources.

Initiate contact with community resources if necessary.

Sustains contact with additional sources

Follow up to assure sustained contact and appropriateness of assistance.

Teach strategies to access and maximize community resources. *Individual/family should be aided in developing a broader base of support to maximize growth potential.*

REFERENCES

Block K, Brandt T, Magyary, D: A nursing assessment standard for early intervention: family coping, *J Ped Nurs* 10:28, 1995.

Bowers JE: Coping, family, potential for growth. In McFarland GK and Thomas MD: *Psychiatric mental health nursing: application of the nursing process,* Philadelphia, 1991, JB Lippincott.

Craft MJ, Willadsen JA: Interventions related to family, *Nurs Clin North Am* 27(2):517, 1992.

McCloskey JC and Bulechek GM (eds): *Nursing interventions classification (NIC),* ed 2, St Louis, 1996, Mosby.

Sims SL, Boland DL, O'Neill CA: Decision making in home health care, *West J Nurs Res* 14(2):186, 1992.

Tunali B, Power TG: Creating satisfaction: a psychological perspective on stress and coping in families of handicapped children, *J Child Psychiatry* 34:945, 1993.

Zerwekh JV: Laying the groundwork for family self-help: locating families, building trust, and building strength, *Pub Health Nurs* 9(1):15, 1992.

Coping, family: potential for growth—cont'd

Coping, ineffective family: compromised

CLINICAL CONDITION/ MEDICAL DIAGNOSIS	RELATED FACTORS
Child with acquired immunodeficiency syndrome (AIDS)	Inadequate understanding by family members; temporary family disorganization

Patient goals
Expected outcomes
    Associated nursing/collaborative interventions *and scientific rationale*

Develop adequate understanding of situation as evidenced by:

Verbalizes need for more information or clearer understanding relating to the situation

Provide adequate and correct information to patient and family members.

Monitor areas in which knowledge or understanding is inadequate in relation to human immunodeficiency virus (HIV)/AIDS.

Provide coordination of services through a case manager *to prevent failure to meet needs or duplication of services.*

Demonstrates understanding of information given

Encourage family to have realistic perspective based on accurate information.

Discusses changes in patient and family as result of health challenge

Encourage family members to discuss usual reactions to HIV/AIDS, such as anger, anxiety, dependency, and depression.

Verbalizes feelings to health care professionals and other family members

Encourage family members to verbalize feelings such as loss, guilt, or anger.

Use communication techniques that confirm legitimacy of both positive and negative feelings, such as reflecting feelings ("You seem frightened") or presenting reality ("Many people feel angry during this situation").

Provide opportunities for patient to discuss need for support with family members.

Clarify communications among family members.

Encourage patient and family members to discuss expectations with each other. *Supportive and informational family education is essential in helping a family that is experiencing ineffective coping. Family growth can be promoted through fostering a sense of "family" within an educational climate.*

Cope with changes in family processes as evidenced by:

Identifies changes in family processes as a result of the child's illness with AIDS

Help family to appraise the situation, including both strengths and weaknesses.

Help family to identify changes in relationships resulting from child's illness with AIDS.

Assumes new roles as necessary to maintain family integrity

Help family members to recognize role changes needed to maintain family integrity.

Refer family member to appropriate additional sources for help in adjusting to changes in family processes. *Encouragement to use sources outside the family may be appropriate to preserve the supportive capacity of family members in assuming new roles over time.*

Family member participates in care of patient

Involve family member in care of patient as much as possible. *Family competence can be increased by restructuring of role relationships.*

REFERENCES

Boland MG, Conviser R: Nursing care of the child, In Flaskerud JH, Ungvarski PJ, eds: *HIV/AIDS: a guide to nursing care,* Philadelphia, 1992, WB Saunders.

Brown MA, Powell-Cope GM: AIDS family caregiving: transitions through uncertainty, *Nurs Res* 40(6):338, 1991.

Brown MA, Powell-Cope GM: Themes of loss and dying in caring for a family member with AIDS, *Res Nurs Health* 16(3):179, 1993.

Fkaskerud, JH: Psychosocial aspects, In Flaskerud JH, Ungvarski PJ, eds: *HIV/AIDS: a guide to nursing care,* Philadelphia, 1992, WB Saunders.

Coping, ineffective family: compromised—cont'd

McCloskey JC, Bulechek GM (eds): *Nursing interventions classification (NIC)*, ed 2, St Louis, Mosby, 1996.

Panel on Women, Adolescents, and Children with HIV Infections and AIDS: Family-centered comprehensive care for children with HIV infection, Washington, DC, 1991, US DHHS.

Stetz KM, Lewis FM, Houck GM: Family goals as indicants of adaptation during chronic illness, *Pub Health Nurs* 11:385, 1994.

Coping, ineffective family: compromised—cont'd

Coping, ineffective family: disabling

CLINICAL CONDITION/ MEDICAL DIAGNOSIS	RELATED FACTORS
Parent with senile dementia, of the Alzheimer's type	Dissonant discrepancy of coping styles; highly ambivalent family relationships

Patient goals
Expected outcomes
 Associated nursing/collaborative interventions *and scientific rationale*

Demonstrate improved coping strategies as evidenced by:

Verbalizes understanding of the health challenge

Provide adequate and correct information about senile dementia of the Alzheimer's type.

Encourage family to develop realistic expectations about prognosis.

Discuss usual reactions to health challenges. *Once the disabling level of anxiety has been reduced, the patient and family should be given sufficient information about the nature and course of the health challenge to aid in the development of alternative coping strategies.*

Verbalizes perceptions of coping styles and areas of conflict

Help family members and patient to verbalize own perceptions of coping styles and areas of conflict.

Identify areas of conflict in coping styles among individuals and within family unit.

Monitor individual and family coping styles.

Identifies alternative coping behaviors that may minimize conflict

Help family members and patient to identify alternative coping behaviors to minimize conflict in adapting to health challenge.

Help family members and patient focus on present feelings.

Incorporates alternative coping behaviors in adapting to health challenge

Assist family members and patient in practicing alternative coping behaviors: relabeling, role playing, contracting, etc. *A family with limited understanding about various coping strategies may need information about alternatives, as well as the potential effect of conflict on coping styles. Assistance in learning alternative coping behaviors may be essential in aiding the family members and patient in incorporating new behaviors.*

Improve level of complementarity in role relationships as evidenced by:

Discusses complementary nature of strengths, needs, and expectations of relationships

Help patient and family members to verbalize individual needs and expectations of relationships as patient's mental status changes.

Help patient and family members to identify individual strengths and weaknesses in adapting to changes in patient's physical and mental health.

Identifies areas where needs and expectations are not being met, leading to feelings of powerlessness

Assist patient and family members to discuss areas where individual strengths, needs, and expectations complement each other in adapting to changes in patient's physical and mental status.

Help patient and family members identify needs and expectations that are not being met.

Identifies strategies to aid developing complementary relationships which can overcome feeling of powerlessness

Help patient and family members identify additional strategies to develop complementary relationships in adapting to changes in patient's physical and mental status.

Incorporates alternative strategies in relationships

Assist patient and family members in practicing new strategies. *A family experiencing disabling anxiety as a result of inability to cope with the changes in role relationships imposed by a health challenge may be assisted by helping them identify the changes that have occurred. Once needs and expectations have been explored, specific strategies to develop complementary relationships in the current situation can be identified and practiced.*

REFERENCES

Alexrod J, Gersmar L, Ross R: Families of chronically mentally ill patients: their structure, coping resources and tolerance for deviant behavior, *Health Soc Week* 19:271, 1994

Butcher LA: A family-focused perspective on chronic illness, *Rehabil Nurs* 19:70, 1994.

Farren CJ and others: Finding meaning: an alternative paradigm for Alzheimer's disease family caregivers, *Gerontologist* 31:483, 1991.

King S and others: Institutionalization of an elderly family member: reactions of spouse and nonspouse caregivers, *Arch Psychiatr Nurs* 5(6):323, 1991.

Knafl KA, Deatrick JA: Family management style: concept analysis and development, *J Pediatr Nurs* 5:4, 1990.

McCubbin H, Patterson J, eds: *Systematic assessment of family stress: resources and coping*, St Paul, 1981, University of Minnesota.

Swearingen PL: *Manual of medical-surgical nursing care: nursing interventions and collaborative management*, ed 3, St Louis, 1994, Mosby, p 765.

Coping, ineffective family: disabling—cont'd

Coping, ineffective individual

CLINICAL CONDITION/ MEDICAL DIAGNOSIS	RELATED FACTORS
Major depressive disorder	Fear of relapse
	Inadequate social support system

Patient goals
Expected outcomes
    Associated nursing/collaborative interventions *and*
      scientific rationale

Has plan for handling a recurrence of depression as evidenced by:

Identifies two or three scenarios in which depressive thoughts and feelings may return

Listen and validate perceptions, as patient recalls the feelings of dissatisfaction, the attempts to live up to expectations of other, the burden of caring for others and not self, and leaving major decisions up to chance. *This assists patient in processing the experience of depression.*

Assist in recalling knowledge of depression (e.g., contributing factors, treatments, outcomes).

Examine with patient what helped in past and what might be helpful in future. *Identification of stressor, strategies to cope, future stressors, and treatments increase adaptation.*

Provide positive reinforcement as hope for the future is expressed and new goals are made.

Establish support system as evidenced by:

Identifies reactions of others to the experience of depression and seeks ways to redesign more supportive relationships

Identify protective, coercive, and collaborative strategies experienced by the patient. *Enhancing the ways to learn about self and others widens a person's definition of what is normal, what is expected, and the scope of resources.*

Coping, ineffective individual

191

Assist patient in working through problems with the support system as they occur.

Promote continued attendance at support group. *Social support provided in groups gives opportunity to learn ways to cope with emotions and to accept self as a person of worth; thereby reducing anxiety, depression, and other emotional distress.*

Acknowledges the human need for others and the consequences for self when isolation occurs

Provide opportunity to discuss fear of intimacy and rejection by others. *Focusing on relationship issues using interpersonal concepts assists patients to solve problems and to use coping resources.*

Instruct about the impact of isolation on thoughts and feelings.

REFERENCES

Badger TA: Living with depression: family members experience and treatment needs, *J Psychosoc Nurs Ment Health Serv* 34(1):21-29, 1996.

Bailey GJ: Mediators of depression in adults with depression, *Clin Nurs Res* 5(1):28-42, 1996.

Freeman A, Dattilio FM, ed: *Cognitive-behavioral strategies in crisis intervention*, New York, 1994, Guilford Press.

Goethe JW, Fischer EH: Functional capabilities of depressed patients one year after hospitalization, *Psychiatr Serv* 46(11):1187-1188, 1995.

Kaplan HI, Sadock BJ, Grebb JA: *Synopsis of psychiatry: behavioral sciences, clinical psychiatry*, ed 7, Baltimore, 1994, Williams & Wilkins.

Rahe RH: Acute stress versus chronic post traumatic stress disorder, *Integr Physiol Behav Sci* 28(1):46-56, 1993.

Schreiber RS: Understanding and helping depressed women, *Arch Psychiatr Nurs* 10(3):165-175, 1996.

Decisional conflict (prenatal genetic testing)

CLINICAL CONDITION/ MEDICAL DIAGNOSIS	
	RELATED FACTORS
Pregnancy	Unclear goals and values; unrealistic expectations; pressure from others

Patient goals
Expected outcomes
 Associated nursing/collaborative interventions *and scientific rationale*

Make and implement an informed choice that is consistent with personal goals and values as evidenced by the following:

Understands what genetic testing can achieve

 Explore patient's goals and clarify alternatives and their possible consequences. *Lack of information or clarity of these items contributes to decisional conflict.*

Expresses realistic expectations of having and not having prenatal testing

 Realign unrealistic expectations. *Distortion in expectations often increases conflict (e.g., anticipating a negative consequence when the likelihood is extremely low) or regret (e.g., anticipating a positive consequence when the likelihood is extremely low).*

Identifies priority of anticipated consequences and implicit tradeoffs in selection process

 With the patient, clarify the patient's views on the desirability of possible consequences and their priority ordering. *Unclear values contribute to decisional conflict.*

 Identify value tradeoffs implicit in making choices. *Having to make tradeoffs often contributes to conflict. Knowing what makes the decision difficult helps in its resolution.*

Selects course of action consistent with personal values

 Facilitate alternative selection consistent with personal values. *Value congruence increases satisfaction with the decision and the likelihood the patient will follow through on the choice.*

Uses self-help skills in implementing selected course of action; expresses satisfaction with the decision made

Teach and reinforce self-help skills required to obtain support from others, to deal with unwanted pressure from others, and to implement the choice. *Individuals have difficulty in implementing decisions made without the resources to do so.*

REFERENCES

Janis H, Mann I: *Decision making,* New York, 1977, The Free Press.

Keeney RL: *Value-focused thinking,* Cambridge, Mass, 1992, Harvard University Press.

O'Connor AM: Validation of a decisional conflict scale, *Med Decis Making* 15:25-30, 1995.

O'Connor AM: Decisional conflict. In McFarland GK, and McFarlane EA, editors: *Nursing diagnosis and intervention: planning for patient care,* ed 3, St Louis, 1997, Mosby.

Pender NJ, Pender AR: *Health promotion in nursing practice,* ed 2, East Norwalk, Conn, 1987, Appleton-Lange.

Rothert ML, Talarczyk GJ: Patient compliance and the decision making process of clinicians and patients, *J Compliance Health Care* 2:55, 1987.

Sjogren B, Vdbenberg N: Decision making during the prenatal diagnostic procedure, *Prenat Diagn* 8:263, 1988.

Denial, ineffective

CLINICAL CONDITION/ MEDICAL DIAGNOSIS	RELATED FACTORS
Myocardial infarction (MI)	Life-threatening event

Patient goals
Expected outcomes
 Associated nursing/collaborative interventions *and scientific rationale*

Maintain appropriate level of denial in relation to life-threatening event as evidenced by the following:

Remains appropriately defended and expresses low to moderate anxiety

 Focus on establishing a trust relationship with patient.

 Assess the nature of the threat. *Assessing the nature of the threat uncovers its presence, its meaning, and whether denial is a deterrent to health and well-being.*

 Consider no intervention if denial is not a deterrent to the patient's health and well-being. *Adaptive denial temporarily protects the patient from psychological harm.*

 Make periodic checks as to patient's stage of denial.

 Do not confront patient's denial *because the patient may not be able to handle the resulting anxiety.*

 Gain insight into the detrimental relationship of denial on health evidenced by statements demonstrating an understanding of the threatening situation.

 Discuss with the patient his or her values, beliefs, and perceptions of the life-threatening situation. *As values and beliefs are discussed, the patient's may gain insight into the use of denial.*

Denial, ineffective

195

Accepts the reality of the life-threatening situation as evidenced by:

Demonstrates health-seeking behavior

Provide patient with the opportunity to express any fears or anxieties of which patient is aware.

Provide patient with specific information about MI and/or reassurance if patient raises any questions or concerns as appropriate to the stage of denial the patient is experiencing. *Factual information presented in a caring, nonjudgemental manner may help the patient focus on his or her behaviors and gain an understanding of the relationship between behaviors and health.*

Do not pressure the patient to raise questions or concerns if patient is not ready. Working with the patient in terms of his or her particular stage of denial at any point in time is important.

REFERENCES

Breznitz S: The seven kinds of denial. In Breznitz S, ed: *The denial of stress,* New York, 1983, International University Press.

Butcher HK, Forchuk C: Ineffective denial. In McFarland GK, McFarJane EA, editors: *Nursing diagnosis and intervention: planning for patient care,* ed 3, St Louis, 1997, Mosby.

Forchuck C, Westwell, J: Denial, *J Psychosoc Nurs Ment Health* 25(6):9, 1987.

Hackett, Cassem NH, Wishnic, HA; The coronary care unit-an appraisal of its psychological hazards, *N Engl J Med* 279:1365, 1968.

Johnson JL, Morse JM: Regaining control: the process of adjustment after myocardial infarction, *Heart Lung* 19(2):126, 1990.

Keckelson ME, Nyamathi AM: Coping and adjustment to illness in the acute myocardial infarction patient, *J Cardiovasc Nurs* 5(1):25, 1990.

Lazarus RS: The costs and benefits of denial. In Breznitz S, ed: *The denial of stress,* New York, 1983, International University Press.

Lowery BJ: Psychological stress, denial and myocardial infarction outcomes, *Image J Nurs Schol* 23:51-55, 1991.

Robinson KR: Developing a scale to measure denial levels of clients with actual or potential myocardial infarctions, *Heart Lung* 23(1):36-44, 1994.

Robinson KR: Denial: an adaptive response, *Dimen Crit Care Nurs* 12(2):102-106, 1993.

Shelp EE, Perl M: Denial in clinical medicine: a reexamination of the concept and its significance, *Arch Intern Med* 145:697, 1985.

Westwell J, Forchuk C: Denial: buffer and barrier, *Canad Nurse* 85(9):16-18, 1989.

Denial, ineffective—cont'd

Diarrhea

CLINICAL CONDITION/ MEDICAL DIAGNOSIS	RELATED FACTORS
Malnutrition and dysphagia; enteral tube feeding with infusion pump	Change in enteral feeding, clogged nasogastric tube

> **Patient goals**
> **Expected outcomes**
> Associated nursing/collaborative interventions *and scientific rationale*

Receive enteral feeding, fluids, medications safely as evidenced by the following:

Body weight increases
Number of liquid, nonformed stools decreases
Fluids/electrolytes gradually return to normal

Consult with physician to replace clogged silicone nasogastric tube with polyurethane nasoduodenal tube, size 10 or 12 Fr. *Polyurethane tubes are coated with a hydrophilic substance that decreases clogging rate.*

Restart feedings at a slower rate until diarrhea is under control; then gradually increase to desired rate.

Keep head of bed elevated during feedings and for 1 half hour after feeding.

Irrigate tube with 30 ml of water every 2 hours, after every intermittent feeding, and after administration of a medication through tube.

Provide extra water (0.5 ml of water for every 1 ml of tube feeding) *to help patient excrete the solute load and keep serum sodium within normal range.*

Check infusion pump every hour.

Refrigerate opened containers of enteral feedings; discard containers and administration sets every 24 hours.

REFERENCES
Bodkin NL, Hansen BC: Nutritional studies in nursing, *Ann Rev Nurs Res* 9:203-220, 1991.

Diarrhea

Gattuso JM, Kamm MA: Adverse effects of drugs used in the management of constipation and diarrhea, *Drug Safety* 10(1):47-65, 1994.

McCloskey JC, Bulechek GM: Diarrhea management. In *Nursing interventions classification (NIC),* ed 2, St Louis, 1996, Mosby.

Metheny N, Eisenberg P, McSweeney M: Effect of feeding tube properties and three irrigants on clogging rates, *Nurs Res* 37(3):165-169, 1988.

Metheny N, Eisenberg P, McSweeney M: The effect of three irrigants on clogging rates of feeding tubes. In Funk SG and others, editors: *Key aspects of recovery: improving nutrition, rest, and mobility,* 1990.

Poyss AS: Fluid therapy. In Bulechek GM, McCloskey JC: *Nursing interventions essential nursing treatments,* ed 2, Philadelphia, 1992, WB Saunders.

Smith CE and others: Diarrhea associated with tube feeding in mechanically ventilated critically ill patients, *Nurs Res* 39(3):148-152, 1990.

Vines SM and others: Research utilization: an evaluation of the research related to causes of diarrhea in tube-fed patients, *Appl Nurs Res* 5(4):64-173, 1992.

Wadle K: Diarrhea. In Maas M, Buckwalter KC, Hardy M (eds): *Nursing diagnosis and intervention for the elderly,* Redwood City, Calif, 1991, Addison-Wesley.

Diarrhea—cont'd

Disuse syndrome, risk for

CLINICAL CONDITION/ MEDICAL DIAGNOSIS	RELATED FACTORS
Paralysis, altered level of consciousness; trauma weakness/ fatigue	Immobility

Patient goals
Expected outcomes
> Associated nursing/collaborative interventions *and scientific rationale*

Maintain joint movement, muscle size and strength, and bone mineralization as evidenced by the following:

Full range of motion (ROM) in joints
Muscle size and strength within normal limits
Ability to bear weight without discomfort
> Perform active/passive ROM exercises *to maintain functional integrity of muscles and joints through use, prevent disuse atrophy of muscles, and prevent contracture development in muscles and joints through stretching of connective tissue.*
>
> Maintain anatomic positioning of limbs *to maintain structural integrity of muscles and joints and prevent contracture development.*
>
> Perform isometric muscle setting exercises *to maintain muscle tone.*
>
> Dangle at bedside as tolerated. Assist patient up to chair as tolerated.
>
> Ambulate as tolerated. *Weight bearing prevents calcium loss through increased bone deposition.*

Maintain adequate systemic and local tissue perfusion as evidenced by the following:

Blood pressure remains normal and no complaint of dizziness during position changes
Peripheral pulses remain intact
No dependent edema formation
No complaint of weakness/fatigue with activity

Perform bed exercises as tolerated *to promote venous return and cardiovascular work capacity.*

Apply antiembolism stockings *to prevent venous pooling in extremities.*

Perform positional change in relation to gravity as tolerated: supine to semi-upright to upright *to prevent decreased orthostatic capacity by enhancing neurovascular tone.*

Actively contract muscles of lower extremities when assuming upright position *to increase muscle pumping of pooled blood to increase venous return and maintain cardiac output.*

Promote feelings of independence and control as evidenced by the following:

Does not verbalize feelings of powerlessness or loss of control

Participates in self-care and activities of daily living (ADLS) to maximum extent possible

Patient and family/significant others express satisfaction with patient's progress and treatment

Allow opportunity for decision making regarding care *to increase patient's sense of control related to situation and environment.*

Encourage participation in ADLs as tolerated.

Encourage independence in self-care activities.

Introduce and encourage use of assistive devices as needed.

Maintain normal skin and tissue integrity as evidenced by the following:

Skin remains dry, pink, warm and intact, especially over bony prominences and pressure points

Reposition frequently, at least every 1 to 2 hours, *to relieve pressure and promote tissue perfusion.*

Inspect all pressure points at least every 2 hours.

Provide clean, dry, and wrinkle-free bedding.

Use assistive pressure-relief devices as needed (e.g., foam mattress, gel flotation pads, air-fluidized bed).

Consider use of continuous mechanical turning or continuous lateral rotation therapy (CLRT)

(oscillating bed or kinetic treatment table) to provide continuous side-to-side positional changes, *which have been found to decrease incidence of pressure ulcer formation in immobilized patients.*

Use of pressure relief interventions should be part of *initial* treatment of underlying condition.

Risk of decubitus formation increases with immobilization time.

Maintains normal tissue turgor, elasticity, and strength

Encourage adequate intake of fluid and diet *to provide tissue hydration and nutrient supply.*

Provide adequate protein in diet *to maintain positive nitrogen balance.*

Maintain normal patterns of elimination as evidenced by the following:

Urine output within normal limits

Urine remains clear, light yellow, and without sediment

Urine specific gravity is 1.010 to 1.025

Bowel movement per regular pattern

Stool soft and formed

Absence of discomfort when urinating or defecating

Absence of urinary frequency or urgency

Encourage adequate fluid intake *to increase volume of urine and water volume of stool.*

Assist patient to get up to bathroom or commode as tolerated. *Anatomic position will facilitate complete emptying of bladder and bowel aided by gravity and muscle contraction.*

Reposition frequently *to prevent pooling and stasis of urine in bladder and promote gastic motility.*

Provide adequate roughage (fiber, fruit, vegetables) in diet as tolerated *to provide bulk and stimulate peristalsis.*

Provide acid-ash diet *to maintain acidity (lower pH level) of urine.*

Give stool softener/laxatives as indicated.

Provide privacy during act of voiding/defecation.

Maintain appropriate and adequate sensory and perceptual status as evidenced by the following:

Remains oriented to time, person, and place

Provide access *to* clock, radio, television, reading materials, and other appropriate diversionary, stimulating activities.

Encourage visits from others.

Maintain normal day/night light patterns.

Avoid monotonous sensory stimuli.

Maintain effective breathing pattern and patent airway as evidenced by the following:

Expectorates secretions

Breath sounds clear

Tidal volume, negative inspiratory force (NIF), and vital capacity within normal limits

Chest excursion is complete and equal bilaterally

Perform deep breathing and coughing exercises every hour *to promote respiratory muscle excursion and mobilize secretions.*

Encourage adequate fluid intake *to provide hydration to keep secretions loose and moist.*

Monitor breath sounds.

Reposition frequently or consider use of continuous mechanical turning or CLRT (oscillating bed or kinetic treatment table) to prevent pooling of secretions and body fluids. *CLRT has been found to decrease incidence of pulmonary complications in immobilized patients.*

REFERENCES

Curry K, Casady L: The relationship between extended periods of immobility and decubitus ulcer formation in the acutely spinal cord-injured individual, *Neurosci Nurs* 24(4):185-189, 1992.

Dettmer DK, Teasell R: Complications of immobility and bedrest: Part I Musculoskeletal and cardiovascular complications, *Can Fam Physician* 39:1428-1432, 1435-1437, 1993.

Hunt AH, Civitelli R, Halstead L: Evaluation of bone resorption: a common problem during impaired mobility, *Sci Nurs*, 12(3):90-94, 1995.

Lentz M: Selected aspects of deconditioning secondary to immobilization, *Nurs Clin North Am* 16(4):729-737, 1981.

MacIntyre NR: Automated lateral rotational therapy in the intensive care unit, *Care Critical Ill* 10(5):210, 212-213, 1994.

Mobily PR, Kelley LS: Iatrogenesis in the elderly; Factors of immobility, *J Gerontal Nurs* 17(9):5-11, 1991.

Olson, EV, Johnson BJ, Thompson, LF: The hazards of immobility, *AJN* 90(3):43-44, 46-48, 1990.

Sahn SA: Continuous lateral rotational therapy and nosocomial pneumonia, *Chest* 99(5):1263-1267, 1991.

Shekleton ME: Impaired physical mobility. In Shekleton M, Litwack K, eds: *Critical care nursing of the surgical patient,* Philadelphia, 1991, WB Saunders.

Titler M and others: Classification of nursing interventions for care of the integument, *Nurs Diagn* 2(2):45-56, 1991.

VonRueden KT, Harris JR: Pulmonary dysfunction related to immobility in the trauma patient, *AACN Clin Iss Adv Pract Acute Crit Care* 6(2):212-228, 1995.

Vorhies D, Riley BE: Deconditioning . . . changes in organ system physiology . . . induced by inactivity and reversed by activity, *Clin Geriatr Med* 9(4):745-763, 1993.

Diversional activity deficit

CLINICAL CONDITION/ MEDICAL DIAGNOSIS	RELATED FACTORS
Elderly patient with a hip replacement	Limited leisure resources; long-term hospitalization

Patient goals
Expected outcomes
  Associated nursing/collaborative interventions *and scientific rationale*

Identify strengths and limitations with respect to engaging in diversional activities as evidenced by the following:

Sets realistic goals for diversional activities

  Review patient's usual pattern of diversional activities *to assess activity level, tolerance and preferences.*

  Assist patient in describing desired or required activity level changes needed because of altered health status.

  Encourage discussion of limitations in usual pattern of diversional activities *to assess impact of stressors and level of adjustment.*

Seeks out realistic opportunities within limited resources for involvement in diversional activities

  Provide opportunities to continue meaningful diversional activities that are realistic within current environment *to support patient's sense of self-worth and productivity.*

  Provide new activities that are age-appropriate *to assure the experience will be as normal as possible.*

  Assist patient in adapting diversional activities to changed health status.

  Include patient in making decisions about varying the daily routine *to promote a sense of control and recognition of personal preferences.*

  Facilitate opportunities for visits from friends and family *to stimulate social interaction and contact with the outside world.*

Diversional activity deficit

Identifies strategies for dealing with limited leisure resources and obtains needed resources as evidenced by the following:

Assumes responsibility for choosing and participating in diversional activities in current environment

Assist patient in identifying realistic resources and energy expenditures required to participate in meaningful activities. *Discussion provides opportunities for mutual goal setting and problem solving.*

Inform patient about options for diversional activities available in current setting (e.g., recreational therapy, occupational therapy, art/music therapy, remotivation therapy, support groups) *to assist in structuring free time and decreasing boredom.*

Support patient's perceptions of resources needed to participate in satisfying diversional activity in individual situation (e.g., confinement).

Engages in satisfactory diversional activities during long-term hospitalization as evidenced by the following:

Initiates participation and demonstrates ongoing interest in diversional activities available in current environment

Help patient assess changes in ability to engage in preferred diversional activities and assist with problem-solving.

Provide feedback to patient about observed level of participation and self-structuring of free time. *Social reinforcement encourages continued efforts by the patient.*

Expresses pleasure and satisfaction with diversional activities in current setting

Integrate diversional activity into patient's daily schedule of care whenever possible.

Adapt daily routine and environment to provide physical and mental stimulation and variety (e.g., change of scenery, creative activities) *to enhance socialization, coping, and involvement in the milieu.*

Encourage patient to provide feedback about satisfaction with choice of activities.

Diversional activity deficit—cont'd

REFERENCES

Abraham IL and others: Therapeutic work with depressed elderly, *Nurs Clin North Am* 26(3):635, 1991.

Badry E, Robins M, Forestier M: Diversional therapy, *Can Nurs* 86(2):33, 1990.

Chin-Sang V, Allen KR: Leisure and the older black woman, *J Gerontol Nurs* 17:30, 1991.

Hutchinson SA, Bondy E: The pals program intergenerational remotivation, *J Gerontol Nurs* 16(12):19, 1990.

Jackson L and others: Age-appropriate activities help residents reach goals, *Provider* 18(6):48, 1992.

Jongbloed L, Morgan D: An investigation of involvement in leisure activities after a stroke, *Am J Occupa Ther* 45(5):420, 1991.

McCloskey JC, Bulechek GM, eds: *Nursing interventions classification (NIC)*, ed 2, St Louis, 1996, Mosby.

Radziewicz RM, Schneider SM: Using diversional activity to enhance coping, *Cancer Nurs* 15(4):293, 1992.

Rubenfeld MG: Diversional activity deficit. In McFarland GK, McFarlane EA: *Nursing diagnosis and intervention*, ed 3, St Louis, 1997, Mosby.

Diversional activity deficit—cont'd

Dysreflexia

CLINICAL CONDITION/ MEDICAL DIAGNOSIS	RELATED FACTORS
Patient has a spinal cord injury (T7 or above) with afferent stimulation below the level of the injury	Distended bladder Cutaneous stimuli below T7

Patient goals
Expected outcomes
  Associated nursing/collaborative interventions *and*
    scientific rationale

Prevent episodes of dysreflexia as evidenced by the following:

Recognizes the signs and symptoms of autonomic dysreflexia

  Teach signs and symptoms of dysreflexia (e.g., elevation of blood pressure >20 mm Hg above patient baseline, pounding headache, visual changes, pallor below level of injury, bradycardia, sweating, piloerection, facial flushing, flushed warm skin above the injury, nasal stuffiness).

Demonstrates understanding of effects of bladder and bowel distention on dysreflexia.

  Teach methods to prevent bladder distention (e.g., Foley care, intermittent catheterization). *Bladder distention is the most common cause of autonomic dysreflexia.*

  Maintain adequate fluid intake. *Adequate fluid intake will help to prevent bladder infection.*

  Adhere to bowel training program. *Bowel distention is the second most common cause of autonomic dysreflexia.*

Recover from episode of dysreflexia without residual effects as evidenced by:

Skin dry without red splotches above the level of the lesion

Dysreflexia

Absence of pallor below lesion
Remove stimuli for dysreflexia by the following:

Examine urinary drainage system for obstruction; eliminate obstruction or remove catheter.

Avoid performing Credé's maneuver.

Catheterize if on intermittent catheterization program.

Assess signs and symptoms of urinary tract infection (UTI).

Loosen tight clothing or restrictive appliances.

Apply topical anesthetic around anus and in rectum; check for and manually remove fecal impaction.

Inspect skin for evidence of pressure sore or rashes. *Sympathetic stimulation below T7 can stimulate an exaggerated, unopposed autonomic nervous system response. The response is exaggerated because the response cannot cross the injured area of the cord and is therefore unopposed by the parasympathetic nervous system.*

Blood pressure and pulse within normal limits for patient

Elevate head of the bed or place patient in sitting position. *Elevation of the head can create orthostatic hypotension and lower the blood pressure.*

Monitor the blood pressure and pulse every 5 minutes during acute episode.

Prepare to administer an antihypertensive agent if bowel and bladder interventions fail.

REFERENCES

Adsit PA, Bishop C: Autonomic dysreflexia—don't let it be a surprise, *Orthopaedic Nursing* 14(3):17-20, 1995.

Bernardez SJ and others: Primary care for the spinal cord injured patient, *Am Acad Phys Assist* 7(7):526-31, 1994.

Ceron GE, Rakowski-Reinhardt AC: Action stat! Autonomic dysreflexia, *Nursing 91* February: 33, 1991.

Dunn, KL: Autonomic dysreflexia: a nursing challenge in the care of the patient with a spinal cord injury, *J Cardiovasc Nurs* 5(4):57, 1991.

Finocchiaro DN, Herzfeld ST: Understanding autonomic dysreflexia, *Am J Nurs* 90(9):56, 1990.

Huston CJ, Boelman R: Emergency! Autonomic dysreflexia, *AJN* 95(6):55, 1995.

Trop CS, Bennett CJ: Autonomic dysreflexia and its urological implications: a review, *J Urol* 146:1461, 1991.

Trop CS, Bennett CJ: The evaluation of autonomic dysrflexia, *Semin Urol* 10(2):95, 1992.

Energy field disturbance

CLINICAL CONDITION/ MEDICAL DIAGNOSIS	RELATED FACTORS
Elderly male with congestive heart failure and recent hip replacement	Substitute caregiver from home health agency is unfamiliar with complexities of care; care recipient experiences difficulty in responding verbally to caregiver queries

Patient goals
Expected outcomes
>   Associated nursing/collaborative interventions *and scientific rationale*

Participate in daily care activities without placing undue burden on caretaker as evidenced by the following:

Follows caretaker's directions

>   Relate reason for substitution and provide information about when previous caretaker will resume care. *Meaning of the event is known only to individual undergoing experience.*

>   Sit with care recipient; use physical touch to reassure him of your concern and willingness to follow care plan. *Reviewing plan of care with recipient will help restore balance in energy field.*

>   Wait for some sign from individual that he is ready to begin daily routine. *It takes time for individual to separate from care expectations and to reconnect with new caregiver.*

Regain verbal ability to communicate fully as evidenced by the following:

Answers telephone and speaks with daughter who visits daily
Carries on conversation with neighbor who brings daily meal
Expresses appreciation to caregiver for attention to needs.

>   Attend to individual's verbal and nonverbal expressions of concerns, and know what is not said.

Presence, how the nurse is with the patient, is respecting the other's human dignity and freedom to choose in a situation.

Collaborate with individual in preparation of written report for next caregiver. *Mutuality in nurse-patient relationship helps to restore energy field. To keep energy field in balance, individual assists with construction of report of event.*

REFERENCES

Cowling WR III: Unitary knowing in nursing practice, *Nurs Sci Quart* 6(4):201-207, 1993.

Eisenhauer LA: A typology of nursing therapeutics, *Image J Nurs Schol* 26(4):261-264, 1994.

Gardner DL. Presence. In Bulechek GM, McCloskey JC (eds): *Nursing interventions: essential nursing treatments,* Philadelphia, 1992, WB Saunders.

Morse JM, Miles MW, Clark DA, Doberneck BM: "Sensing" patient needs: exploring concepts of nursing insight and receptivity used in nursing assessment, *Schol Inq Nurs Pract* 8(3):233-254, 1994.

Parse RR. Quality of life: sciencing and living the art of human becoming, *Nurs Sci Quart* 7(1):16-21, 1994.

Younger JB: The alienation of the sufferer, *Adv Nurs Sci* 17(4):53-72, 1995.

Energy field disturbance—cont'd

Environmental interpretation syndrome, impaired

CLINICAL CONDITION/ MEDICAL DIAGNOSIS	RELATED FACTORS
Eighty-year-old male has experienced increased confusion over the last year.	Ongoing incidents of disorientation and cognitive impairment
During a recent clinical evaluation of injury related to a fall, a diagnosis of multi-infarct dementia was established.	
Discharged to a foster home.	

Patient goals
Expected outcomes
  Associated nursing/collaborative interventions *and scientific rationale*

Participate in a structured environment as evidenced by the following:

Returns to room that he/she identifies as "home"

  Establish a consistent daily routine.

  Provide a constant caregiver(s). *Patients experience increased security when cared for by people they recognize.*

  Approach and communicate with the patient in a positive manner. *Verbal and nonverbal communication are important in establishing a relationship with a person who is cognitively impaired.*

  Collaborate with family to determine meaningful personal items.

  Incorporate personal items that the patient recognizes as his or her own into the patient's environment (i.e., photographs, furniture, special possessions). *Meaningful possessions provide a familiar context and sense of security to the environment.*

Environmental interpretation syndrome, impaired

211

Modify room environment to personal preference (i.e., bed placement, hygiene items, room lighting).

Avoid changes in room environment such as re-arrangement of furniture or other items, holiday decorations. *Frequent environmental change may produce conflicting cues.*

Staff members refer to and treat room as patient's home.

No attempts to leave foster home

Select room away from usual exit areas. *Cognitively impaired individuals are at risk to either wander or follow others out of the environment and become lost.*

Select room assignment in area of low environmental stimuli. *Disturbing visual images or loud noise can precipitate a catastrophic reaction.*

Plan activities according to patient's stimulus toleration level. *With increased stimulation there is increased risk for agitated behavior.*

Camouflage exits as appropriate so they appear as a portion of the environment (curtain, wall, bookshelf).

Redirect patient activities when he or she attempts to exit: diversional activities such as going for a walk, sorting magazines, folding towels or recycling may be appropriate.

Prepare a plan to use in event that patient elopes from the environment: Ensure that identification bracelet with current information is worn by the patient at all times; keep a recent full body photograph on file; identify community resources to assist with locating the patient; and develop a search process.

REFERENCES

Abraham IL and others: Multidisciplinary assessment of patients with Alzheimer's disease, *Nurs Clin North Am* 29(1):113-128, 1994.

Armstrong-Esther CA, Browne KD, McAfee JG: Elderly patients: still clean and sitting quietly, *J Adv Nurs* 19:264-271, 1994.

Barry PP: Medical evaluation of the demented patient, *Med Clin North Am* 78(4):779-784, 1994.

Beck CK, Shue VM: Interventions for treating disruptive behavior in demented elderly people, *Nurs Clin North Am* 29(1):143-155, 1994.

Bowie P, Mountain: Using direct observation to record the behavior of long-stay patients with dementia, *Internat Geriat Psychiatry* 8:857-864, 1993.

Fisher JE, Fink CM, Loomis CC: Frequency and management difficulty of behavioral problems among dementia patients in long-term care facilities, *Clin Gerontologist* 13(1):3-12, 1993.

Goldsmith SM, Hoeffer B, Rader J: Problematic wandering behavior in the cognitively impaired elderly, *J Psychosoc Nurs* 33(2):6-12, 1995.

Hall GR: Caring for people with Alzheimer's disease using the conceptual model of progressively lowered stress threshold in the clinical setting, *Nurs Clin North Am* 29(1):129-141, 1994.

Loewenstein DA: Neuropsychological assessment in Alzheimer's disease, *Med Clin North Am* 78(4):789-793, 1994.

Nelson J: The influence of environmental factors in incidents of disruptive behavior, *J Gerontol Nurs* 21(5):19-24, 1995.

Rantz MJ, McShane RE: Nursing interventions for chronically confused nursing home residents, *Geriatric Nurs* 16(1):22-27, 1995.

Shedd PP, Kobokovich LJ, Slattery MJ: Confused patients in the acute care setting: Prevalence, interventions, and outcomes, *J Gerontol Nurs* 21(4):5-12, 1995.

Stolley JM and others: Managing the care of patients with irreversible dementia during hospitalization for comorbidities, *Nurs Clin North Am* 28(4):767-782, 1993.

Family processes, altered: alcoholism

CLINICAL CONDITION/ MEDICAL DIAGNOSIS	RELATED FACTORS
Wife of a public figure admitted to acute hospital with alcoholic liver disease	Resistance to treatment; strained relationships between wife and nondrinking husband and between husband and children age 10 and 12.

Patient goals
Expected outcomes
> Associated nursing/collaborative interventions *and scientific rationale*

Family will create conditions that enable drinking family member to enter substance abuse treatment program as evidenced by the following:

Recognizes and acknowledges that family problem is alcoholism

Makes decision to enter alcohol abuse treatment program

Locates and accesses needed child care services

> Challenge family to use the acute illness as impetus to deal with the real problem.

> Explore willingness to recognize and acknowledge the problem as alcoholism. *Since alcoholism is a stigma, family may masquerade situation as another health problem.*

> Confront patient and family when denial is evident. *A sustained state of alcoholic denial prevents the voluntary seeking of treatment.*

> Provide information about medical and social resources. *Knowing that a solution to a problem exists makes it easier to acknowledge.*

> Alert family to the possibility of emergence of alcohol-related interpersonal problems during the transition to recovery. *Transition to recovery is a long process and a series of related difficulties may require identification and problem-solving.*

> Discuss importance of accessing reliable child care services to facilitate continuing in treatment

Family processes, altered: alcoholism

program. *Lack of child care facilities is one of main reasons for not entering or staying in treatment.*

Family will acquire insight into the association among family functioning, role demands, role expectations, and alcoholism as evidenced by the following:

Participates in long-term family counseling
Reports improved family relationships

Assist family to identify specific areas of needed emotional and social support.

Encourage expression of feelings about specific areas of need.

Refer to family therapist and/or recovered alcoholism counselor with experience in dealing with alcoholic families. *An experienced family therapist or counselor will be alert to emergence of alcohol-related difficulties and will assist with problematization and interventions.*

Help family to focus on improving problem-solving skills using nonthreatening example, such as planning a family vacation.

REFERENCES

Allan CA: Acknowledging alcohol problems: the use of a visual analogue scale to measure denial, *Nerv Ment* 179:620-625, 1991.

Hall JM: How lesbians recognize and respond to alcohol problems: a theoretical model of problematization, *Adv Nurs Sci* 16(3):46-63, 1994.

Hughes TL: Research on alcohol and drug use among women: a review and update. In McElmurry BJ, Parker RS (eds): *Annual review of women's health*, New York, 1993, National League for Nursing.

Johnson SK et al: Perceived changes in adult family members roles and responsibilities during critical illness, *Image J Nurs Schol* 27(3):238-243, 1995.

Lindeman M, Hawks JH, Bartek JK: The alcoholic family: a nursing diagnosis validation study, *Nurs Diagn* 5(2):65-73, 1994.

Rosenfield SN, Stevenson JS: Perception of daily stress and oral coping behaviors in normal, overweight and recovering alcoholic women, *Res Nurs Health* 11:166-174, 1988.

Sullivan EJ, Handley SM: Alcohol and drug abuse, *Annu Rev Nurs Res* 11:166-174, 1993.

Watson WL: Family therapy. In Bulechek GM, McCloskey JC: *Nursing interventions: essential nursing treatments*, ed 2, Philadelphia, 1992, WB Saunders.

Whall AL, Loveland-Cheery CJ: Family unit-focused research: 1984-1991, *Annu Rev Nurs Res* 11:227-247, 1993.

Wing DM: Transcending alcoholic denial. *Image: Nurs Scholar* 27(2):121-126, 1995.

Family processes, altered: alcoholism—cont'd

Family processes, altered

CLINICAL CONDITION/ MEDICAL DIAGNOSIS	RELATED FACTORS
Somatization	Role disruption
	Hispanic social support system disrupted

Patient goals
Expected outcomes
   Associated nursing/collaborative interventions *and scientific rationale*

Family will achieve stabilized functioning as evidenced by:

Views problem as having meaning for members of the family unit

   Help family refine (reframe) situation in terms that have increased options and possibilities for change. The family member having the health problem is not labeled as "bad" or "of the devil"; others are not perceived as denying, blaming, being hostile, overprotective, not help-ful, or "making matters worse." *Redefinition assists in reexamining the situation as a response to multiple stressors (e.g., new culture, loss of extended family, job instability, inadequate housing).*

   Assist family to clarify its own resources, especially strengths. *Accurate information on conditions in environment helps prevent negative perceptions of situation that impedes adaptation. Valuing own coping strategies assist group in dealing with issues facing them.*

   Identify possible/potential issues (e.g., male domi-nance versus more equality, individual needs versus family needs, risk for depression).

Demonstrate problem-solving skills from the identifi-cation of problem to the evaluation of the action taken and effective responsiveness to members

   Support efforts of family to clarify the who, what, when, and how of the stress, and to identify

Family processes, altered

their responses as a family unit. *Consensus of problems and actions to be taken can result in creative, helpful solutions to health problems.*

Assist family in problem solving by providing information, raising questions, assisting to summarize progress, helping to reallocate important functions of family during crisis period.

Support family leader to resume his or her role by giving prompts, clarifying tasks and offering suggestions.

Model and validate ways to express emotions in a supportive, nonthreatening, less-critical manner.

Family will use knowledge about somatization and its own internal resources to promote wellness of its members as evidenced by:

Attempts to understand how physical symptoms represent ways to express distress (i.e., anger, grief, loss, family conflict, worry)

Assist members to express feelings or emotional distress directly.

Support family involvement in treatment process.

Refer to self-help groups that address women's issues, culture-specific issues, and/or group problem-solving processes.

Focus on helping members understand ways to decrease anxiety.

Teach stress management skills or refer to stress management group.

Demonstrate ways for family members to express appropriate concern and support for each other.

Identify situations, public attitudes, nonverbal messages which increase stress for family members.

REFERENCES

DeSiante LM: The Mexican-American migrant farm worker family: mental health issues, *Nurs Clin North Am* 29(1):65-72, 1994.

Doornbos MM: The strength of families coping with serious mental illness, *Arch Psychiatr Nurs* 10(4):214-220, 1996.

Escobar JI: Transcultural aspects of dissociation and somatization disorders, *Psychiatr Clin North Am* 18(3):555-569, 1995.

Family processes, altered—cont'd

Guarnaccia PJ, Good BJ, Kleinman A: Epidemiologic studies of Puerto Rican mental health. In Mezzick JE, Jorge MR, Salloum IM, eds: *Psychiatric epidemiology: assessment concepts and methods,* Baltimore, 1994, John Hopkins University.

Kaplan HI, Sadock BJ, Grebb JA: *Synopsis of psychiatry: behavioral science, clinical psychiatry,* ed 7, Baltimore, 1994, Williams & Wilkins.

Roberts SJ: Somatization in primary care: The common presentation of psychosocial problems through physical complaints, *Nurse Pract* 19(5):50-56, 1994.

Rogler LH, Cortes DE, Malgady RS: The mental health idioms of distress. Anger and perceptions of injustice among New York Puerto Ricans, Hispanic Research Center, Fordham University, Bronx, NY, *J Nerv Ment Dis* 182(6):327-330, 1994.

Rose LE: Families of psychiatric patients: a critical review and future research directions, *Arch Psychiatr Nurs* 10(2):67-76, 1996.

Solomon P, Draine J: Adaptive coping among family member of persons with serious mental illness, *Psychiatr Serv* 46(11):1156-1160, 1995.

Fatigue

CLINICAL CONDITION/ MEDICAL DIAGNOSIS	RELATED FACTORS
Business executive with lung cancer	Role demands; increased metabolic demands

Patient goals
Expected outcomes
 Associated nursing/collaborative interventions *and scientific rationale*

Establish a pattern of rest/activity that enables fulfillment of role demands as evidenced by the following:

Negotiates realistic goal expectations

Help patient to identify excessive demands of various role obligations.

Instruct patient to maintain a fatigue diary for a 1-week period.

Exercises 3 times a week within own tolerance
Engages in preferred leisure 2 to 3 times a week
Verbalizes decreased sense of fatigue

Monitor level of fatigue using Rhoden Fatigue Scale and Fatigue Severity Scale. *Analysis of the relationship between activities and levels of fatigue will help define areas in which to reduce role demands and energy losses.*

Formulate with patient options for decreasing work demands (e.g., reduction in work hours, delegation of selected tasks).

Help patient to plan a daily schedule that includes pacing leisure activities, rest, and exercise.

Verbalizes feeling well-rested on arising

Monitor sleep pattern.

Teach patient to eliminate/reduce physical activities 1 hour before bedtime. *A function of sleep is to restore both mental and physical energy.*

Improve nutritional status as evidenced by the following:

Stabilizes body weight
Consumes well-balanced diet based on individual needs

Teach use of food diary to monitor eating habits.

Review food diary/food preferences with patient.

Help patient to identify foods high in protein and complex carbohydrates.

Provide information on use of high-calorie food supplements.

Teach patient/significant other short-cuts to meal planning/preparation. *Role demands and coping with the effects of illness increase energy demand and requirement for nutrients.*

Restore mental energy as evidenced by the following:

Uses a relaxation technique at least once a day
Verbalizes an increased sense of control

Teach and monitor relaxation techniques agreeable to patient (e.g., progressive music relaxation, creative imagery, and music).

Negotiate use of meditation or prayer. *Stress depletes energy, which contributes to fatigue. Relaxation techniques can be effective in stress management.*

REFERENCES

Blesch KS and others: Correlates of fatigue in people with breast or lung cancer, *Oncol Nurs Forum* 18(1):81-87, 1991.

Fryback PB: Health for people with a terminal diagnosis, *Nurs Sci Q* 6(3):147-159, 1993.

Grandjean E: Fatigue: its physiological and psychological significance, *Ergonomics* 11(5):427, 1988.

Hegyvary ST: Patient care outcomes related to management of symptoms, *Annu Rev Nurs Res* 11:145-168, 1993.

Lee KA: Fatigue: A prevalent symptom in need of nursing management strategies. In Larson P, ed: *Symptom management proceedings,* San Francisco, 1992, University of California School of Nursing.

Potempa KM: Chronic fatigue, *Annu Rev Nurs Res* 11:57-76, 1993.

Sheppard KC: The relationships among nursing diagnoses in discharge planning for patients with lung cancer. *Nurs Diag* 4(4):148-155, 1993.

Sheppard KC: The relationships among nursing diagnoses and community agencies and services required for lung cancer patients at discharge. In Carroll-Johnson RM, Paquette M, eds: *Classification of nursing diagnoses: proceedings of the tenth conference,* Philadelphia, 1994, JB Lippincott.

Fear

CLINICAL CONDITION/ MEDICAL DIAGNOSIS	RELATED FACTORS
Bowel cancer	Impending surgery with possible pain, loss of control, and disfigurement

Patient goals
Expected outcomes
  Associated nursing/collaborative interventions *and scientific rationale*

Identify specific aspects of impending surgery that are sources of fear as evidenced by the following:

Verbalizes specific fears relating to surgery, such as possible pain, realistic perception of danger, own coping ability, and need for assistance

  Using techniques of therapeutic communication, encourage patient to verbalize feelings such as those related to potential personal perception of danger, perception of own coping skills or limitations, and need for assistance from nursing staff. *Specificity in identifying the causes of fear facilitates specificity in intervention strategies. Verbalizing feelings can lessen the intensity and duration of fear.*

Acquire knowledge/skills for dealing with specific fears as evidenced by the following:

Verbalizes perceptions that are consistent with reality

  Provide information to reduce distorted perceptions. Encourage specifics rather than generalizations. *A realistic appraisal promotes effective problem solving to decrease danger.*

Verbalizes and displays comfort with unit environment, procedure, and staff

  Initiate teaching about surgery, including colostomy. For unfamiliar environment, orient patient to unit and staff.

Demonstrates effective coughing, deep breathing, and leg exercises

  Teach rationale and procedure for turning, coughing,

Fear

221

deep breathing, and leg exercises; allow time for practice and return demonstration.

Explains events expected to occur before and after surgery

Teach specifics for type of surgery, as appropriate for patient.

Verbalizes realistic expectations for postoperative period

Teach what to expect after surgery, especially sensations that will be experienced (e.g., recovery room, wound dressings, pain, colostomy, irrigation). *Knowledge of what to expect, particularly on a sensory level, decreases fear of the unknown.*

Identify and teach specifics of the surgical experience that the patient would like to know.

Teach about postoperative analgesia, and encourage patient to request analgesic when needed *to cope with fear of pain.*

Teach ways of enhancing control (e.g., include patient in planning care; share test results as appropriate) *to deal with fear of loss of control.*

Consider visit by someone who has successfully experienced and is well adjusted to the surgery (e.g., colostomy) *to deal with fear of disfigurement. Fear decreases when one identifies with someone who has successfully dealt with a similar fearful situation.*

Engage in adaptive coping as evidenced by the following:

Verbalizes increased psychological comfort and coping skills

Use available support system to increase comfort and relaxation.

Include family and significant others in teaching *so that they are supportive and knowledgeable, rather than fearful.*

Encourage comforting measures (e.g., music, religious objects, own pajamas, pillow). *Familiar sources of comfort can alleviate the distress that accompanies fear.*

Arrange a visit with clergy, if desired by patient.

Verbalizes positive attitude toward outcome of surgery and adjustment to disfigurement

Adopt a positive attitude that patient can cope and have a positive surgical experience.

Experiences a restful sleep

Facilitate a good night's sleep preoperatively.

Experience reduced fear as evidenced by the following:

Has normal pulse and respiration rates

Has normal blood pressure

Verbalizes decreased fear

Continually monitor level of fear (many surgeons will cancel surgery if patient is especially fearful). *The neuroendocrine physiologic response to fear may precipitate life-threatening arrhythmias during stressful situations.*

REFERENCES

Caldwell LM: The influence of preference for information on preoperative stress and coping in surgical outpatients, *Appl Nurs Res* 4(4):177, 1991.

Grainger RD: Conquering fears and phobias, *Am J Nurs* 91(5):15, 1991.

Marks M, De Silva P: The "Match/Mismatch" model of fear: empirical status and clinical implications, *Behav Res Ther* 32(7):759, 1994.

McFarland GK, Thomas MD: *Psychiatric mental health nursing: application of the nursing process,* Philadelphia, 1991, JB Lippincott.

Mock VL: Fear. In McFarland GK and McFarlane EA: *Nursing diagnosis and intervention: planning for patient care,* ed 3, St Louis, 1997, Mosby.

Salmon P: Psychological factors in surgical stress; implications for management, *Clin Psych Rev* 12:681, 1992.

Tarsitano BP: Structured preoperative teaching. In Bulecheck GM, McCloskey JC: *Nursing interventions: essential nursing treatments,* ed 2, pp 168-178, Philadelphia, 1992, WB Saunders.

Taylor-Loughran AE and others: Defining characteristics of the nursing diagnosis fear and anxiety: a validation study, *Appl Nurs Res* 2(4):178, 1989.

Teasdale K: Information and anxiety: critical reappraisal, *J Adv Nurs* 18:1125, 1993.

Whitley GG: Expert validation and differentiation of the nursing diagnoses, anxiety and fear, *Nurs Diagn* 5(4):143, 1994.

Whitney GG: Concept analysis of fear, *Nurs Diagn* 3(4):155, 1992.

Fear—cont'd

Fluid volume deficit (1)

CLINICAL CONDITION/ MEDICAL DIAGNOSIS	RELATED FACTORS
Hyperglycemic hyperosmotic nonketotic coma	Failure of regulatory mechanism

Patient goals
Expected outcomes
  Associated nursing/collaborative interventions *and
  scientific rationale*

Achieve fluid volume and electrolyte balance as evidenced by the following:

Has vital signs and lab values within normal limits

Monitor vital signs every 15 minutes until stable;
  monitor level of consciousness.

Administer insulin per order according to blood
  glucose levels; *insulin is required to reverse hyperglycemia.*

Has balanced intake and output, stable weight

Monitor intake and output every hour and weigh
  patient daily; *these provide a good measure of body
  fluid balance.*

Maintain intravenous therapy for replacement of
  fluid per order.

Monitor for circulatory overload during fluid replacement (e.g., neck vein distention, rales,
  dyspnea, S_3, increase in CVP or PAP, and tachycardia).

Administer electrolyte replacement therapy (particularly potassium, chloride, magnesium, and
  phosphorus) as appropriate; *osmotic diuresis
  causes electrolyte depletion and insulin administration causes electrolytes to shift intracellularly.*

Continue to monitor and report to physician worsening fluid volume deficit/electrolyte imbalance
  signs and symptoms (e.g., dilute urine, increased
  urine output, hypotension, increased pulse rate,
  decreased skin turgor, increased body temperature, weakness).

Fluid volume deficit (1)

REFERENCES

Cullen L: Interventions related to fluid and electrolyte balance, *Nurs Clin North Am* 27(2):569, 1992.

Graves L: Diabetic ketoacidosis and hyperosmolar hyperglycemic nonketotic coma, *Crit Care Nurse* 13(3):50, 1990.

Jones, T: From diabetic ketoacidosis to hyperglycemic hyperosmolar nonketotic syndrome, *Crit Care Nurs Clin North Am* 6(4):703, 1994.

Leske JS: Hyperglycemic hyperosmolar nonketotic coma: a nursing-care plan, *Crit Care Nurse* 5(5):49, 1985.

Pflaum S: Investigation of intake-output as a means of assessing body fluid balance, *Heart Lung* 8(3):495, 1979.

Fluid volume deficit (1)—cont'd

Fluid volume deficit (2)

CLINICAL CONDITION/ MEDICAL DIAGNOSIS	RELATED FACTORS
Hypovolemic shock	Active loss of body fluid

Patient goals
Expected outcomes
> Associated nursing/collaborative interventions *and scientific rationale*

Maintain fluid volume and electrolyte balance as evidenced by:

Has blood pressure and pulse within his/her normal limits

> Monitor vital signs every hour; monitor level of consciousness; monitor hemodynamic status, including CVP, MAP, PAP, and PCWP if available.*
>
> Determine cause of active loss and use nursing actions to prevent further loss.

Has balanced intake and output, stable weight

> Monitor intake and output every hour and report urine output of less than 30 to 60 ml/hr. *Urine volume decreases in hypovolemia because decreased plasma volume results in decreased renal blood flow.*
>
> Weigh patient at the same time daily. *Weights with intake and output provide a good measure of body fluid balance.*
>
> Maintain intravenous therapy for replacement of fluid using colloids, crystalloids, or blood products per order. *Colloids hydrate the intravascular space and pull fluids from the interstitium into the blood stream; crystalloids replace intracellular fluid and are distributed to the interstitium and intravascular space, and blood replacement must be given to*

*CVP: Central Venous pressure
MAP: Mean arterial pressure
PAP: Pulmonary arterial pressure
PCWP: Pulmonary capillary wedge pressure

Fluid volume deficit (2)

provide oxygen-carrying capacity if hemoglobin is significantly decreased.

Push oral fluids to 2600 ml/day if appropriate.

Monitor skin condition: color, moisture, turgor.

Monitor for possible circulatory overload during fluid replacement (e.g., neck vein distention, rales, dyspnea, S_3 increase in CVP or PAP, and tachycardia).

Has urine specific gravity and lab results within normal limits.

Monitor urine specific gravity every 2 hours; *concentrated urine (specific gravity >1.030) is response to water deficit as ADH is released in response to increased osmolarity of body fluids).*

Monitor lab results relevant to fluid balance (Hct, blood urea nitrogen (BUN), albumin, total protein, serum osmolarity).

Monitor and report worsening fluid volume deficit and/or electrolyte imbalance including signs and symptoms of decreased urine output, concentrated urine, output greater than intake, hypotension, increased pulse rate, increased body temperature, weakness, and change in mental status.

REFERENCES

Cullen L: Interventions related to fluid and electrolyte balance, *Nurs Clin North Am* 27(2):569, 1992.

Meyers K, Hickey MK: Nursing management of hypovolemic shock, *Crit Care Nurse* 11(1):57, 1988.

Pflaum S: Investigation of intake-output as a means of assessing body fluid balance, *Heart Lung* 8(3):495, 1979.

Fluid volume deficit (2)—cont'd

Fluid volume deficit, risk for

CLINICAL CONDITION/ MEDICAL DIAGNOSIS	RELATED FACTORS
Congestive heart failure and hypertension	Daily use of diuretics

Patient goals
Expected outcomes
    Associated nursing/collaborative interventions *and scientific rationale*

Maintain adequate fluid volume and electrolyte balance as evidenced by:

Patient/family verbalizes knowledge of monitoring fluid status

Teach patient/significant other the following:

Monitor weights and intake and output; *these provide a good measure of body fluid balance.*

Record blood pressure.

Monitor congestive heart failure weekly by assessing exercise tolerance, symptom relief and quality of life.

Teach maintaining of regular schedule for taking diuretics, K^+ supplements, and eating K^+ rich foods, such as bananas, oranges, and raisins; *thiazide diuretics may result in potassium depletion.*

Teach about importance of good nutrition and fluid intake; *adequate fluid intake is important to prevent dehydration, in elderly patients thirst is decreased and drinking is less.*

Change positions slowly *to minimize orthostatic hypotension.*

Monitor skin turgor and avoid excessive dryness; *poor skin turgor and dryness may indicate dehydration.*

Avoid very hot environments; *heat may cause excessive water loss.*

Teach importance of calling physician with weight loss accompanied by headache, lightheadedness, fatigue, low urinary output, irritability and rapid pulse; weight gain of 2 lbs. or more in one day; signs and symptoms of electrolyte imbalance (i.e., unusual fatigue, abdominal distention, anorexia, vomiting, constipation, muscle cramps, paresthesia or confusion).

REFERENCES

Cullen L: Interventions related to fluid and electrolyte balance, *Nurs Clin North Am* 27(2):569, 1992.

Cuny J, Enger E: Medical management of chronic heart failure: direct-acting vasodilators and diuretic agents, *Crit Care Nurs Clin North Am* 5(4):575, 1993.

Lapinski ML: Cardiovascular drugs and the elderly population, *Heart Lung* 11(5):430, 1982.

Mendyka B: Fluid and electrolyte disorders caused by diuretic therapy *AACN Clin Iss* 3(3):672, 1992.

Pflaum S: Investigation of intake-output as a means of assessing body fluid balance, *Heart Lung* 8(3):495, 1979.

Porth C, Erickson M: Physiology of thirst and drinking: implication for nursing practice, *Heart Lung* 21(3):273, 1992.

Fluid volume excess

CLINICAL CONDITION/ MEDICAL DIAGNOSIS	RELATED FACTORS
Heart failure	Impaired myocardial contractility, decreased cardiac output

Patient goals
Expected outcomes
> Associated nursing/collaborative interventions *and scientific rationale*

Achieve normal level of fluid volume as evidenced by the following:

Has body weight within his/her normal range

Weigh patient daily and consult physician to adjust diuretic dosage as necessary.

Monitor intake and output.

Restrict fluid intake in presence of dilutional hyponatremia with serum Na^+ level below 130 mEq/L and monitor intake and output daily; *excessive water intake will cause further dilution of Na^+ in the blood.*

Signs of fluid volume excess are eliminated; the risks of further complications (e.g., pulmonary edema/ shock) are reduced

Assess neck veins for jugular venous distention (JVD); auscultate lungs for presence of crackles; assess liver for increased size and hepatojugular reflux (HJR); assess legs and dependent areas for symmetrical bilateral swelling; laterally displaced apical impulse. *Patients with heart failure may have an increase in intravascular and extravascular fluid volume.*

Auscultate heart for presence of S_3 and S_4 sounds. *An S_3 may indicate decreased compliance or increased ventricular diastolic volume; an S_4 may indicate decreased compliance or increased volume of filling.*

Hemodynamic status is restored to normal/ acceptable range for this patient

Monitor mean arterial pressure (MAP) and pulse

Fluid volume excess

pressure (through arterial line if available) to determine hemodynamic status. *MAP indicates overall perfusion of tissues/organs. Pulse pressure provides an estimate of the heart's stroke volume or pumping ability and is an index of the resistance to left ventricular emptying (afterload).*

Monitor pulmonary artery (PA) pressures (through PA catheter if available). *Central venous pressure (CVP) detects hemodynamic changes in the right side of the heart; pulmonary artery diastolic pressure (PAD) and pulmonary capillary wedge pressure (PCWP) secure an accurate evaluation of the volume of blood in the left ventricle before contraction (preload); cardiac output (CO) (indirect determination via the PA catheter) serves as a means to evaluate therapy; systemic vascular resistance (SVR) is an index of afterload or the pressure of blood in the arterial circulation against which blood in the heart must be ejected.* Consult physician if values exceed acceptable ranges and discuss therapeutic options.

Administer diuretics (e.g., furosemide, bumetanide, metolazone as ordered. *Diuretics increase the effective circulating blood volume to normal/ acceptable range, thus decreasing preload.*

Administer angiotensin converting enzyme (ACE) inhibitors (captopril, enalapril, lisinopril) as ordered. *ACE inhibitors effectively block angiotensin II production which reduces Na^+ and water retention by the kidneys, therefore reducing preload.*

Administer inotropic agents (e.g., digoxin, dobutamine, amrinone, milrinone) as ordered. *Inotropic agents increase myocardial contractility, decrease preload, and therefore increase cardiac output.*

Administer vasopressor agents (e.g., dopamine) as ordered. *Dopamine at low dosages (1 to 2 mcg/kg/min) increases renal blood flow, promoting diuresis.*

Administer vasodilator agents (e.g., sodium nitroprusside, hydralazine, nitrates) as alternatives to ACE inhibitors if ordered. *Sodium nitroprusside has a dual action, dilating both arterioles and veins, with a dramatic decrease in preload and afterload. Vasodilators, in general, reduce peripheral resistance (afterload) and secondarily augment cardiac output and renal blood flow.*

Monitor response to drug therapy, report untoward reactions, and discuss with the physician alternative therapies.

Electrolyte levels are within normal range for this patient

Monitor serum level of electrolytes, particularly K^+ and Mg^{++}. *Hypokalemia and hypomagnesemia predispose the patient to the development of arrhythmias. If patient's heart rate and rhythm are being monitored, observe for PVCs, flat or inverted T wave, or a prominent U wave. These ECG changes are warning signs of hypokalemia.* The nurse may need to provide a K^+ rich diet as appropriate; consult physician for K^+ or Mg^{++} supplement as necessary.

Monitor laboratory results (e.g., increased specific gravity; increased urine osmolality; presence of protein, urea, and granular casts in urine; increased blood urea nitrogen (BUN) and creatinine; increased mean corpuscle volume (MCV); and decreased hematocrit) *relevant to fluid retention.*

Provide reduced Na^+ diet (2 gm or less, if indicated).

Experience less discomfort due to excessive fluid volume as evidenced by the following:

Verbalizes less dyspnea on exertion, orthopnea, and paroxysmal nocturnal dyspnea and experiences more comfort

Provide position that will promote venous return and allow fluid shift (e.g., semi-Fowler's position).

Provide support to edematous areas (e.g., pillow under arms and scrotal support).

Teach passive and active range-of-motion exercises as appropriate. Advance activity to patient's individual tolerance level.

Assist with activities of daily living, as indicated, and have patient's personal items within easy reach *to preserve energy level.*

Provide high-protein and high-calorie diet *to improve nutritional status and enhance the healing of waterlogged body tissue, if present.*

Monitor serum albumin level. *Patients with heart failure may have low albumin levels secondary to a malnourished and/or dilutional state. Adequate serum albumin levels are necessary to maintain plasma oncotic pressure and maintain fluid in the intravascular spaces.*

Counsel patient if concerns are expressed about body image and self-esteem as a result of excessive fluid retention.

Provide appropriate skin care if edematous and monitor potential for infection.

Maintain an acceptable level of fluid volume as evidenced by the following:

Sets realistic goals for maintaining optimal fluid level

Collaborate with patient/significant other to determine mutually agreeable goals of therapy if feasible.

Complies with treatment plan, appropriate referrals for therapy related to personal fears/concerns as indicated, scheduled clinic appointments

Provide information about the nature of heart failure and prescribed therapy.

Clarify patient responsibilities including self-monitoring and what to do if symptoms worsen. *Noncompliance is a major cause of worsening symptoms, readmission, and reduced life expectancy.*

Initiate psychological, dietary, and spiritual counseling as indicated.

Reinforce importance of regular follow-up care.

Provide individualized patient teaching appropriate to age, reading level, and cultural background.

Teach patient the purpose of prescribed medications, medication schedule, and common side effects.

Keeps written record of fluctuations of weight and reports abnormal excess

Teach patient the importance of continuing daily weight measurement after discharge.

Encourage patient to report a weight gain in excess of 4 lbs. to physician or nurse.

Describes dietary/fluid restrictions

Teach patient that high Na^+ level induces fluid retention.

Teach patient the importance of eliminating table salt and offer alternatives to salt (e.g., herbs/spices).

Teach patient the importance of timing fluid intake and avoidance of alcohol.

Sleeps 6 hours or more a night

Discuss measures to promote uninterrupted sleep (e.g., use of additional pillows, recliner chair, taking of diuretics more than 6 hours before bedtime).

Discuss alternative patterns of sleep times.

Exercises regularly as tolerated

Encourage regular exercise such as walking or cycling: *Regular exercise may improve functional status and symptoms.*

REFERENCES

Dracup K and others: Management of heart failure, II Counseling, education, and lifestyle modifications, *JAMA* 272(18):1442.

English MA, Mastrean MB: Congestive heart failure: public and private burden, *Crit Care Nurs Q* 18(1):1, 1995.

Konstam M, Dracup K, Baku D and others: *Heart failure: evaluation and care of patients with left-ventricular systolic dysfunction.* Clinical practice guideline No. II. AHCPR Publication No. 94-0612, Rockville, Md, 1994, Agency for Health Care Policy and Research, Public Health Service, U.S. Department of Health and Human Services.

Navas JP, Marinez-Maldonado M: Pathophysiology of edema in congestive heart failure, *Heart Dis Stroke* 2(4):325, 1993.

Poyss AS: Fluid therapy. In Bulechek GM, McCloskey JC, eds: *Nursing interventions: essential nursing treatments,* ed 2, Philadelphia, 1992, WB Saunders.

Prizant-Weston M, Castiglia K: Hemodynamic regulation in nursing interventions. In Bulechek GM, McCloskey JC, eds: *Nursing interventions: essential nursing treatments,* ed 2, Philadelphia, 1992, WB Saunders.

Sherman A: Critical care management of the heart failure patient in the home, *Crit Care Nurs Q* 18(1):77, 1995.

Wright JM: Pharmacologic management of congestive heart failure, *Crit Care Nurs Q* 18(1):32, 1995.

Wright SM: Pathophysiology of congestive heart failure, *J Cardiovasc Nurs* 4(3):1, 1990.

Yusef S: Clinical experience in protecting the failing heart, *Clin Cardiol* 6:(Suppl. II):25, 1993.

Fluid volume excess—cont'd

Gas exchange, impaired

CLINICAL CONDITION/ MEDICAL DIAGNOSIS	RELATED FACTORS
Acute respiratory failure, after anesthesia	Altered oxygen supply, alveolar hypoventilation

Patient goals
Expected outcomes
    Associated nursing/collaborative interventions *and scientific rationale*

Maintain adequate oxygen supply and alveolar ventilation as evidenced by the following:

Hypoxemia is resolved or improved with or without oxygen supplement or mechanical ventilation
Eucapnia or usual compensated $PaCO_2$ and pH levels
Impairment of mental status and restlessness are absent or reduced

Maintain patent airway while patient is both awake and asleep.

Encourage patient to take deep breaths (see Airway Clearance, Ineffective).

Position patient to facilitate ventilation/perfusion matching ("good side down"). *Positioning affects distribution of pulmonary circulation and ventilation. Position patient so that most normal area of lung is dependent.*

Remove secretions by coughing or suctioning (see Airway Clearance, Ineffective).

Consult physician regarding supplementary oxygen during rest, activity and/or sleep. If ordered, select devices that enable the patient to perform activities of daily living.

If hypoxemia persists, consult physician for possible mechanical assistance or ventilation.

If mechanical ventilation is prescribed, monitor ventilator settings, endotracheal and tracheal tube function, and function of ventilator and breathing circuits. Assess patient's ability to wean daily.

Gas exchange, impaired

Initiate weaning and support oxygenation requirements as described above. *Weaning is the titration of the intervention of mechanical ventilation. A patient's ability to wean depends on a number of physiological and psychological variables such as control of breathing, respiratory muscle strength and endurance, lung mechanics, gas exchange, as well as the patient's psychological readiness to be separated from the ventilator.*

If mechanical ventilation becomes long-term, assess for home management by self or significant other. (see Ventilation, inability to sustain spontaneous).

Performs techniques that maximize ventilation and perfusion matching

Teach patient and significant other about treatments, medications, oxygen therapy, and equipment.

Counsel patient who has chronic hypoxemia to obtain supplementary oxygen prescription from physician before air travel or trips to high altitude.

REFERENCES

Brook-Brunn JA: Postoperative atelectasis and pneumonia: risk factors, *Am J Crit Care* 4(5):340-349, 1995.

Chailleux E and others: Predictors of survival in patients receiving domiciliary oxygen therapy or mechanical ventilation, *Chest* 109(3):741-749, 1996.

Chochesy JM, Daly BJ, Montenegro HD: Weaning chronically critically ill adults from mechanical ventilatory support: A descriptive study, *Am J Crit Care* 4(2):93-99, 1995.

Evans A, Winslow E: Oxygen saturation and hemodynamic response in critically ill, mechanically ventilated adults during intrahospital transport, *Am J Crit Care* 4(2):106-111, 1995.

Glass C and others: Nurses' ability to achieve hyperinflation and hyperoxygenation with a manual resuscitation bag during endotracheal suctioning, *Heart Lung* 22(2):158-165, 1993.

Hoffman LA and others: Nasal cannula and transtracheal oxygen delivery. A comparison after 6 months of each technique, *Am Rev Respir Dis* 145(4 Pt 1):827-831, 1992.

Melendez JA and others: Post thoracotomy respiratory muscle mechanics during incentive spirometry using respiratory inductance plethysmography, *Chest* 101(2):432-436, 1992.

Nocturnal oxygen therapy trial group: Continuous or nocturnal oxygen therapy in hypoxemic chronic obstructive lung disease: a clinical trial, *Ann Intern Med* 93:391-398, 1980.

Slutsky AS and others: American College of Chest Physicians' Consensus Conference—Mechanical ventilation, *Chest* 104:1833-1859, 1993.

Traver GA and others: Continuous oscillation: outcome in critically ill patients, *J Crit Care* 10(3):97-103, 1995.

Grieving, anticipatory

CLINICAL CONDITION/ MEDICAL DIAGNOSIS	RELATED FACTORS
Wife of spouse with non-Hodgkin's lymphoma	Perceived potential loss of spouse

Patient goals
Expected outcomes
Associated nursing/collaborative interventions *and scientific rationale*

Wife participates in constructive anticipatory grief work as evidenced by the following:

Discusses thoughts and feelings related to potential loss of spouse

Encourage wife to describe perceptions of potential loss *to identify specific aspect of grieving process wife is experiencing.*

Encourage verbalization of fears, concerns, and other emotions; *recognize that the expression of intense emotions, such as anger, is common, and should not be taken as a personal attack; verbalization of thoughts and feelings facilitates the grieving process.*

Provide assurance that experiencing intense, chaotic feelings and reactions is normal *to minimize wife's concerns that she is experiencing abnormal reactions.*

Avoid judgmental and defensive responses to criticisms of health care providers. *It is important to keep in mind the difference between criticism generated as a result of displaced anger related to potential loss of spouse and valid criticism of providers.*

Provide wife with ongoing information of husband's diagnosis, prognosis, progress, and plan of care for husband's diagnosis of non-Hodgkin's lymphoma.

Meets ongoing self-care needs

Determine current sources of social support, such as family, friends, and church, and disruptions in current lifestyle related to potential loss of spouse, such as finances, living arrangements, and transportation. *Social support is an important resource to assist wife/patient/children during this health crisis, and it can influence the extent to which wife is able to meet self-care needs.*

Encourage wife to attend to her own self-care needs such as rest, sleep, nutrition, leisure activities, and time away from patient. *This will help her maintain her own health, have the ability to devote time to the children, if any, and continue to provide support to patient.*

Maintains constructive family functioning as a family unit

Help wife, spouse, and children to share mutual fears, concerns, plans, and hopes with each other.

Evaluate need for referral to resources, such as mental health professional for wife, husband, and/or children; referral to school counselor, Social Security representative, legal consultant, or grief support groups. *Parents' preoccupation with their own grief may affect their ability to recognize their children's distress: uncertainties about finances and legal worries can have an adverse effect on family closeness. Early intervention can reduce the likelihood of dysfunctional grieving.*

Enlist support from others such as family, friends, and clergy.

Encourage wife to describe desires and information needs in caring for patient.

Facilitate wife's assistance with patient's physical care; include children as appropriate.

Facilitate flexible visiting hours that include the children.

Discuss indicators of change in physical condition of patient with wife and children, *to minimize undue anxiety and to help prepare them for the loss of their loved one.*

Provide comforting measures for patient; encourage wife, children, additional significant others to assist if they wish.

Demonstrate competence by meeting patient's psychosocial and physical needs promptly and with empathy.

Encourage wife, children and additional significant others to maintain verbal communication and touch with their loved one during times when he may be unable to respond, *to maintain closeness for the patient and to decrease family's sense of helplessness.*

Provide as much privacy as possible for wife, children, and others to be alone with patient *for them to share freely.*

REFERENCES

Cowles KV, Rodgers BL: The concept of grief: a foundation for nursing research and practice, *Res Nurs Health* 14:119, 1991.

Curry LC, Stone JG: The grief process: a preparation for death, *Clin Nurse Special* 5(1):17, 1991.

Dobratz MC: Causal influences of psychological adaptation in dying, *West J Nurs Res* 15(6):708, 1993.

Glass BC: The role of the nurse in advanced practice in bereavement care, *Clin Nurse Special* 7(2):62, 1993.

Hampe SO: Needs of the grieving spouse in a hospital setting, *Nurs Res* 24:113, 1975.

Lohnes KL, Kalter N: Preventive intervention groups for parentally bereaved children, *Am J Orthopsychiatry* 64(4):594, 1994.

Rosenheim E, Reicher R: Children in anticipatory grief: the lonely predicament, *J Clin Child Psychol* 15(2):115, 1986.

Siegel K and others: Perceptions of parental competence while facing the death of a spouse, *Am J Orthopsychiatry* 60(4):567, 1990.

Grieving, dysfunctional

CLINICAL CONDITION/ MEDICAL DIAGNOSIS	RELATED FACTORS
Elderly widower whose wife recently died from cancer; exacerbation of chronic obstructive pulmonary disease (COPD)	Absence of anticipatory grieving, loss of health

Patient goals
Expected outcomes
  Associated nursing/collaborative interventions *and scientific rationale*

Experience resolution of dysfunctional grieving as evidenced by the following:

Acknowledges awareness of losses

Encourage verbalization of thoughts and feelings related to death of spouse and loss of health. *Aging survivors have an increased tendency to deny their own feelings as well as deny the death of a loved one.*

Monitor for suicidal ideation/intent. *Initial known risk factors include age, marital status, and health problems.*

Encourage description of current and anticipated problems related to loss of spouse and loss of health.

Evaluate need for referral to resources, such as brief psychotherapy, spiritual counseling.

Differentiate between helpful and maladaptive use of denial associated with wife's death as well as own health. *Initial denial protects from emotional pain; prolonged denial inhibits grief recovery.*

Gradually present patient with more facts *to facilitate awareness of losses and to lay groundwork for adaptive behaviors.*

Facilitate working through feelings by demonstrating tolerance for expression of negative feelings, supporting verbalizations of ambivalence, and helping patient to understand reasons for feelings. *Working through intense feelings facilitates resolution of grief and allows for engagement in problem solving.*

Point out universality of need for normal grieving.

Allow for death review to be repeated as often as necessary. *It is cleansing to repeat parts of the dying process and the death and may take many such death reviews to allow grieving persons to begin to move toward reorganization.*

Develops appropriate goals for COPD management

Monitor patient's current level and pattern of mood, energy, concentration, appetite, sleep. *Newly bereaved may experience a diminished immune response; there is a higher incidence of chronic disease among this population. It is important to differentiate from signs and symptoms of dysfunctional grieving and COPD exacerbation.*

Encourage description of current and anticipated problems related to loss of health.

Clarify and offer factual information about COPD exacerbation.

Offer realistic hope for positive coping in the present, as well as the future.

Facilitate patient's developing a daily schedule that addresses dietary management, exercise, sleep and rest periods, diversional and recreational activities. *Dysfunctional grieving may result in inadequate attention to health maintenance activities.*

Make referral to Behavioral Medicine Clinic Better Breathers Club.

Identifies alternate plans for meeting goals that were significant before loss of spouse

Assist patient to develop realistic goals and lifestyle changes.

Promote patient's recognition of past and present strengths that can be used for coping with current losses *to reinforce confidence in grief recovery.*

Monitor patient's perception of current adaptation to loss of spouse and loss of health, patient's perception of use of coping skills/problem solving abilities, and perception of available social support. *Perception of the existence of social support is a positive indicator for successful grief recovery.*

Encourage family and friends to offer support by visiting patient frequently on a regular basis. *Weekly visits by family have been found to be related to constructive grief resolution.*

Provide guidance about available community resources (e.g., senior citizens activity center, grief recovery groups). *Facilitating, encouraging, and teaching patient about use of resources will assist adjustment to changes resulting from current losses.*

REFERENCES

Bateman A and others: Dysfunctional grieving, *J Psychosoc Nurs* 30(12):5, 1992.

Curry LC, Stone JG: Moving on: recovering from the death of a spouse, *Clin Nurs Special* 6(4):180, 1992.

Gabriel RM, Kirschling JM: Assessing grief among the bereaved elderly: a review of existing measures, *Hosp J* 5(1):29, 1989.

Herth K: Relationship of hope, coping styles, concurrent losses, and setting to grief resolution in the elderly widow(er), *Res Nurs Health* 13(2):109, 1990.

Parry JK: Death review: an important component of grief resolution, *Soc Week Health Care* 20:97, 1994.

Steele L: Risk factor profile for bereaved spouses, *Death Stud* 16(5):387, 1992.

Steele LL: The death surround: factors influencing the grief experience of survivors, *Oncol Nurs Forum* 17(2):235, 1990.

Worden JW: *Grief counseling and grief therapy,* ed 2, New York, 1991, Springer.

Growth and development, altered

CLINICAL CONDITION/ MEDICAL DIAGNOSIS	RELATED FACTORS
Fetal alcohol syndrome (FAS)	Prenatal exposure to teratogens, inadequate caretaking, poor support system

---

Patient goals
Expected outcomes
  Associated nursing/collaborative interventions *and scientific rationale*

Reach maximum potential in mental and physical development as evidenced by the following:

Meets physical and emotional needs as a result of adequate maternal caretaking

At regular intervals, monitor child's cognitive, social and psychomotor development; monitor height and weight. *Diagnosis of FAS requires manifestations in three categories:*
  1. *Prenatal or postnatal growth retardation (below 10th percentile for gestational age)*
  2. *Central nervous system dysfunction (neurological impairment; cognitive or developmental delay)*
  3. *Presence of at least two characteristic dysmorphic facial features*

Assist mother in providing adequate care

Support mother with praise for each accomplishment. *Nurturing of mother increases self-esteem and promotes nurturing of infant.*

Involve significant others in the care of the infant. *Addictive mothers have limited coping skills and may need help to adequately care for their baby.*

Facilitate access to health care, monitor compliance. *Children with FAS may have recurrent otitis media, eye, and dental problems, as well as needs related to associated birth defects such as cleft palate, kidney and heart defects, and neural tube defects.*

Monitor the child's safety within the home environment; involve Child Protective Services as

Growth and development, altered

243

necessary. *Use of alcohol lowers inhibitions and impairs judgment. This results in compromised parenting abilities, which places the child at greater risk of physical and sexual abuse and neglect.*

Provide support and reinforce appropriate parenting activities; educate concerning physical and psychosocial needs of child with FAS; suggest ways to provide appropriate environment and stimulation based on infant's cues. *FAS infants are irritable, have abnormal sleep patterns, agitation, increased crying, and resistance to cuddling or holding. This behavior may frustrate mother, causing her to withdraw, or may result in failure to thrive or abuse.*

Monitor nutritional status: in collaboration with nutritionist, assess mother's feeding technique, provide guidance related to feeding problems, and assist/encourage mother to select foods that will provide calories and nutrition. *FAS infants have delays in the normal progression of oral feeding development. Many have a weak suck, poor muscle tone, and feed poorly. They may have difficulty coordinating sucking and swallowing with breathing, and show little interest in food.*

Achieve adequate support system as evidenced by the following:

Family obtains and uses appropriate supportive services

Refer mother to alcohol dependency treatment program for help with alcohol addiction and to FAS support group; refer to early intervention program/physical therapist to support motor and cognitive development, nutritionist to ensure adequate caloric intake, and agency providing day care or respite care for special-needs children.

Collaborate with involved professionals. *Care for child with FAS is similar to care for children with other chronic conditions requiring multidisciplinary approach: needs are long-term; neurological prob-*

lems continue through lifespan and can include delays in fine and gross motor, cognitive functioning, expressive and receptive language, vision deficits, learning disabilities, psychosocial problems, and difficulties in adaptive functioning.

REFERENCES

Applebaum MG: Fetal alcohol syndrome: diagnosis, management, and prevention, *Nurse Pract* 20(10), 1995.

Coles CD: Impact of prenatal alcohol exposure on the newborn and the child, *Clin Obstetr and Gynecol* 36(2), 1993.

Flandermeyer AA: The drug-exposed neonate. In Kenner C, Brueggenmeyer A, Gunderson LP: *Comprehensive neonatal nursing,* Philadelphia, 1993, WB Saunders.

Harris SR and others: Effects of prenatal alcohol exposure on neuromotor and cognitive development during early childhood: a series of case reports, *Phys Ther* 73(9), 1993.

Olson HC: The effects of prenatal alcohol exposure on child development, *Inf Young Childr* 6(3), 1994.

Olson HC, Burgess DM, Streissguth AP: Fetal alcohol syndrome (FAS) and fetal alcohol effects (FAE): a lifespan view with implications for early intervention, *Zero to Three* 13(Aug/Sept), 1993.

Spohr HL, Willms J, Steinhausen, HC: Prenatal alcohol exposure and long-term consequences, *Lancet* 341(8850), 1993.

Wekselman K and others: Fetal alcohol syndrome from infancy through childhood: a review of the literature, *J Pediatr Nurs* 10(5), 1995.

Growth and development, altered—cont'd

Health maintenance, altered

CLINICAL CONDITION/ MEDICAL DIAGNOSIS	RELATED FACTORS
Diabetes mellitus	Impaired ability to make deliberate and thoughtful judgments; insufficient material resources

Patient goals
Expected outcomes
  Associated nursing/collaborative interventions *and scientific rationale*

Seek help as needed to maintain diabetic control as evidenced by the following:

Clarifies needs related to maintaining diabetic control

Assist patient in identifying and clarifying needs related to maintaining diabetic control including meal planning, exercise and medication regimen. *Accurate needs assessment will enhance the success of the diabetic care and aid in preventing complications.*

Provide opportunity for discussion of health alteration and related self-care needs. *Adult learning principles guide practice including assessing readiness to learn and using experiential learning.*

Assist patient in understanding how choice of health care practices will affect diabetic control. *Educational plans should include current, relevant information and be geared to patient's educational level, interest level, and cultural practices. Ethnicity affects food choices, health beliefs, and health behaviors.*

Defines type of help needed for diabetic control

Assist patient in defining what help is needed to maintain diabetic control by monitoring blood glucose levels. *Patients should establish individual blood glucose goals with health care team.*

Help patient identify potential risk factors including hypoglycemia and cardiovascular changes. *Assessment of patient's perceived risk can enhance relevant health maintenance behaviors.*

Consult with significant others in defining diabetic control needs.

Discuss with patient how significant others may be helpful. *Family and caregiver's involvement will support control maintenance activities.*

Assist patient in determining approaches to obtaining help from significant others.

Support significant others with their role in helping patient maintain diabetic control. *Involving significant others can enhance and reinforce the practice of health maintenance behaviors.*

Describes resources available to facilitate diabetic control behaviors

Teach patient/significant others about helpful resources available in the family and community. *Knowledge of resources facilitates action.*

Facilitate patient and family contact with relevant resources; initiate referrals as necessary. *Diabetes control may be better if patient and support persons are actively involved in care decisions.*

Selects helping resources based on evaluation in relation to needs

Discuss with patient perceived needs and aim to match with available resources.

Help patient evaluate potential of helpfulness of available resources. *To be useful resources must be readily accessible, economical, and responsive to specific needs.*

Contacts resources as appropriate

Assist patient in determining ways to make contact and discuss needs.

Reinforce patient's contact with appropriate resources. *The more involved the patient is in self-care, the more likely they are to feel in control.*

Reports use of help as needed to maintain diabetic control

Discuss with patient outcomes of resource contacts.

Assist patient to evaluate usefulness of resources.

Help patient to identify factors affecting the maintenance of diabetic control. *Active learning leads to more effective interpretation and integration of knowledge.*

Establish ability to maintain diabetic control as evidenced by the following:

Identifies factors affecting present altered health maintenance ability

> Help patient to evaluate personal strengths and weaknesses that affect ability to maintain diabetic control. *Helping the patient make adjustments needed will depend on where the patient started and how he/she moves along in identified tasks.*

> Support patient in organizing and using strengths to maintain diabetic control. *Individuals all have unique strengths that can be used to maintain health. Individual values will affect decision making.*

> Teach patient about safety precautions related to diabetes (Medical alert identification, foot care, response to hypoglycemia).

Uses community resources appropriately

> Assist patient to evaluate the effectiveness of use of community resources.

Monitor and identify future diabetic control needs as evidenced by the following:

Develops effective behavior to support maintaining diabetic control

> Monitor patient's progress in establishing diabetic control and maintaining health. *Individuals can be helped to modify lifestyle and control health behaviors.*

> Help patient to develop behaviors that support continued diabetic control. *A person's perspective of health, locus of control, self-esteem, and health status influence health prevention behavior.*

> Continue to educate patient to recognize altered health state including signs and symptoms to report to health professionals.

> Recommend regular follow-up with health professional. *Follow-up is important to prevent complications and unhealthy behavior.*

Health maintenance, altered—cont'd

Participates actively in diabetic control behaviors

Discuss with patient and provide positive feedback on behaviors that are effective in maintaining diabetic control. *Increased commitment and participation by patient will enhance effectiveness of behavior.*

Assist patient to evaluate effectiveness of behaviors selected to maintain diabetic control at specific intervals.

Collaborate with patient to determine additional behaviors needed to maintain diabetic control. *Interpersonal interactions support a person's tendency to be self-actualizing.*

REFERENCES

Boehm S and others: Behavioral analysis and behavioral strategies to improve self-management of type II diabetes, *Clin Nurs Res* 2(3):327-344, 1993.

Boynton P: Health maintenance alteration: a nursing diagnosis of the elderly, *Clin Nurs Spec* 3(1):5, 1989.

Carlson SL: Altered health maintenance. In McFarland GK, McFarlane EA: *Nursing diagnosis and intervention,* ed 3, St Louis, 1997, Mosby.

Funnell MM, Hall LB: National standards for diabetes management education programs, *Diabetes Care* 18(1):100-116, 1995.

Funnell MM, Merritt JH: The challenges of diabetes in older adults, *NCNA* 28(1):45, 1993.

Hinnen D: Issues in diabetes education, *NCNA* 28(1):113, 1993.

Pender NJ, Pender AR: Attitudes, subjective norms and intentions to engage in health behaviors, *Nurs Res* 35(1):15, 1986.

Peret KK, Stachowiak B: Alteration in health maintenance: conceptual bases, etiology, and defining characteristics. In Kim MJ, McFarland GK, McLane AM, eds: *Classification of nursing diagnosis: proceedings of the fifth national conference,* St Louis, 1984, Mosby.

Redland AR, Stuifbergen AK: Strategies for maintenance of health-promoting behaviors, *Adv Clin Nurs Res* 28(2):427-442, 1993.

Tripp SL, Stachowiak B: Health maintenance, health promotion: is there a difference? *Pub Health Nurs* 9(3):155-161, 1992.

Wierenga, M.E.: Lifestyle modification for weight control to improve diabetes health status, *Patient Educ Couns* 23:33-40, 1994.

Health-seeking behaviors (stress management)

CLINICAL CONDITION/ MEDICAL DIAGNOSIS	RELATED FACTORS
History of irritable bowel syndrome	Desire for improved quality of life

Patient goals
Expected outcomes
> Associated nursing/collaborative interventions *and scientific rationale*

Experience a trusting relationship as evidenced by the following:

Identifies present state of wellness and areas in lifestyle that require attention

> Introduce client to Travis Wellness Inventory and Crumbaugh and Maholick's Purpose in Life Test.
> Promote client's interest in completing Inventory and Life Test.
> Assist client in interpreting findings.
> Help client to identify factors that threaten personal wellness and action that can be taken.
> Discuss with client the interdependent and interactive relationship of present state of well-being to daily behaviors, thinking, attitudes, and beliefs.

Identifies realistic goals and plans for enhancing health

> Facilitate verbalization of desire for change, fears, excitement, priorities, goals, and possible action.

Experience enhanced self-awareness as evidenced by the following:

Verbalizes present patterns of response to stress and use coping strategies

> Assist client in identifying present stressors: internal processes and external events.
> Assist client in identifying behavioral responses to stress. *The immune system weakens under conditions of chronic stress, increasing susceptibility to illness.*
> Explore client's use of coping strategies and degree of effectiveness.

Health-seeking behaviors (stress management)

250

Assist client in assessing quality of dietary intake and physical activity program. Share with client the relationship of nutritional status, exercise, and stress management.

Examine with client the feasibility of using conscious relaxation as a means of taking positive personal control. *Learning internally oriented relaxation techniques (e.g., autogenic training or meditation) helps patient gain/maintain a sense of control.*

Consistently engages in one self-training approach
Communicates outcomes of engaging in program(s) of choice and modifies approach as desired

Elicit client's willingness and interest in expanding self-awareness through self-training programs: self-hypnosis, creative visualization, meditation, sound therapy, etc.

Share with client the process of integrating selected/desired programs. Provide client with follow-up resource material.

Emphasize importance of consistency, patience, working within unique capacity in carrying out self-training program.

REFERENCES

Adams JD: *Understanding and managing stress; instruments to assess your life style,* San Diego, 1989, University Associates.

Crumbaugh JC, Maholick LT: *Purpose in life test.* Available from Psychometric Affiliates, PO Box 3167, Munster, Ind 46231.

Duffy ME: Determinants of health promoting lifestyles in older persons, *Image* 25(1):23-28, 1993.

Girdano DA, Everly GS, Dusek DE: *Controlling stress and tension: a holistic approach,* ed 2, Englewood Cliffs, NJ, 1993, Prentice Hall.

Goldberg ML: The relationship between the health-promotion model and health-seeking behaviors, In Carroll-Johnson RM, Paquette M: *Classification of nursing diagnosis: proceedings of the tenth conference,* Philadelphia, 1992, JB Lippincott.

Kabat-Zinn J: *Wherever you go, there you are: mindfulness meditation in everyday life,* New York, 1994, Hyperion.

Kelly J: A trifocal model of nursing diagnosis: wellness reinforced, *Nurs Diagn* 6(3):123-128, 1995.

McCloskey JC, Bulechek GM: Self-modification assistance. *Nursing interventions classifications (NIC),* ed 2, St Louis, Mosby, 1996.

Payne RA: *Relaxation techniques: a practical handbook for the health care professional,* New York, 1995, Churchill Livingstone.

Scandrett-Hibdon S, Uecker S: Relaxation training. In Bulechek GM, McCloskey JC, eds: *Nursing interventions: essential nursing treatments,* ed 2, Philadelphia, 1992, WB Saunders.

Travis J, Ryan R: *Wellness workbook: a guide to attaining high level wellness,* Berkeley, Calif, 1986, Ten Speed Press.

Home maintenance management, impaired

CLINICAL CONDITION/ MEDICAL DIAGNOSIS	RELATED FACTORS
Total hip replacement	Inadequate knowledge about postoperative home management; impaired functional status

Patient goals
Expected outcomes
    Associated nursing/collaborative interventions *and scientific rationale*

Integrate hip precautions into activities of daily living (ADLs) as evidenced by the following:

Maintains proper hip alignment (i.e., avoid extreme flexion, abduction and internal rotation)

Collaborate with physical therapist about hip precaution teaching. *An interdisciplinary approach enhances teaching.*

Provide written instructions to reinforce learning about hip precautions. *Written instructions ensure a consistent resource.*

Encourage use of adaptive equipment (e.g., elevated toilet seat, abduction wedge, or pillows).

Monitor integration of hip precautions into performance of ADLs as independence progressively increases. *This ensures that patient incorporates teaching into practice.*

Instruct patient about signs and symptoms of dislocation. *Ensure that patient has knowledge of potential complications.*

Progress toward independence in ADLs as evidenced by the following:

Uses assistive devices correctly and consistently to facilitate ADLs

Monitor patient's use of assistive devices and correct performance as indicated.

Participates actively in performance of ADLs with less assistance over time

Promote gradual independence in ADLs. *Attaining maximal independence fosters successful reintegration into home environment.*

Encourage use of analgesics before activities. *Comfort is conducive to compliance with medical regimen.*

Teach patient to pace activities. *This enhances healing of involved hip joint and muscle.*

Encourage progressive increase in activities inside/outside the home, with physician approval. *Progressive activity increase allows for healing and strengthening.*

Verbalizes knowledge of treatment plan and community resources

Collaborate with patient/significant other to arrange for home health services (e.g., home health aide and/or registered nurse). *Such services promote return to independent living situation.*

Collaborate with patient/significant other or household member to arrange for continuing rehabilitative services (e.g., physical therapy provided in outpatient department or in the home setting). *These services promote return to independent living situation.*

Plan for adapting home environment to promote maximal safety as evidenced by the following:

Begins adaptation of environment to promote safety

Collaborate with patient/significant other to plan for a safe home environment (e.g., move furniture to clear pathway for walker, remove loose scatter rugs). *Mutual planning enhances compliance.*

Instruct patient to keep environment well-lighted. *This enhances safe mobility.*

Encourage use of cordless telephone *to ensure ability to summon emergency assistance.*

Encourage patient to wear nonskid shoes. *This enhances safe mobility.*

Provide patient/significant other or household member with 24-hour emergency number for health services *to ensure ability to summon emergency assistance.*

Begins adaptation of environment for optimal daily functioning

Instruct patient to use chair with firm seat and armrests. *This maintains correct hip alignment at no more than 90 degrees flexion and facilitates safe transfer activities.*

Assist patient in negotiating rental/purchase and installation of bathtub rails, tub bench, elevated toilet seat, and grab bars *to promote independence and safety with ADLs.*

REFERENCES

Brown JS, Furstenberg AL: Restoring control: empowering older patients and their families during health crisis, *Soc Work Health Care* 17(4):81-97, 1992.

Browning MA: Discharge planning. In Hogstel MO: *Clinical manual of gerontological nursing* St Louis, 1992, Mosby.

Bull MJ: Managing the transition from hospital to home, *Qualitat Health Res* 2(1):27-41, 1992.

Erickson B, Perkins M: Interdisciplinary team approach in the rehabilitation of hip and knee arthroplasties, *Am J Occupa Ther* 48(5):439-445, 1994.

Hough D, Crossat S, Nye P: Patient education for total hip replacement, *Nurs Manag* 22(3):801-J, 80N-80P, 1991.

Kadushin J and others: Patient and family involvement in discharge planning, *J Gerontolog Soc Work* 22(3/4):171-199, 1994.

Lindstrom CC and others: High quality and lower cost: they can coexist, *Sem Nurse Manag* 3(3):133-136, 1995.

Orr P: An educational program for total hip and knee replacement patients as part of a total arthritis center program, *Orthop Nurs* 9(5):61-69, 89, 1990.

Rothman NL and others: Establishing a home care protocol for early discharge of patients with hip and knee arthroplasties, *Home Healthcare Nurses* 12(1):24-30, 1994.

Snyder PE: Fractures. In Sr. Maher AB, Salmond SW and Pellino TA: *Orthopaedic nursing,* Philadelphia, 1994, WB Saunders.

Wong J and others: Affects of an experimental program in post hospital adjustment of early discharged patients, *Int Nurs Studies* 26(1):7-20, 1990.

Hopelessness

CLINICAL CONDITION/ MEDICAL DIAGNOSIS	RELATED FACTORS
Chronic obstructive pulmonary disease	Isolation from prolonged activity restriction

Patient goals
Expected outcomes
    Associated nursing/collaborative interventions *and scientific rationale*

Identify choices available to mobilize energy on own behalf as evidenced by the following:

Reduces isolation from the environment

Establish contact and rapport with patient.

Assist patient in identifying enjoyable diversional activities.

Provide opportunities for patient to spend time with one other person; gradually increase amount of time and number of persons.

Discuss with patient options for increasing support network. *Hope depends on interaction with significant others and thrives in an atmosphere of trust.*

Expresses feelings

Provide opportunity for patient to express feelings verbally and nonverbally (e.g., writing or drawing).

Facilitate expression of feelings by active listening, open-ended questions, and reflection.

Provide opportunity for physical expression of feelings (e.g., punching bag or exercise), when possible, and within physical capabilities.

Express empathy while communicating belief that patient can act contrary to the way he or she feels.

Offer realistic hope through communicating belief that patient has or can learn skills needed to cope with problems and physical limitations.

Hopelessness

Assist patient in identifying person(s) with whom he/she is comfortable expressing feelings. *Expressing feelings abates hopelessness.*

Observe for signs of suicidal intent (e.g., sudden behavior or mood change, conversations about the futility of life).

Reports increased feelings of self-confidence

Demonstrate unconditional positive regard for patient.

Assist patient in identifying those roles that can consistently be carried out successfully within physical limitations.

Assist patient in developing self-care skills that contribute to mastery of the environment.

Encourage patient to identify and participate in satisfying experiences. *Developing self-confidence depends on repetitive positive interactions and mastery of the environment.*

Encourage positive self-statements by patient.

Provide honest praise about patient's accomplishments.

Verbalizes ability to control or influence self and environment

Involve patient in decisions about activities of daily living (ADLs) and health care.

Teach patient how to discriminate between controllable and uncontrollable events. *The perception of control over self and environment is enhanced through expanding the patient's ability to cope, problem-solve, and communicate.*

Assist patient in determining realistic goals.

Assist patient in identifying alternative ways to cope.

Assist patient in identifying consequences of implementing identified alternatives.

Teach patient new coping strategies.

Demonstrate and teach effective communication techniques (e.g., active listening).

REFERENCES

Bulechek G, McCloskey J: *Nursing interventions: essential nursing treatments*, Philadelphia, 1992, WB Saunders.

Naschinski C: Hopelessness. In Thompson J, McFarland G, Hirsch J, Tucker S: *Mosby's clinical nursing,* ed 3, St Louis, 1993, Mosby.

Range L, Penton S: Hope, hopelessness and suidicidality in college students, *Psych Reports* 75:456-458, 1994.

Rickelman B, Houfek: Toward an interactional model of suicidal behaviors: cognitive rigidity, attributional style, stress, hopelessness and depression, *Arch Psych Nurs* 9(3):158-167, 1995.

Rifai A and others: Hopelessness in suicide attempters after acute treatment of a major depression in late life, *Am J Psych* 151(1):1687-1690, 1994.

Thackston-Hawkins L, Compton W, Kelly D: Correlates of hopelessness on the MMPI-2, *Psych Reports* 75:1071-1074, 1994.

Hyperthermia

CLINICAL CONDITION/ MEDICAL DIAGNOSIS	RELATED FACTORS
Heat stroke	Exposure to a hot environment

> **Patient goals**
> **Expected outcomes**
>> Associated nursing/collaborative interventions *and scientific rationale*

Establish normothermia as evidenced by:

Maintains temperature within normal range

Monitor temperature by continuous rectal or pulmonary artery method.

Respiration, pulse and blood pressure within normal limits for patient

Monitor vital signs every 15 minutes until stable.

Absence of hyperthermia signs and symptoms, such as tachycardia, hyperventilation, flushed skin, and seizures

Apply external cooling measures.

Apply cooling blankets at a temperature of 23.9° C; *this temperature causes less shivering and is effective in reducing febrile temperatures.*

Apply ice packs in axillae and groin; *axillae and groin are close to large blood vessels that will lose heat readily by conduction.*

Wrap hands and feet in terry-cloth toweling to prevent shivering; *hands and feet have many nerve endings sensitive to heat loss; shivering should be avoided as it causes increases in metabolic rate, CO_2 production, oxygen consumption, and myocardial work and decreases in O_2 saturation and glycogen stores.*

Provide intravenous fluid therapy per order.

Provide fluids, 3000 ml/day or as ordered; *dehydration may be present due to loss of fluid from diaphoresis and increased ventilation.*

Administer antipyretics as ordered and note response; *antipyretics reduce fever by affecting hypothalamic response to pyrogens.*

Hyperthermia

258

REFERENCES

Bruce J, Grove S: Fever: pathology and treatment, *Crit Care Nurse* 12(1):40, 1992.

Caruso C and others: Cooling effects and comfort of four cooling blanket temperatures in humans with fever, *Nurs Res* 41(2):68, 1992.

Holtzclaw B: Shivering, *Nurs Clin North Am* 25(4):977, 1990.

Holtzclaw B: The febrile response in critical care: state of the science, *Heart Lung* 21(5):482, 1992.

Stevens T: Managing postoperative hypothermia, rewarming and its complications, *Crit Care Nurs* 16(1):60, 1993.

Hypothermia

CLINICAL CONDITION/ MEDICAL DIAGNOSIS	RELATED FACTORS
Cold injury	Exposure to a cold environment

> **Patient goals**
> **Expected outcomes**
> > Associated nursing/collaborative interventions *and scientific rationale*

Establish normothemia as evidenced by:

Maintains temperature within normal range

Monitor temperature using tympanic, pulmonary artery, esophageal rectal or urinary bladder method; *these best reflect the temperature of deep body tissues.*

Maintains pulse, respiration, and blood pressure within normal limits for patient

Monitor vital signs every 15 minutes until stable; monitor electrocardiogram continuously; report arrhythmias, such as bradycardia, and treat per order; *during hypothermia, circulating volume decreases causing decreased cardiac output and resulting in decreased oxygen delivery and arrhythmias.*

Monitor for hypotension; *if rapid rewarming occurs sudden vasodilitation may cause severe hypotension.*

Absence of signs and symptoms of hypothermia: shivering, cool skin, pallor, decreased level of consciousness

Use passive techniques to increase environmental temperature to 27° to 30° C.

- Warm blankets *to prevent convective heat loss and transfer heat to peripheral tissues.*
- Cover the head; *60% of total body heat loss occurs through top of head.*

Use active external techniques.

- Fluid circulating/forced warm air blankets, heat lamps; *patients report comfort, and shivering may be reduced.*

Use active internal techniques.

- Warm crystalloids at 37° to 39° C and use blood warmer for blood transfusions.
- Morphine sulfate or meperidine per order to control shivering; *shivering causes increases in metabolic rate, CO_2 production and decreases in O_2 saturation and glycogen stores.*
- Monitor arterial blood gas levels; *because of medullary respiratory depression, respiratory acidosis may result.*

REFERENCES

Augustine S: Hypothermia therapy in the postanesthesia unit: a review, *J Postanesthesia Nurs* 5(4):254, 1990.

Erickson R, Yount S: Effect of aluminized covers on body temperature in patients having abdominal surgery, *Heart Lung* 20(3):255, 1991.

Fritsch D: Hypothermia in the Trauma patient, *AACN Clinical Iss* 6(2):196, 1995.

Giuffre M and others: Rewarming postoperative patients: lights, blankets or forced warm air, *J Postanesthesia Nurs* 6(6):387, 1991.

Heffline M: A comparative study of pharmacological versus nursing interventions in the treatment of postanesthesia shivering, *J Postanesthesia Nurs* 6(5):311, 1991.

Heidenreich T and others: Temperature and temperature measurement after induced hypothermia, *Nurs Res* 41(5):296, 1992.

Holtzclaw B: Shivering, *Nurs Clin North Am* 25(4):977, 1990.

Lawson L: Hypothermia and trauma injury; temperature monitoring and rewarming strategies, *Crit Care Nurse* 15(1):21, 1992.

Oliver S, Fuessel E: Control of postoperative hypothermia in cardiovascular surgery patients, *Crit Care Nurse* 12(4):63, 1990.

Stevens T: Managing postoperative hypothermia, rewarming and its complications, *Crit Care Nurse Q* 16(1):60, 1993.

Whitman G: Hypertension and hypothermia in the acute postoperative period, *Crit Care Nurs Clin North Am* 3(4):661, 1991.

Hypothermia—cont'd

Incontinence, functional

CLINICAL CONDITION/ MEDICAL DIAGNOSIS	RELATED FACTORS
Congestive heart failure	No established toileting regimen; impaired mobility requiring use of a walker

> **Patient goals**
> **Expected outcomes**
> Associated nursing/collaborative interventions *and scientific rationale*

Establish/adhere to toileting routine as evidenced by the following:

Attempts voiding every hour, gradually increases to every 3 to 4 hours
Voids before retiring
Uses voiding log to record voiding and attempts to void

> Collaborate with patient to establish a 1-hour prompted voiding schedule; gradually increase to 3 to 4 hours if tolerated.
>
> Teach and monitor use of voiding record *to identify changes in pattern of urination.*

Achieve continence as evidenced by the following:

Reports gradual decrease in episodes of incontinence
Records episodes of involuntary loss of urine
Performs pelvic floor exercises (PFEs) 3 times a day
Takes afternoon diuretic 4 to 5 hours before bedtime

> Teach progressive use of PFEs. Provide written instructions. Sit or stand without tensing muscles of legs, buttocks, or abdomen. Contract and relax circumvaginal muscles and urinary and anal sphincters for 3 to 4 seconds and repeat in a staccato fashion. Do PFEs 25 to 30 times, 3 times daily. *PFEs strengthen the circumvaginal muscles, urinary sphincter, and external anal sphincter.*
>
> Develop with patient a schedule for taking diuretic.

Incontinence, functional

262

Monitor medications for drugs that influence bladder tone (e.g., *low K⁺ level decreases bladder tone*).

Modify environment to facilitate continence as evidenced by the following:

Accepts use of commode on a temporary basis
Keeps walker, supplies, and telephone nearby
Wears clothing easy to manage for toileting
Uses continence aids to protect skin and clothing

Collaborate with patient to establish a self-care system for managing urinary incontinence.

Assist patient with selection and creation of a private area for commode and supplies. *Private area for commode will facilitate patient-initiated voiding attempts.*

Demonstrate sensitivity to patient's feelings about incontinence.

Provide information about continence aids. *Use of continence aids helps to alleviate patient's anxiety and contributes to continence.*

REFERENCES

Agency for Health Care Policy and Research: *Clinical practice guidelines for urinary incontinence in adults* (AHCPR 92-0038), Rockville, Md, 1992, US Department of Health and Human Services.

Baker J, Norton P: Evaluation of absorbent products for women with mild to moderate urinary incontinence, *Appl Nurs Res* 9(1):29-36, 1996.

Dowd TT: Discovering older women's experience of urinary incontinence, *Res Nurs Health* 14(3):179-186, 1991.

Jirovec MM: Effect of individualized prompted toileting on incontinence in nursing home residents, *Appl Nurs Res* 4(4):188-191, 1991.

McCloskey JC, Bulechek GM: Urinary habit training. In *Nursing interventions classification (NIC)*, ed 2, St Louis, 1996, Mosby.

McCloskey JC, Bulechek GM: Urinary incontinence care. In *Nursing interventions classification (NIC)*, ed 2, St Louis, 1996, Mosby.

Ouellet LL, Ruch KL: A synthesis of selected literature on mobility: a basis for studying impaired mobility, *Nurs Diagn* 3(2):72-80, 1992.

Palmer MH and others: Detecting urinary incontinence in older adults during hospitalization, *Appl Nurs Res* 5(4):174-180, 1992.

Palmer MH, German PS, Ouslander JG: Risk factors for urinary incontinence one year after nursing home admission, *Res Nurs Health* 14(6):405-412, 1991.

Sampselle CM, DeLancey JO: The urine stream interruption test and pelvic muscle function, *Nurs Res* 41(2):73-77, 1992.

Talbot LA: Coping with urinary incontinence: development and testing of a scale, *Nurs Diagn* 5(3):127-132, 1994.

Wyman JF and others: Influence of functional, urological, and environmental characteristics on urinary incontinence in community-dwelling older women, *Nurs Res* 42(5):270-275, 1993.

Incontinence, reflex

CLINICAL CONDITION/ MEDICAL DIAGNOSIS	RELATED FACTORS
Spinal cord lesion above the level of the reflex arc	No sensation of voiding; incomplete emptying of the bladder

> **Patient goals**
> **Expected outcomes**
> > Associated nursing/collaborative interventions *and scientific rationale*

Achieve continence as evidenced by the following:

Expresses willingness to try manual voiding techniques

Participates in selection of reminders to void

Episodes of incontinence are rare

> Assist in selection, teaching, and trial of manual voiding facilitation techniques (e.g., stimulation of anus, tapping lower abdomen, doing push-ups on commode). *A reflex bladder contraction occurs in response to perineal or lower abdominal stimulation.*
>
> Establish reminders to void.
>
> Monitor amount of residual urine.

Participates in learning clean intermittent catheterization (CIC)

Participates in development of manual voiding on schedule

Monitors signs and symptoms for evidence of bladder and/or urinary tract infection

> Demonstrate and have patient/significant other return demonstrate CIC. *Patient/significant other must learn CIC to monitor residual urine: knowing CIC gives patient greater sense of control.*
>
> Teach and monitor use of appropriate hygienic measures, cleaning and storage of catheters.
>
> Teach patient/significant other signs and symptoms of bladder urinary tract infection.

Determine need for use of urinary containment device at night.

Establish a manual voiding and/or catheterization schedule, usually every 4 to 6 hours.

REFERENCES

Agency for Health Care Policy and Research: *Clinical practice guidelines for urinary incontinence in adults* (AHCPR 92-0038), Rockville, Md, 1992, US Department of Health and Human Services.

Baker J, Norton P: Evaluation of absorbent products for women with mild to moderate urinary incontinence, *Appl Nurs Res* 9(1):29-36, 1996.

Clark A, Romm J: Effect of urinary incontinence on sexual activity in women. *J Reprod Med* 38(9):679-683, 1993.

Dowd TT: Discovering older women's experience of urinary incontinence, *Res Nurs Health* 14(3):179-186, 1991.

Jirovec MM. Effect of individualized prompted toileting on incontinence in nursing home residents, *Appl Nurs Res* 4(4):188-191, 1991.

McCormick KA, Palmer MH: Urinary incontinence in older adults, *Am Rev Nurs Res* 10:25-53, 1992.

Palmer MH and others: Detecting urinary incontinence in older adults during hospitalization, *Appl Nurs Res* 5(4):174-180, 1992.

Specht J and others: Urinary incontinence. In Maas M, Buckwalter KC, Hardy M, eds: *Nursing diagnosis and interventions for the elderly,* Redwood City, Calif, 1991, Addison-Wesley.

Incontinence, stress

CLINICAL CONDITION/ MEDICAL DIAGNOSIS	RELATED FACTORS
Postpartum 5 weeks with 5 children	Weak pelvic muscles with sphincter incompetence; displacement of urethra and bladder neck during exertion

Patient goals
Expected outcomes
> Associated nursing/collaborative interventions *and scientific rationale*

Increase pelvic floor muscle tone and sphincter function as evidenced by the following:

Performs pelvic floor exercises (PFEs) 3 times a day for 6 months

> Teach patient a method for doing PFEs and provide written instructions. Sit or stand without tensing muscles of legs, buttocks, or abdomen. Contract and relax circumvaginal muscles and urinary and anal sphincters for 3 to 4 seconds and repeat in a staccato fashion. Do PFEs 25 to 30 times, 3 times daily. *PFEs strengthen the circumvaginal muscles, urinary sphincter, and external anal sphincter.*

Implement a voiding routine as evidenced by the following:

Keeps a voiding record
Uses timer to provide cue to void every 2 hours
Reduces episodes of incontinence
Drinks 6 to 8 glasses of water a day
Uses continence aids

> Teach patient to keep a voiding log.
> Instruct patient to void by the clock, beginning with 2-hour intervals; gradually lengthen interval between attempts to void.
> Collaborate with patient to establish a fluid intake pattern to maintain hydration, e.g., 200 ml every 2 hours during day.

Teach use of incontinence aids. *Use of incontinence aids will help decrease anxiety.*

REFERENCES

Agency for Health Care Policy and Research: *Clinical practice guidelines for urinary incontinence in adults* (AHCPR 92-0038), Rockville, Md, 1992, US Department of Health and Human Services.

Baker J, Norton P: Evaluation of absorbent products for women with mild to moderate urinary incontinence, *Appl Nurs Res* 9(1):29-26, 1996.

Brink CA and others: A digital test for pelvic muscle strength in women with urinary incontinence, *Nurs Res* 43(6):352-356, 1994.

Clark A, Romm J: Effect of urinary incontinence on sexual activity in women, *J Reprod Med* 38(9):679-683, 1993.

McCloskey JC, Bulechek GM. Urinary habit training. *Nursing interventions (NIC),* ed 2, St Louis, 1996, Mosby.

McCormick KA, Palmer MH: Urinary incontinence in older adults, *Am Rev Nurs Res* 10:25-53, 1992.

Mitteness LS: Urinary incontinence: a perspective on symptom management. In Larson PJ (ed) *Symptom management proceedings,* San Francisco, 1992, University of California San Francisco.

Sampselle CM, Delancey JO: The urine stream interruption test and pelvic muscle function, *Nurs Res* 41(2):73-77, 1992.

Skoner MM, Thompson WD, Caron VA, Factors associated with risk of stress urinary incontinence in women, *Nurs Res* 43(5):301-306, 1994.

Specht J and others: Urinary incontinence. In Maas M, Buckwalter KC, Hardy M, eds: Nursing diagnosis and interventions for the elderly, Redwood City, Calif, 1991, Addison-Wesley.

Woodtli A: Stress incontinence: clinical identification and validation of defining characteristics, *Nurs Diagn* 6(3):115-122, 1995.

Woodtli A: Mixed incontinence; a new nursing diagnosis? *Nurs Diagn* 6(4):135-142, 1995.

Incontinence, total

CLINICAL CONDITION/ MEDICAL DIAGNOSIS	RELATED FACTORS
Pelvic trauma/fistula	No established toileting regimen; self-care limitations (functional level 3)

> **Patient goals**
> **Expected outcomes**
>> Associated nursing/collaborative interventions *and scientific rationale*

Achieve a complete, regular bladder evacuation as evidenced by the following:

Incontinent episodes are contained
Residual urine is less than 50 ml

Provide urinary containment device for immediate use because *most routine treatment modalities are ineffective.*

Develop with patient/caregiver strategies for coping with use of urinary containment devices.

Monitor residual urine.

Avoid urological complications as evidenced by the following:

Makes and keeps appointment with urologist for fistula closing
Returns demonstration of intermittent catheterization

Refer patient for medical evaluation.

Monitor color, odor, and amount of urine.

Demonstrate/monitor clean intermittent catheterization *to prevent urinary infection.*

Implement written plan for fluid intake (e.g., 200 ml every 2 hours from 8 AM to 6 PM).

Achieve desired level of independence in self-care as evidenced by the following:

Establishes a plan to gain independence in self-care consistent with limitation

Monitors own fluid intake/voiding patterns and makes adjustments
Sets goals for increase in self-care activities
Identifies problems/potential problems related to use of urinary containment devices

Maintain skin integrity as evidenced by the following:

Skin remains intact
Uses continence aids to keep self dry
> Implement written plan for keeping skin clean/dry.
> Monitor skin for signs of redness, abrasions, etc.
> Demonstrate use of easy-to-remove protective clothing.

Maintain patient's/caregiver's dignity and feelings of self-worth as evidenced by the following:

Increases number of positive self-statements
> Monitor nurse/patient interactions for negative self-statements.
> Teach patient thought-stopping and thought-substitution techniques.
> Use behavioral approaches acceptable to patient and caregiver.

Primary caregiver participates in outside recreational/social activities weekly
> Evaluate caregiver's perceived health, sense of well-being, and feelings of burden.
> Discuss with patient/caregiver importance of planning for caregiver's participation in desired recreational/social activities.

REFERENCES

Agency for Health Care Policy and Research: *Clinical practice guidelines for urinary incontinence in adults,* (AHCPR 92-0038), Rockville, Md, 1992, US Department of Health and Human Services.

Baker J, Norton P: Evaluation of absorbent products for women with mild to moderate urinary incontinence, *Appl Nurs Res* 9(1):29-36, 1996.

Dowd TT: Discovering older women's experience of urinary incontinence, *Res Nurs Health* 14(3):179-186, 1991.

Jirovec MM: Effect of individualized prompted toileting on incontinence in nursing home residents, *Appl Nurs Res* 4(4):188-191, 1991.

Lewis-Abney K, Rosenkranz CF: Content validation of impaired skin integrity and urinary incontinence in the home health setting, *Nurs Diagn* 5(1):36-42, 1994.

Incontinence, total—cont'd

McCloskey JC, Bulechek GM: Urinary incontinence care. *Nursing interventions classification (NIC),* ed 2, St Louis, 1996, Mosby.

McCormick KA, Palmer MH: Urinary incontinence in older adults, *Am Rev Nurs Res* 10:25-53, 1992.

Specht J and others: Urinary incontinence. In Maas M, Buckwalter KC, Hardy M, eds: *Nursing diagnoses and interventions for the elderly* pp 181-204, Redwood City, Calif, 1991, Addison-Wesley.

Wyman JF and others: Influence of functional, urological, and environmental characteristics on urinary incontinence in community-dwelling older women, *Nurs Res* 42(5):270-275, 1993.

Incontinence, total—cont'd

Incontinence, urge

CLINICAL CONDITION/ MEDICAL DIAGNOSIS	RELATED FACTORS
Interstitial cystitis	No established toileting routine; inadequate intake of noncaffeine liquids

Patient goals
Expected outcomes
    Associated nursing/collaborative interventions *and scientific rationale*

Establish and adhere to toileting routine as evidenced by the following:

Attempts voiding every 2 hours; gradual increase to every 3 to 4 hours
Exercises pelvic floor muscles regularly
Records voiding attempts, pelvic floor exercises, and episodes of incontinence in voiding log
Voids before going to bed
    Collaborate with patient to develop and implement toileting regimen.
    Teach and monitor use of voiding record.
    Teach pelvic floor exercises (PFEs) *to strengthen circumvaginal muscles.*
    Monitor change in voiding pattern.

Alter pattern of response to urge to void as evidenced by the following:

Avoids rushing to the toilet
Responds to urge to void by pausing and relaxing abdominal muscles, then proceeding at a normal pace
    Teach patient to alter pattern of response to urge to void, including avoiding rushing to toilet; responding to urge to void by pausing to relax abdominal muscles; and proceeding at a normal pace. *Relaxation of abdominal muscles decreases sense of urgency and helps patient remain continent.*

Modify fluid intake to maintain acid urine as evidenced by the following:

Drinks concentrated cranberry juice daily

271

**Takes superphysiological amounts of vitamin C, at
least 1000 mg per day**
Substitutes herbal tea for caffeine-containing liquids
**Drinks 8 oz of water with meals, between meals, and
in early evening**

Teach patient to drink concentrated cranberry juice
and/or take superphysiological doses of vitamin
C. *In very large doses some vitamin C is excreted in
urine as ascorbic acid. The acidity of urine helps to
prevent bacterial growth.*

Teach patient to drink 8 oz of water with and between meals and in early evening.

Provide patient with written information about
caffeine-containing liquids; teach to substitute
caffeine-free liquids.

REFERENCES

Agency for Health Care Policy and Research: *Clinical practice guidelines
for urinary incontinence in adults* (AHCPR 92-0038), Rockville, Md,
1992, US Department of Health and Human Services.

Baker J, Norton P: Evaluation of absorbent products for women with
mild to moderate urinary incontinence, *Appl Nurs Res* 9(1):29-36,
1996.

Brink CA and others: A digital test for pelvic muscle strength in
women with urinary incontinence. *Nurs Res* 43(6):352-356, 1994.

Clark A, Romm J: Effect of urinary incontinence on sexual activity in
women. *J Reprod Med* 38(9):679-683, 1993.

Dowd TT: Discovering older women's experience of urinary incontinence, *Res Nurs Health* 14(3):179-186, 1991.

McCloskey JC, Bulechek GM: Urinary bladder training. In *Nursing interventions classification (NIC),* ed 2, St Louis, 1996, Mosby.

McCloskey JC, Bulechek GM: Urinary habit training. In *Nursing interventions classification (NIC),* ed 2, St Louis, 1996, Mosby.

McCormick KS, Palmer MH: Urinary incontinence in older adults, *Am
Rev Nurse Res* 10:25-53, 1992.

Mitteness LS. Urinary incontinence: a perspective on symptom management. In Larson PJ, ed: *Symptom management proceedings,* San
Francisco, 1992, University of California, San Francisco.

Skoner MM, Thompson WD, Caron VA: Factors associated with risk of
stress urinary incontinence in women, *Nurs Res* 43(5):301-306, 1994.

Specht J and others: Urinary incontinence. In Maas M, Buckwalter
KC, Hardy M, eds: *Nursing diagnoses and interventions for the elderly,*
Redwood City, Calif, 1991, Addison-Wesley.

Woodtli A: Stress incontinence: clinical identification and validation
of defining characteristics, *Nurs Diagn* 6(3):115-122, 1995.

Woodtli A: Mixed incontinence; a new nursing diagnosis? *Nurs Diagn*
6(4):135-142, 1995.

Wyman JF and others: Influence of functional, urological, and environmental characteristics on urinary incontinence in community-
dwelling older women, *Nurs Res* 42(5):270-275, 1993.

Infant behavior, disorganized

CLINICAL CONDITION/ MEDICAL DIAGNOSIS	RELATED FACTORS
Painful procedures for the premature infant	Excessive environmental stimulation; long-term hospitalization requiring painful procedures

Patient goals
Expected outcomes
Associated nursing/collaborative interventions *and scientific rationale*

Experience less pain as evidenced by the following:

Fewer, less intense episodes of crying

Assess infant's responses, on a routine basis, to painful stimuli and pharmacologic soothing techniques.

Premedicate infant before painful procedures. *Reducing pain level will reduce physiologic and behavioral stress in the infant.*

Reduce number of routine blood drawing events; group blood drawing episodes and conduct on a once daily or weekly basis as indicated by health status.

Create one long-term access route when frequent blood drawing is indicated.

Allow only precertified and experienced personnel to perform painful procedures, including insertion of IV's, PCVC, or central lines.

Apply minimal amount—and the least irritating type—of tape; remove tape carefully for all equipment requiring tape for stabilization.

Administer pharmacologic agents as indicated.

Use nonpharmacologic techniques to enhance the therapeutic effects of pharmacologic agents. *Employing soothing techniques may comfort and/or distract the infant and reduce irritability.*

Swaddle the infant.

Place hand on the infant to contain the infant's extremities.

Infant behavior, disorganized

Decrease the excessive environmental stimulation.

Reposition the infant to maximize infant comfort.

Help the infant to console itself by freeing hands so the infant may put hands to mouth.

Provide pacifier. *Sucking on the pacifier may decrease irritability and improve oxygenation.*

Hold the infant and provide soothing verbal cues.

Soothe the infant by lightly stroking the infant on the back, abdomen, or extremities.

Experience less distress during procedures as evidenced by the following:

Fewer and less intense episodes of crying and other nonverbal cues of distress such as body language.

Facilitate motor stability and function by the following strategies:

- Provide pacifier. *Sucking on the pacifier may console the infant and reduces irritability.*
- Contain the infant by placing two hands on the infant and holding extremities close to the infant.
- Swaddle the infant. *Swaddling may comfort the infant and reduce irritability.*
- Position infant prone or side-lying with hands and extremities in flexion. *Positioning with proper body alignment will promote motor development.*
- Free infant's hands when swaddling so that the infant may put hands to mouth. *Allowing the infant access to his/her hands will assist the infant to learn how to console self and reduce level of stress.*
- *Providing motor stability reduces stress and irritability and promotes motor development.*

Facilitate autonomic stability and function by the following strategies:

- Monitor physiologic responses to procedures.
- Allow time for the infant to recover physiologically between procedures.
- Swaddle the infant.
- Position infant prone or side-lying with hands and extremities in flexion.

- Provide soft verbal cues to the infant by talking softly to the infant.
- Reduce sound and light to the lowest levels.

REFERENCES

Als H and others: Individualized behavioral and environmental care for very low birth weight infants at high risk for bronchopulmonary dysplasia: neonatal intensive care unit and developmental outcome, *Pediatrics,* 78(6):1123, 1986.

Field TM, Goldson E: Pacifying effects on nonnutritive sucking on term and preterm neonates during heelstick procedures, *Pediatrics,* 74(6):1012, 1984.

Franck LS: A new method to quantitatively describe pain behavior in infants, *Nurs Res* 35:28, 1986.

OGN Nursing practice resource: Prevention, recognition and management of neonatal pain, Washington, DC, 1991, NAACOG:3.

Stevens, BJ, Franck L: Special needs of preterm infants in the management of pain and discomfort *J Obstetr Gynecolog Neonatal Nurs* 24(9):856-862, 1995.

VandenBerg K, Franck LS: *Bronchopulmonary dysplasia: strategies for total patient care,* Petaluma, Calif, 1990, Neonatal Network.

Infant behavior, disorganized—cont'd

Infant behavior, disorganized: risk for

CLINICAL CONDITION/ MEDICAL DIAGNOSIS	RELATED FACTORS
Prematurity; intraventricular hemorrhage	Excessive environmental stimulation; autonomic instability

Patient goals
Expected outcomes
    Associated nursing/collaborative interventions *and scientific rationale*

Experience reduction in environmental stimuli as evidenced by the following:

Sleeps for appropriate periods of time

Demonstrate fewer episodes of irritability.

Regulate the nursery environment by the following strategies:

- Maintain low noise levels in the nursery, not greater than 60 decibel, 40 decibel optimal. *Elevated sound levels may induce stress in the premature infant and affect physiologic function.*
- Decrease movement of personnel around incubator.
- Train ancillary support hospital staff to decrease noise levels during their work.
- Conduct rounds away from the incubator.
- Remove sources of noise, such as garbage cans, hospital tube system, ancillary equipment.
- Lower the sound levels of the intercom and the telephone within the unit.
- Keep all objects such as thermometers or glass bottles off the top of the incubator.
- Close incubator portholes quietly.
- Cover the open bassinet or incubator with an adult bath blanket to absorb sound.
- Evaluate potential equipment purchases for sound levels.
- Decrease light levels in the nursery. *Excessive light levels may affect the development of vision.*

Infant behavior, disorganized: risk for

- Reduce overhead lighting to no greater than 25 footcandles.
- Provide day/night rotation of light.
- Cover the incubator with a receiving blanket during sleep.

Experience less distress during procedures as evidenced by the following:

Fewer and less intense episodes of crying and other nonverbal cues of distress such as body language.

Cluster nursing care around feedings and divide procedures over the 24-hour period to distribute them evenly.

Procedures such as suctioning or chest physical therapy should not be routine; infants should be carefully assessed for need and response to these procedures.

Facilitate motor stability and function by the following strategies:

- Provide pacifier *to assist with modulation of state and reduce irritability.*
- Contain the infant by placing two hands on the infant and holding extremities close to the infant.
- Swaddle the infant. *Swaddling may comfort the infant and reduce irritability.*
- Position infant prone or side-lying with hands and extremities in flexion. *Positioning with proper body alignment will promote motor development.*
- *Providing motor stability reduces stress and promotes motor development.*

Facilitate autonomic stability and function by the following strategies:

- Monitor physiologic responses to procedures.
- Allow time for the infant to recover physiologically between procedures.
- Swaddle the infant.
- Free infant's hands when swaddling so that the infant may put hands to mouth. *Allowing the infant access to his or her hands will assist the*

infant to learn how to console self and reduce level of stress.

- Position infant prone or side-lying with hands and extremities in flexion. *Prone or side-lying position improves oxygenation.*
- Provide soft verbal cues to the infant by talking softly to him or her.
- Further reduce sound levels and light levels.

Experience complete sleep cycles as evidenced by the following:

Sleeps for appropriate periods of time

Facilitate complete sleep cycles by the following strategies:
- Do not allow the infant's sleep to be disrupted for routine physical examinations, radiographs, or blood drawing.
- Construct boundaries (nesting) around the infant during sleep.
- Administer oral tactile stimulation by a lemon glycerine swab when central apnea occurs during sleep. *Administration of the lemon glycerine swab during central apnea will promote reinitiation of respiratory effort without altering the infant's sleep state.*
- *Completion of sleep cycles promotes growth, including brain growth.*

Experience social interaction as evidenced by the following:

Demonstrates responsive body language
Cries less frequently

Promote parental visits by including parents in the planning and implementation of their infant's care.

Promote opportunities for social interaction by the following strategies:
- Modulate behavioral state to the quiet alert state after feeding by administering verbal stimulation (soft human voice), eye-to-eye contact (when the infant is alert), touch (light stroking or skin-to-skin contact) and vestibu-

lar stimulation (rocking) as tolerated by the infant. *Modulating the behavioral state will promote alertness and behavioral responsiveness in the infant while providing the opportunity for interaction between parent (or caregiver) and infant.*

- Stroke infant and talk to infant softly during routine assessments.
- Swaddle and hold infant outside incubator or bassinet during feeding and talk to the infant with eye-to-eye contact during feeding.

Progress with oral feeding as evidenced by the following:

Demonstrates tolerance for more breastfeeding sessions

Demonstrates more effective sucking reflex

Facilitate progression of oral feeding by providing nonnutritive sucking before oral feeding and during gavage feeding; support mother in frequent breastfeeding sessions.

Modulate behavioral state from sleep to active alert before feeding by administering verbal stimulation (soft human voice), eye-to-eye contact (when the infant is alert), touch (light stroking or skin-to-skin contact), and vestibular stimulation (rocking). *Modulating behavioral state to the active alert state just prior to feedings may enhance feeding behaviors.*

Experience age-appropriate sensory stimulation as evidenced by the following:

Demonstrates appropriate sensory responses

Provide age-appropriate infant sensory stimulation by the following strategies:

- Select sensory intervention based on the infant's health status, postconception age, extent of perinatal injury, and individual response patterns. *Providing appropriate sensory interventions in a nursery that has a stress reduction program in place will promote optimal development.*

- Initiate constant vestibular stimulation at birth for infants less than 34 weeks' gestation at birth and wean to intermittent vestibular stimulation at 32 to 34 postconception weeks.
- Maintain boundaries (nesting) for infants during sleep and alertness.
- Teach parents about their infant's responses to environmental stimuli and promote parental provision of age-appropriate sensory stimuli.
- Place visual stimuli more than 8 inches away from the infant's face. *Placing visual stimuli more than 8 inches away from the infant's face will promote optimal visual development.*

REFERENCES

Als H and others: Individualized developmental care for the very-low-birth-weight preterm infant: medical and neurofunctional effects, *JAMA* 21(11):853, 1994.

Becker PT and others: Effects of developmental care on behavioral organization in very-low-birth-weight infants, *Nurs Res* 42(4):214, 1993.

Burns KC, and others: Infant stimulation: modification of an intervention based on physiologic and behavioral cues, *JOGNN* 23(7):581, 1994.

Garcia AP, White-Traut RC: Preterm infants' responses to taste/smell and tactile stimulation during an apneic episode, *J Ped Nurs* 8(4):245, 1993.

Gill NE and others: Effect of nonnutritive sucking on behavioral state in preterm infants before feeding, *Nurs Res* 37(6):347, 1992.

Holditch-Davis D: The development of sleeping and waking states in high risk preterm infants, *Inf Beh Dev* 13(513), 1990.

Mann NP, Haddow R, Stokes L, Goodley S, Rutter N: Effect of night and day on preterm infants in a newborn nursery: randomized trial, *Br Med J* 293(15):1265. 1986.

White-Traut RC and others: Environmental influences on the developing premature infant: theoretical issues and applications to practice, *JOGNN* 23(5):393, 1994.

White-Traut RC and others: Patterns of physiologic and behavioral response of intermediate care preterm infants to intervention, *Ped Nurs* 19(6):625, 1993.

White-Traut RC, Pate CH: Modulating infant state in premature infants, *J Ped Nurs* 2(2):96, 1987.

Infant behavior, disorganized: risk for—cont'd

Infant behavior, organized: potential for enhanced

CLINICAL CONDITION/ MEDICAL DIAGNOSIS	RELATED FACTORS
Prematurity; periventricular leukomalacia	Excessive environmental stimulation; long-term hospitalization

Patient goals
Expected outcomes
  Associated nursing/collaborative interventions *and scientific rationale*

Experience reduction in environmental stimuli as evidenced by the following:

Sleeps for appropriate periods of time
Demonstrates fewer episodes of irritability

Regulate the nursery environment by the following strategies:

- Maintain low noise levels in the nursery, not greater than 60 decibel, less than 40 decibel optimal. *Elevated sound levels may induce stress in the premature infant and affect physiologic function.*
- Decrease movement of personnel around incubator.
- Train ancillary support hospital staff to decrease noise levels during their work.
- Conduct rounds away from the incubator.
- Remove sources of noise, such as garbage cans, hospital tube system, ancillary equipment.
- Lower the sound levels of the intercom and the telephone within the unit.
- Keep all objects such as thermometers or glass bottles off the top of the incubator.
- Close incubator portholes quietly.
- Close the open bassinet or incubator with an adult bath blanket to absorb sound.
- Evaluate potential equipment purchases for sound levels.

- Decrease light levels in the nursery. *Excessive light levels may affect the development of vision.*
- Reduce overhead lighting to no greater than 25 footcandles.
- Provide day/night rotation of light.
- Cover the incubator or open bassinet with a receiving blanket during sleep.

Experience complete sleep cycles as evidenced by the following:

Sleeps for appropriate periods of time

Facilitates complete sleep cycles:

- Do not allow the infant's sleep to be disrupted for routine physical examinations, radiographs, blood drawing.
- Construct boundaries (nesting) around the infant during sleep.
- Administer oral tactile stimulation with a lemon glycerine swab when central apnea occurs during sleep. *Administration of the lemon glycerine swab during central apnea will promote reinitiation of respiratory effort without altering the infant's sleep state.*
- *Completion of sleep cycles promotes growth, including brain growth.*

Experience social interaction as evidenced by the following:

Demonstrates responsive body language
Cries less frequently

Promote parental visits by including parents in the planning and implementing of their infant's care.

Promote opportunities for social interaction:

Modulate behavioral state to the quiet alert state after feeding by administering verbal stimulation (soft human voice), eye-to-eye contact (when the infant is alert), touch (light stroking or skin-to-skin contact), and vestibular stimulation (rocking) as tolerated by the infant. *Modulating the behavioral state will promote alertness and behavioral responsiveness in the infant while providing the opportunity for interaction between parent (or caregiver) and infant.*

282

Progress with oral feeding as evidenced by the following:

Demonstrates tolerance for more breastfeeding sessions

Demonstrates more effective sucking reflex

Facilitate progression of oral feeding by providing nonnutritive sucking before oral feeding and during gavage feeding; support mother in frequent breastfeeding sessions.

Modulate the behavioral state from sleep to active alert prior to feeding by administering verbal stimulation (soft human voice), eye-to-eye contact (when the infant is alert), touch (light stroking or skin-to-skin contact), and vestibular stimulation (rocking). *Modulating the behavioral state to the active alert state just prior to feeding may enhance feeding behavior.*

Experience age-appropriate sensory stimulation as evidenced by the following:

Demonstrates appropriate sensory responses

Promote opportunities for social interaction by the following strategies:

- Modulate the behavioral state to quiet alert state after feeding by administering verbal stimulation (soft human voice), eye-to-eye contact (when the infant is alert), touch (light stroking or skin-to-skin contact), and vestibular stimulation (rocking) as tolerated by the infant. *Modulating the behavioral state will promote alertness and behavioral responsiveness in the infant while providing the opportunity for interaction between parent (or caregiver) and infant.*

- Stroke infant and talk to infant softly during routine assessments.

- Swaddle and hold infant outside incubator or bassinet during feeding and talk to the infant with eye-to-eye contact during feeding.

Provide age-appropriate infant sensory stimulation.

- Select sensory interventions based on the infant's health status, postconception age, extent of perinatal injury, and individual response patterns. *Providing appropriate sensory interventions in a nursery that has a stress-reduction program in place will promote optimal development.*

- Initiate constant vestibular stimulation at birth for infants less than 34 weeks' gestation at birth and wean to intermittent vestibular stimulation at 32 to 34 postconception weeks.
- Maintain boundaries (nesting) for infants during sleep and alertness.
- Teach parents about their infant's responses to environmental stimuli and promote parental provision of age-appropriate sensory stimuli.
- Place visual stimuli more than 8 inches away from the infant's face. *Placing visual stimuli more than 8 inches away from the infant's face will promote optimal visual development.*

Experience less distress during procedures as evidenced by the following:

Fewer and less intense episodes of crying and other nonverbal cues of distress such as body language

Cluster nursing care around feedings and divide procedures over the 24-hour period to evenly distribute them.

Procedures such as suctioning or chest physical therapy should not be routine; infants should be carefully assessed for need and response to these procedures.

Facilitate motor stability and function by the following strategies:

- Provide pacifier.
- Contain the infant by placing two hands on the infant and holding extremities close to the infant.
- Swaddle the infant. *Swaddling may comfort the infant and reduce irritability.*
- Position infant prone or side-lying with hands and extremities in flexion. *Positioning with proper body alignment will promote motor development.*
- Free infant's hands when swaddling so that the infant may put hands to mouth. *Allowing*

the infant access to his or her hands will assist the infant to learn how to console self.

- *Providing motor stability reduces stress and promotes motor development.*

Facilitate autonomic stability and function by the following strategies:

- Monitor physiologic responses to procedures.
- Allow time for the infant to recover physiologically between procedures.
- Swaddle the infant. *Swaddling may comfort the infant and reduce irritability.*
- Position infant prone or side-lying with hands and extremities in flexion. *Positioning with proper body alignment will promote motor development.*
- Provide soft verbal cues to the infant by talking softly to him or her.
- Further reduce sound levels and light levels.

REFERENCES

Als H and others: Individualized developmental care for the very low-birth weight preterm infant: medical and neurofunctional effects, *JAMA* 21(11):853, 1994.

Becker PT and others: Outcomes of developmentally supportive nursing care for very low birth weight infants, *Nurs Res* 40(3):150, 1991.

Burns KC and others: Infant stimulation: modification of an intervention based on physiologic and behavioral cues, *JOGNN* 23(7):581, 1994.

Garcia AP, White-Traut RC: Preterm infant's responses to taste/smell and tactile stimulation during an apneic episode, *J Ped Nurs* 8(4):245, 1993.

Gill NE and others: Effect of nonnutritive sucking on behavioral state in preterm infants before feeding, *Nurs Res* 37(6):347, 1992.

Holditch-Davis D: The development of sleeping and waking states in high risk preterm infants, *Inf Beh Dev* 13:513, 1990.

Holditch-Davis D and others: Effect of standard rest periods on convalescent preterm infants, *JOGNN* 24(5):424-432, 1995.

Mann NP, Haddow R, Stokes L, Goodley S, Rutter N: Effect of night and day on preterm infants in a newborn nursery: randomized trial, *BMJ* 293(15):1265, 1986.

White-Traut RC, Nelson MN, Burns KC, Cunningham NA: Environmental influences on the developing premature infant: theoretical issues and applications to practice, *JOGNN* 23(5):393, 1994.

White-Traut RC and others: Patterns of physiologic and behavioral response of intermediate care preterm infants to intervention, *Ped Nurs* 19(6):625, 1993.

White-Traut RC, Pate CH: Modulating infant state in premature infants, *J Ped Nurs* 2(2):96, 1987.

Infant behavior, organized: potential for enhanced—cont'd

Infant feeding pattern, ineffective

CLINICAL CONDITION/ MEDICAL DIAGNOSIS	RELATED FACTORS
Prematurity	Uncoordinated sucking, swallowing, and breathing mechanisms

Patient goals
Expected outcomes
   Associated nursing/collaborative interventions *and scientific rationale*

Recognize the methods to deliver expressed mother's milk (EMM) to the high-risk preterm infant as evidenced by the following:

Knows why gavage method is to be used
   Provide information to the mother that most small, preterm infants cannot be breastfed directly. Therefore they receive EMM by artificial feeding such as gavage infusion until they have demonstrated the ability to feed orally. *Preterm infant's ability to coordinate sucking, swallowing, and breathing varies from 32 to 36 weeks of gestation, depending on feeding method.*

Knows the types of gavage feeding
   Discuss possible adverse, short-term, physiological, and biochemical responses to intermittent bolus gavage feeding, such as apnea, bradycardia, and hypoxemia *to determine whether to use continuous or intermittent gavage feeding.*
   Use intermittent bolus gavage infusion of EMM at a slow rate for all preterm infants whenever possible *to minimize or prevent adverse sequelae of rapid gastric filling.*

Achieve adequate nutritional state as evidenced by the following:

Infant gains weight and grows within expected limits
   Administer EMM by continuous nasogastric (CNG) infusion, if needed, by using following safeguards:

Infant feeding pattern, ineffective

Perform routine bacteriologic surveillance of EMM so that EMM contains only skin flora in concentration not exceeding 10^3 colony-forming units (cfu) per ml.

Infuse the EMM at the highest possible rate that is safe for the infant, *to minimize the bacterial growth and nutrient loss.*

Use syringe pump placed at 45-degree angle and small-lumen infusion tubing *to minimize nutrient loss.*

Measure lipid content of EMM by creamatocrit at the distal end of the infusion system. *If lipid adheres to the infusion syringe and tubing, infant may receive a more dilute, low-calorie milk and subsequently demonstrate suboptimal growth.*

Change syringe and tubing every 4 hours *to minimize bacterial growth.*

REFERENCES

Brennan-Behm M and others: Caloric loss from expressed mother's milk during continuous gavage infusion, *Neonatal Netw* 13(2):26-33, 1994.

Meier PP: Bottle and breast feeding: effects of transcutaneous oxygen pressure and temperature in preterm infants, *Nurs Res* 37:36, 1988.

Meier PP, Wilks SO: The bacteria in expressed mother's milk, *MCN* 12:420, 1987.

Meier PP and others: Bottle and breastfeeding: physiologic effects on preterm infants (abstract), *Neonatal Netw* 10:78, 1991.

Symington A and others: Indwelling versus intermittent feeding tubes in premature neonates, *JOGNN* 24(4):321, 1995.

Infant feeding pattern, ineffective—cont'd

Infection, risk for

CLINICAL CONDITION/ MEDICAL DIAGNOSIS	RISK FACTORS
Cancer chemotherapy-induced immunosuppression; neutropenia	Suppressed immune system

> **Patient goals**
> **Expected outcomes**
>> Associated nursing/collaborative interventions *and scientific rationale*

Experience no infection as evidenced by the following:

Has no signs and symptoms of infection

Monitor temperature every 4 hours; report any change of 1° F above or below the patient's normal diurnal variation, an elevation of 100.2° F that endures for 24 hours or a one-time reading of 101° F.

Auscultate lungs daily; have patient report sore throat or perianal tenderness. *Typical signs of inflammation may be absent in neutropenia.*

Weigh patient daily.

Check body fluids for alterations in color, odor, or consistency.

Limit use of aspirin/acetaminophen, *because these can mask a fever.*

Obtain cultures per order and report abnormalities.

Wash hands before each contact with patient.

Use gloves as necessary.

Discontinue invasive lines as soon as possible.

Avoid invasive procedures.

Use strict aseptic technique when performing invasive procedures.

Prevent patient exposure to infected visitors/staff.

Avoid fresh flowers and plants in room and raw vegetables/fruits in diet; *organisms in these may cause a problem in neutropenia.*

Monitor results of CBC and report WBC abnormalities. Use reverse isolation if indicated; *neutropenia of 500 to 1000 increases risk of infection.*

Patient/significant other verbalizes knowledge of infection prevention

Teach patient to choose high-calorie, high-protein, high-vitamin foods especially vitamins C and E; *such foods will promote cellular repair and regeneration and help produce lymphocytes.*

Teach patient to drink fluids, 2600 ml/day, *because this helps avoid UTI/constipation.*

Administer and teach patient about colony-stimulating factors.

Teach patient to increase dietary fiber; *this will help prevent infection by preventing trauma from constipation.*

Teach patient to follow steps for prevention of impaired skin integrity.

Teach patient to shower daily and use good oral hygiene.

Begin stress management counseling; *the prolonged effects of stress inhibit the function of the immune system.*

REFERENCES

Camp-Sorrell D: Controlling adverse effects of chemotherapy, *Nursing* 21(4):34, 1991.

Carter L: Influences of nutrition and stress on people at risk for neutropenia: nursing implications, *Oncol Nurs Forum* 208(8):1241, 1993.

Fazio MT, Glaspy JA: The impact of granulocyte colony-stimulating factor on quality of life in patients with severe chronic neutropenia, *Oncol Nurs Forum* 18(8):1411, 1991.

Flyge HA: Meeting the challenge of neutropenia, *Nursing* 93 23(7):60, 1993.

Griffin J: Nursing care of the critically ill immunocompromised patient, *Crit Care* 9(1):25, 1986.

Reheis C: Neutropenia, *Nurs Clin North Am* 20(1):219, 1985.

Injury, perioperative positioning: risk for

CLINICAL CONDITION/ MEDICAL DIAGNOSIS	RISK FACTORS
General surgery	Neuromuscular deficits; immobilization

Patient goals
Expected outcomes
  Associated nursing/collaborative interventions *and scientific rationale*

Become mobile and maintain tissue perfusion as evidenced by the following:

Moves all extremities without complaints of paresthesia

Pad neuromuscular junctions pertinent to each surgical position by the following strategies:

- Pad ulnar site when patient is in supine, Trendelenburg, and reverse Trendelenburg positions. *Compression of ulnar nerves will cause intermittent to continuous paresthesia.*
- Pad ulnar site when patient is in sitting position; provide pillow across abdomen to rest forearms.
- Pad brachial plexus site when patient is in prone and lateral positions; place axillary rolls bilaterally to eliminate compression upon plexus.

Avoid acutely hyperextending or abducting extremities.

- Avoid abducting the upper extremities more than 90 degrees when patient is in the following positions: supine, Trendelenburg, reverse Trendelenburg, lithotomy, and prone. *This causes compression of the brachial plexus between the scapula and the first rib.*
- Avoid acute flexion of the patient's thigh because it *causes compression of the peroneal nerve in the lithotomy position.*

Place safety strap 2 inches above the patella to negate the incidence of falls.

Specific anatomic tissue sites exhibit decreased erythema

Pad and protect all bony prominences pertinent to each surgical position by the following techniques:

- Pad occiput, scapula, olecranon and ulna, sacrum, and ischial tuberosities when patient is in supine, Trendelenburg and reverse Trendelenburg positions. *After short periods of vascular occlusion, erythema will occur. This is reactive hyperemia, which is a sudden increase of blood flow as a result of a sudden release of compression.*
- Elevate and lower extremities simultaneously while in patient lithotomy position to *facilitate venous return and eliminate back strain.*
- Avoid strapping the popliteal spaces tightly when knee-padded stirrups are used, to avoid compressing the popliteal artery, or the osseofascial compartment. *After prolonged pressure, damaged tissue liberates large quantities of histamine into the surrounding fluid. This increases capillary permeability, thereby causing more fluid to leak into surrounding tissues. This increase in pressure within the small osseofascial compartment causes additional compression of nerves and blood vessels, leading to obliteration of blood flow, neuromuscular dysfunction, and tissue ischemia.*
- Pad the occiput, scapula, olecranon, ulna, sacrum, ischial tuberosity, and calcaneus when patient is in sitting position.
- Pad the eyes, ear, and cheeks when patient is in prone position, using a Mayfield headrest or doughnut; place long rolls parallel with the torso from the nipples to the iliac crests to protect the breasts; check the male genitals for pressure and anatomic alignment; use pillows to pad patellas and toes; place arms alongside

the body, tucked in with palmar surfaces up or on armboards alongside the head, flexed at the elbow.

- Pad the ear, acromion process, iliac crest, greater trochanter, and malleoli when patient is in lateral position; place a pillow between the legs to decrease the pressure of skin surfaces on one another; flex the leg that comes in contact with the table *for stability*; place 4- to 6-inch wide adhesive across the hips *for stability*, but do not have the tape in direct contact with skin because this can cause abrasions or allergic reactions.
- Pad the footboard to decrease shearing force of the patient's posterior surface caused by sliding when patient is in reverse Trendelenburg position.
- Pad the tissue extending past or in direct contact with the metal table surface for obese patients. *Adipose tissue has little or no vascularity.*

REFERENCES

Agency for Health Care Policy and Research: *Clinical practice guideline number 3, pressure ulcers in adults,* Pub. No. 92-0047, May, 1992.

Agency for Health Care Policy and Research: *Clinical practice guideline number 3, pressure ulcers in adults: Prediction and prevention,* Pub. No. 92-0050, May, 1992.

Association of Operating Room Nurses: *Standards, recommended practices,* Denver, 1994.

Guyton: *Medical physiology,* ed 3, Philadelphia, 1994, WB Saunders.

Hagisawa and others: Assessment of skin blood content and oxygenation in spinal cord injury subjects during reactive hyperemia, *J Rehab Res Develop* 31(1):1-14, 1994.

Kneedler: *Perioperative nursing care,* ed 3, Boston, 1994, Blackwell Scientific.

Phippen ML, Wells MP: *Perioperative nursing practice,* Philadelphia, 1994, Saunders.

Rothrock M, Meeker M: *Alexander's care of the patient in surgery,* ed 10, St Louis, 1994, Mosby.

Sabisten DC: *Textbook of surgery,* Philadelphia, 1991, WB Saunders.

Schubert V, Heraud J: The effects of pressure and shear on skin microcirculation in elderly stroke patients lying in supine or semirecumbent positions, *Age Aging* 23(5):405-410, 1994.

Slater RR, Weiner TM, Karuda MJ: Bilateral leg compartment syndrome complications from prolonged lithotomy position, *Orthopedics* 17(10):954-959, 1994.

Spector WD: Correlates of pressure sores in nursing homes—evidence from the National Expenditure Survey, *J Invest Dermatol* 102(6):542-545, 1994.

Injury, perioperative positioning: risk for—cont'd

Injury, risk for

CLINICAL CONDITION/ MEDICAL DIAGNOSIS	RISK FACTORS
Borderline personality disorder	Emotional lability

> **Patient goals**
> **Expected outcomes**
> Associated nursing/collaborative interventions *and scientific rationale*

Experience no self-destructive impulses and maintain appropriate judgment, as evidenced by the following:

Demonstrates decreased emotional lability along with appropriate impulse control

Foster interpersonal trust with patient.

Identify personal or environmental risk factors *to assess and quantify safety needs and level of vulnerability for self-injury.*

Monitor emotional state (e.g., depression, anxiety, anger, suspiciousness) *to determine level of arousal and early signs of escalation.*

Monitor mental status to assess for the possibility of cognitive impairment and *decreased impulse control related to organic mental disorders.*

Examine physical environment for possible risks and remove hazardous objects or make modifications in setting *to promote safety.*

Assess suicidal risk *to determine the need for increased surveillance.*

Contract with patient about desired responses to stressors and acceptable behaviors (e.g., "no-harm" contract) *to facilitate consistency, set limits and identify therapeutic goals.*

Avoid power struggles with patient by demonstrating affective involvement plus allowing opportunities for reasonable choices *to enhance moderation of state anger in limiting setting situation, regardless of patient's diagnosis or level of impulsivity.*

Injury, risk for

Administer medications to calm patient, if appropriate.

Plan for unpredictable behaviors toward self or others.

Recognizes stressors that may increase risk of self-injury

Assist patient in identifying specific stressors within self or the environment that may increase risk of injury *to obtain patient's perception of threat and to assess coping capacity.*

Encourage patient to seek a protective environment when needed.

Monitor stress level of patient (observation and patient self-report).

Reduce environmental overstimulation (e.g., excessive noise, crowding, invasion of personal space, frustrating situations) *to minimize sense of threat.*

Determine appropriate interpersonal boundaries and nonverbal communication *to minimize anxiety, dependence, and patient's fear of abandonment by staff.*

Evaluate social network and role of significant others in affecting patient's behavior. *Social pressure and support may facilitate positive coping and reinforce appropriate responses.*

Learns new strategies to cope with stress and experiences no self-destructive impulses

Encourage patient to express feelings *to decrease escalation and build-up of negative emotions.*

Teach patient about self-monitoring emotional state *to promote greater awareness of personal threshold for stress.*

Teach patient constructive physical and mental strategies to channel emotions *to provide appropriate outlets for tensions.*

Assist patient in planning and rehearsing coping strategies *to reduce stress and maintain control during crisis.*

Refer patient to individual or group psychotherapy, or other resources as appropriate.

Injury, risk for—cont'd

REFERENCES

Barstow DG: Self injury and self mutilation: nursing approaches, *J Psychosoc Nurs Ment Health Serv* 33(2):19, 1995.

Dulit RA and others: Clinical correlates of self-mutilation in borderline personality disorder, *Am J Psychiatry* 151(9):1305, 1994.

Gainer MJ, Torem MS: Ego-state therapy for self-injurious behavior, *Am J Clin Hypnosis* 35(4):257, 1993.

Lancee WJ and others: The relationship between nurses' limit setting styles and anger in psychiatric inpatients, *Psychiatr Serv* 46(6):609, 1995.

Paris J: The etiology of borderline personality disorder: a biopsychosocial approach, *Psychiatry* 57(4):316, 1994.

Knowledge deficit (home IV therapy)

CLINICAL CONDITION/ MEDICAL DIAGNOSIS	RELATED FACTORS
Pancreatic cancer	New treatment experience
	Delayed readiness for learning

Patient goals
Expected outcomes
  Associated nursing/collaborative interventions *and scientific rationale*

Develop trusting relationship as evidenced by the following:

Discusses with caregiver fears and concerns about health state, previous experiences with health care delivery, and therapeutic regimen

  Allow sufficient time during each visit for one-to-one interaction.

  Engage in active listening.

  Inform patient about time of each scheduled visit.

Seeks assistance for financial insecurities

  Instruct patient as to caregiver's availability through phone contact and between visits and types of concerns/questions that could be discussed.

  Leave contact person's name for patient to call about financial information.

  Document patient's phone calls: time, date, content, and action taken.

  Capitalize on opportunities to compliment and/or praise.

Develop readiness for learning as evidenced by the following:

Identifies past pattern of effective learning

  Determine competency and comprehension regarding home IV therapy.

Seeks information through active dialogue

  Monitor readiness to learn and determine best methods for teaching/learning. *Certain aspects of current/ongoing health situation may alter a patient's ability to learn and retain information.*

Uses printed information pieces as reinforcement to learning

Provide specific instructions including pictures for home IV therapy.

Establish best approach for teaching: structured, unstructured, or both.

Use patient teaching flow sheet.

Increase knowledge and skill of basic IV therapy as evidenced by the following:

Demonstrates handwashing procedure and use of aseptic technique

Demonstrate and have patient return demonstration on handwashing technique and aseptic technique.

Inspect site of IV puncture at each visit.

Demonstrates correct preparation of IV fluids (i.e., attaching tubing and cleaning the line)

Evaluate home setting for an area to store supplies and for preparing solutions.

Label needle device with data, time, size, and length of catheter.

Change tubing and give complete site care in keeping with standard.

Give complete site care every 48 hours.

Demonstrate and have patient return demonstration of how to add IV solution.

Demonstrate and have patient return demonstration of use of infusion pump.

Demonstrates correct discontinuance of IV fluid

Demonstrates correct method of capping line

Demonstrate and have patient return demonstration of discontinuance of IV solution and capping of line.

Disposes of equipment as demonstrated

Evaluate patient's disposal of IV equipment.

Demonstrate disposal of IV equipment in home setting.

Demonstrates correct recording on IV sheet

Demonstrate method for recording IV therapy.

Evaluate entries made by patient on IV record.
Teaching/learning effectiveness is enhanced when patient becomes actively engaged in the learning process.

Offset potential complications as evidenced by the following:

Identifies signs and symptoms of infiltration and phlebitis

Describe signs and symptoms of infiltration and how it occurs.

Describe signs and symptoms of phlebitis and basis of its occurrence.

Verbalizes action to take if evidence of infiltration or phlebitis is noted

Instruct actions to be taken if evidence of either infiltration or phlebitis is noted.

Checks IV site and flow rate at designated intervals during infusion

Verbalizes rationale for regulation of flow

Verbalizes action to take if uncertain about events

Instruct patient to check IV site and flow rate at regular intervals.

REFERENCES

Christman NJ, Kirchoff KT, Oakley MG: Concrete objective information. In Bulechek GM, McCloskey JC, eds: *Nursing interventions—essential nursing treatment,* ed 2, Philadelphia, 1992, WB Saunders.

LaRocca JC: *Handbook of home care IV therapy,* St Louis, 1994, Mosby.

Markel S: PIC/PICC and extended peripheral catheters; five years experience in home care, *J Home Health Care Pract* 7(1):35-40, 1994.

McCloskey JC, Bulechek GM: *Nursing interventions classification (NIC),* ed 2, St Louis, 1996, Mosby.

Meredith D: Patient selection criteria for home IV therapies: from A to Z, *Caring* 14(5):40-42, 1995.

Michela NJ: High tech home care infusion therapy, *Geriatr Nurs* 16(5):249-250, 1995.

Rakel B: Knowledge deficit. In Maas M, Buckwalter KC, Hardy M, eds: *Nursing diagnosis and interventions for the elderly,* Redwood City, Calif 1991, Addison-Wesley.

Redman BK, Thomas ESN: Patient teaching. In Bulechek GM, McCloskey JC: *Nursing interventions: essential nursing treatments,* Philadelphia, 1992, WB Saunders.

Smith CE: A model of caregiving effectiveness for technologically dependent adults residing at home, *Adv Nurs Sci* 17(2):27-40, 1994.

Loneliness, risk for

CLINICAL CONDITION/ MEDICAL DIAGNOSIS	RISK FACTORS
Transition to widowhood after recent move to retirement area of the country	Lives alone in own home in semirural area; retired recently after 30 years of teaching.

Patient goals
Expected outcomes
   Associated nursing/collaborative interventions *and scientific rationale*

Learn to accept and enjoy living alone as evidenced by the following:

Searches for meaning in sudden transition to widowhood

Monitors tasks required to continue living in own home

Paces daily activities to decrease risks such as falling and fatigue

Negotiates reliance on others for tasks beyond physical capability

Exercises three times per week to increase or maintain body strength

   Refer patient to counselor for help in searching for meaning in sudden loss of spouse. *Finding meaning enables individuals to seek new opportunities for personal growth.*

   Provide information about process of transition. *Knowing what to expect helps to decrease stress. Stress and emotional distress can be expected during the transition.*

   Monitor transition to see if expectations are congruent with reality. *Development of a timeline that shows process of transition may help validate a healthy transition.*

   Determine need for new knowledge and skill, and for resources in the community.

Develop a network of friends and companions, as evidenced by the following:

Volunteers to assist teacher in local school two mornings a week

Participates in church-related activities (e.g., plays bridge, joins guild)

Invites new acquaintances to attend a concert or other activity

Attends class at community college to learn a new craft, such as quilting

Verbalizes subjective sense of well-being

Assist patient to create conditions conducive to a healthy transition.

Provide opportunities for development of new relationships; for example, discuss local needs for volunteers in schools, libraries, and hospitals. *New relationships help to prevent bouts of loneliness that accompany widowhood.*

Provide information about educational institutions in the community. *Attending classes together helps individuals make new friends with common interests.*

Monitor indicators of a healthy transition and provide feedback to client; examples are mastery of new behaviors and well-being that comes with making new friends.

REFERENCES

Adlersberg M, Thorne S: Emerging from the chrysalis: older widows in transition, *Gerontolog Nurs* 16:4-8, 1990.

Elsen J, Blegen M: Social isolation. In Maas M, Buckwalter KC, Hardy M, eds: *Nursing diagnoses and interventions for the elderly,* Redwood City, Calif, 1991, Addison-Wesley.

Lien-Gieschen T: Validation of social isolation related to maturational age: elderly, *Nurs Diagn* 1993, 4(1):37-44.

Lopata HZ, Heinemann GD, Baum J: Loneliness: antecedents and coping strategies in the lives of widows. In Peplau LA, Perlman D: *Loneliness: a sourcebook of current theory, research and therapy,* New York, 1982, Wiley and Sons.

McCloskey JC, Bulechek GM: Socialization enhancement. In *Nursing interventions classification (NIC),* ed 2, St Louis, 1996, Mosby.

Peplau LA and others: Being old and living alone. In Peplau LA, Perlman D: *Loneliness: a sourcebook of current theory, research and therapy,* New York, 1982, Wiley and Sons.

Porter EJ: Older widows' experience of living alone at home, *Image J Nurs Scholarship* 26(1):19-24, 1994.

Porter EJ: "Reducing my risks:" a phenomenon of older widows' lived experience, *Adv Nurs Sci* 17(2):54-65, 1994.

Russel D: The measurement of loneliness. In Peplau LA, Perlman D: *Loneliness: a sourcebook of current theory, research and therapy,* New York, 1982, Wiley and Sons.

Schumacher KL, Meleis AI: Transitions: a central concept in nursing, *Image J Nurs Schol* 1994, 26(2):119-127.

Management of therapeutic regimen, community: ineffective

CLINICAL CONDITION/ MEDICAL DIAGNOSIS	RELATED FACTORS
Cognitively impaired older adults living with family members in rural communities	Limited personal and community resources; increasing evidence of neglect and abuse of elderly.

Patient goals
Expected outcomes
> Associated nursing/collaborative interventions *and scientific rationale*

Community will experience increased awareness of the extent of the problems as evidenced by the following:

Establishes a task force of representatives of health care and social agencies concerned with the problem

Gathers data from community agencies to determine the extent of the problems and inventory of resources

Disseminates information about findings through public service announcements (PSAs) and other media

> Collaborate with regional council on aging to obtain funding from regional agencies and foundations to support appointment of an ombudsman and work of task force. *Staff of council will have access to funding sources and could serve as liaison to funding agencies.*

> Recruit applicants for position of ombudsman and make a recommendation to the task force.

> Recruit task force members from health and social agencies; include representatives from funding sources when possible. *Funding sources like to know status of ongoing work and may be more generous when included.*

> Prepare bulletins and informational pamphlets for PSAs, newspapers, and other media. *Keeping the public informed of progress of task force will help ensure citizens' support for additional resources.*

Management of therapeutic regimen, community: ineffective

Community will mobilize existing resources to provide immediate assistance to any families in a crisis situation as evidenced by the following:

Recruits volunteers from local service organizations to provide respite time for caregivers

Makes discretionary funds from the departments of social services (DSSs) available

Publicizes emergency assistance numbers

Urges caregivers to report families needing immediate assistance

Contact service organizations and offer to provide information about needs of families. *A personal contact will meet with success more often than a letter, especially when that contact is made by a recognized leader, such as a community health nurse.*

Meet with personnel in DSS to review known cases of need and obtain information about financial resources.

Work with task force to provide accurate PSAs that include a reminder to respect an individual's right to privacy. *Some individuals and families do not want any assistance from a social agency regardless of the situation.*

Weigh privacy issues with the need to expedite services.

Assist the informal support systems in the community: neighbors, friends, and family members. *In rural communities caregivers receive most of their support from informal networking.*

Community will develop a long-term plan for dealing with care of cognitively impaired adults and with issues of neglect and abuse as evidenced by the following:

Collaborates with regional council on aging to prepare grant proposals to obtain funds from community block grants to meet needs of the rural cognitively impaired elderly

Reviews policies for adult protection in each community and identifies need for adult protection teams where none exist

Develops an elder abuse training program
Offers training to formal and informal caregivers

Serve as patients' advocate on task force, regional council, and with DSSs. *Providing patients with information about their rights in particular situations enables them to make informed decisions.*

Inform individuals and family members about adult protection services available in the local community.

Provide consultation and assistance with development of elder abuse training program. *The professional expertise of the nurse is valued by colleagues.*

Develop and implement plan for ongoing assessment and evaluation of services available to and used by families of cognitively impaired older adults.

REFERENCES

Bull MJ: Factors influencing family caregiver burden and health, *West Nurs Res* 12:758-776, 1990.

Burgener SC, Shimer R: Variables related to caregiver behaviors with cognitively impaired elders in institutional settings. *Res Nursing Health* 16(3):193-202, 1993.

Fulmer TT: Elder mistreatment, *Annu Rev Nurs Res* 12:51-64, 1994.

Given BA, Given CW: Family caregiving for the elderly, *Annu Rev Nurs Res* 9:77-101, 1991.

Magilvy JK, Congdon JAG, Martinez R: Circles of care: home care and community support for rural older adults, *Adv Nus Sci* 16(3):22-33, 1994.

Segesten K: Patient advocacy—an important part of the daily work of the expert nurse, *Schol Inq Nurs Pract* 7(2):129-135, 1993.

Weinert C, Burman ME: Rural health and health-seeking behaviors, *Annu Rev Nurs Res* 12:65-92, 1994.

Management of therapeutic regimen, community: ineffective—cont'd

Management of therapeutic regimen, families: ineffective

CLINICAL CONDITION/ MEDICAL DIAGNOSIS	RELATED FACTORS
Wife and mother with malnutrition and dehydration 2 months after a stroke, living with elderly husband and dependent daughter with chronic fatigue syndrome.	Sudden inception of caregiving role by husband and daughter; neglect of wife and mother

Patient goals
Expected outcomes
   Associated nursing/collaborative interventions *and scientific rationale*

Family will improve quality of care delivered to wife and mother as evidenced by the following:

Expresses desire to give required care to wife/mother
Expresses willingness to attend classes to master skills needed to manage caregiving tasks
Participates in development of plan of care
Prepares and provides nutritionally balanced meals
Supplements meals with high-calorie drinks and up to 8 glasses of liquids a day

   Determine husband's and daughter's motivation to manage care of wife and mother in the home. *Sudden inception of caregiving role may have led to unrealistic expectations of their ability to provide care.*

   Monitor situation for signs of abuse and neglect; for example, administer Risk of Elder Abuse in the Home (REAH) test. *Abuse is often perpetrated by a dependent person.*

   Teach husband and daughter to include wife and mother with the problem-solving, especially how to frame problems so that reasonable solutions can be found. *Values, experience, and emotions are central to framing a problem; information alone is insufficient.*

Visit family two or three times a week until plan of care is fully implemented and support services are in place. *Family members may have desire to care for ill member but lack skills and physical capability.*

Teach daughter to keep a written record of mother's food intake and to monitor body weight twice a week. *Food diary provides feedback to mother and daughter about adequacy of food intake.*

Family will accept assistance from outside medical and social resources as evidenced by the following:

Makes and keeps appointments with physicians and representatives of home health care agencies
Contacts volunteer services to locate individual willing to help with weekly shopping and housekeeping

Determine need for assistance in managing tasks of daily living; locate and access required services in the community. *There may not be sufficient energy and ability within the family to provide needed care.*

Refer daughter to physician to treat chronic fatigue syndrome.

Provide information about volunteer services in community that could assist with shopping and housekeeping. *Volunteers may provide sufficient supportive services to prevent excessive caregiver burden.*

Confer with wife's physician to request in-home services of physical therapist. *Physical therapists provide programs of daily exercises and activities that would increase her strength, and decrease caregiving burden.*

REFERENCES

Cartwright JC and others: Enrichment processes in family caregiving to frail elders, *Adv Nurs Sci* 17(1):31-43, 1994.

Given BA, Given CW: Family caregiving for the elderly, *Annu Rev Nurs Res* 9:77-101, 1991.

Bowers BJ: Intergenerational caregiving: adult caregivers and their aging parents, *Adv Nurs Sci* 9(2):21-31, 1987.

Brandriet LM, Lyons M, Bentley J: Perceived needs of poststroke elders following termination of home health services, *Nurs Health Care* 15(10):514-520, 1994.

Congdon JAG: Managing the incongruities: the hospital discharge experience for elderly patients, their families, and nurses, *Appl Nurs Res* 7(3):125-131, 1994.

Davis LL, Grant JS: Constructing the reality of recovery: family home care management strategies, *Adv Nurs Sci* 17(2):66-76, 1994.

Fulmer TT: Elder mistreatment, *Annu Rev Nurs Res* 12:51-64, 1994.

Kison C: Health beliefs and compliance of cardiac patients, *Appl Nurs Res* 5(4):181-185, 1992.

McCloskey JC, Bulechek GM: Family integrity promotion. *Nursing interventions classification (NIC),* ed 2, St Louis, 1996, Mosby.

Robinson KM: A social skills training program for adult caregivers, *Adv Nurs Sci* 10(2):59-72, 1988.

Sims S, Boland D, O'Neill CA: Decision-making in home health care, *West J Nurs Res* 14(2):186-200, 1992.

Management of therapeutic regimen, individual: effective

CLINICAL CONDITION/ MEDICAL DIAGNOSIS	RELATED FACTORS
Insulin-dependent older female with arthritis and obesity	Wishes to improve overall health status; expresses interest in seeking services of alternative health physician

Patient goals
Expected outcomes
> Associated nursing/collaborative interventions *and scientific rationale*

Negotiate collaboration between an internist and a physician who offers alternative health care as evidenced by the following:

Discusses plan to locate and access services of a physician who offers alternative health care
Makes and keeps appointment with both physicians
Continues to participate in diabetes education classes
Monitors own responses to new regimen

> Help patient to locate and access services of alternative health practitioner *to demonstrate confidence in patient's ability to improve health status.*
> Teach importance of continued monitoring of health status as advised by both physicians.
> Serve as advocate for patient in negotiation with health care providers.
> Acquaint patient with strategies to improve self-monitoring of sensations, symptoms, and power components of self-care. *Knowledge of theoretical underpinnings of self-care will increase patient's ability to become own advocate.*

Implement new health practices into activities of daily living as evidenced by the following:

Makes decision with family members to follow a vegetarian diet to bring down blood sugar and to decrease body weight.
Joins local health club to engage in water exercises, swimming, and walking on treadmill.

Modifies recreational and volunteer activities to free time for health-related activities.

Provide information about risks associated with very low calorie diets (VLCD). *VLCDs should not be used for longer than 12 to 16 weeks; risks include nitrogen losses, increased tendency to develop gallstones, and cardiovascular problems.*

Provide information about metabolic changes associated with dieting, such as decrease in resting metabolic rate (RMR). *The decrease in RMR results from more efficient metabolism; that is, fewer calories are needed to support energy needs at rest. The decrease for women ranges from 10% to 30%.*

Discuss metabolic changes associated with dieting and exercise. *During periods of dieting, the energy requirement for a given activity decreases by 25%; therefore, weight loss is slower.*

Provide support to remain on dietary regimen to avoid yo-yo syndrome, that is, repeated dieting and refeeding with increases in body weight. *Repeated dieting and refeeding increase risks associated with dieting, and weight loss is more difficult to achieve.*

REFERENCES

Gast HL and others: Self-care agency: conceptualizations and operationalization *Adv Nurs Sci* 12(1):26-38, 1989.

Hartweg DL: Self-care actions of healthy middle-aged women to promote well-being, *Nurs Res* 42(4):221-227, 1993.

Keeling and others: Noncompliance revisited: a disciplinary perspective of a nursing diagnosis, *Nurs Diag* 4(3):91-98, 1993.

Keller ML, Ward S, Baumann LJ: Processes of self-care: monitoring sensations and symptoms, *Adv Nurs Sci* 12(1):54-66, 1989.

Olson A: Women and weight control. In McElmurry BJ, Parker RS: *Annual review of women's health,* New York, 1993, National League for Nursing.

McWilliam CL and others: Creating health with chronic illness, *Adv Nurs Sci* 18(3):1-15, 1996.

Perry JA, Woods NF: Older women and their images of health: a replication study, *Adv Nurs Sci* 18(1):51-61, 1995.

Weinert C, Burman ME: Rural health and health-seeking behaviors, *Annu Rev Nurs Res* 12:65-92, 1994.

Management of therapeutic regimen, individuals: ineffective

CLINICAL CONDITION/ MEDICAL DIAGNOSIS	RELATED FACTORS
Male police officer newly diagnosed with non–insulin-dependent diabetes	Powerlessness Perceived barriers versus perceived benefits

---

Patient goals
Expected outcomes
    Associated nursing/collaborative interventions *and scientific rationale*

Make effective choices in ADLs and achieve goals of treatment program as evidenced by the following:

Increases sense of control in making choices about treatment program

Encourage patient to identify actual and/or potential barriers (e.g., food and family customs, ethnic health care practices, religious preferences, work schedule) that prevent him from engaging in treatment plan and feeling a sense of control over outcomes.

Evaluate patient's attitudes, cultural beliefs, and values about current health state and treatment regimen. *Attitudes, beliefs, and values can serve as barriers or supports for further interventions in patient's management of therapeutic regimen.*

Evaluate impact of diabetes regimen on current level of function, life-style, and employment.

Explore with patient past experiences, strengths, problems in illness, threats to health, and other stressful situations in which patient has experienced powerlessness.

Discuss patient's perspectives on his future health status, life-style, and career. *It is important to determine patient's perspectives of current health status and treatment regimen to collaborate with him in developing a practical plan for participating in treatment and in meeting treatment goals.*

Discuss patient's sense of responsibility for management of his disease. *Awareness contributes to a heightened sense of responsibility.*

Recognizes and accepts benefits of treatment

Discuss with patient consequences of not adhering to treatment regimen and possible negative outcomes. *Adequate understanding of illness, involvement in a treatment regimen and outcomes, serves as a basis for developing a plan for behavior change.*

Encourage patient to discuss perceived benefits of following prescribed regimen. *There is an increase in effective management of diabetes when patients perceive the benefits of following the treatment program.*

Provide feedback to patient on assessment of and choice of options *to facilitate making informed decisions and choices, thereby increasing feelings of control and adherence to treatment regimen.*

Collaborate with patient to develop plan that focuses on selected areas *to maximize patient's feelings of control. Capitalizing on strengths and starting with selected behavioral target areas for change are important beginning steps in developing a plan for patient to participate effectively in treatment program and to meet specific health goals.*

Meets goals of treatment program

Encourage patient to focus on single area and set small goals for a "trial period" *so that patient can obtain feedback on how to be successful in his plan.*

Collaborate with patient in setting mutual goals that are short-term, realistically manageable, and progressive *to reach ultimate, long-range goals.*

Support patient as he begins with plan, giving positive feedback and focusing on small achievements. *Small achievements and reaching short-term goals will decrease patient's sense of powerlessness and increase a sense of control over his health status and involvement in the treatment plan.*

Encourage patient to discuss and seek out additional resources and other social supports that will help him obtain positive feedback on adherence to treatment regimen and enhance his feelings of satisfaction and achievement. *Social support may help or hinder patient's adherence to treatment regimen and may depend on the patient's perception of the influence that others may have on their life.*

Monitor patient's progress at regular, scheduled intervals. Encourage patient to discuss setbacks as well as progress. *Management of chronic illness requires the nurse to keep in mind long-range planning with patient on more short-term, achievable goals that will contribute to the patient's ultimate long-term success.*

REFERENCES

Anderson RM, Fitzgerald JT, Oh MS: The relationship between diabetes-related attitudes and patient's self-reported adherence *Diabetes Educ* 19(4):287, 1993.

Anderson RM and others: A comparison of the diabetes-related attitudes of health care professionals and patients, *Patient Educa Couns* 21:41, 1993.

Bakker RH, Kastermans MC, Dassen TW: An analysis of the nursing diagnosis ineffective management of therapeutic regimen compared to noncompliance and Orem's self-care deficit theory of nursing, *Nurs Diagn* 6(4):161-166, 1995.

Burckhardt CS: Coping strategies of the chronically ill, *Nurs Clin North Am* 22(3):543, 1987.

Lubkin IM: *Chronic illness: impact and intervention,* ed 2, Boston, 1991, Jones & Bartlett.

Jensen L, Allen M: Wellness: the dialectic of illness, *Image: J Nurs Schol* 25(3):220, 1993.

Raymond NR, D'Eramo-Melkus G: Non–insulin-dependent diabetes and obesity in the Black and Hispanic population: culturally sensitive management, *Diabetes Educ* 19(4):313, 1993.

Seley JJ: Is noncompliance a dirty word? *Diabetes Educ* 19(5):386, 1993.

Thorne SE: Constructive noncompliance in chronic illness, *Holistic Nursing Practice* 5(1):62-69, 1990.

Wierenga ME, Browning JM, Mahn JL: A deceptive study of how clients make life-style changes, *Diabetes Educ* 16(6):469-473, 1990.

Memory, impaired

CLINICAL CONDITION/ MEDICAL DIAGNOSIS	RELATED FACTORS
Forty-year-old female with diagnosis of mild head injury	Temporary neurologic disturbance

Patient goals
Expected outcomes
> Associated nursing/collaborative interventions *and scientific rationale*

Recognize the need for cognitive rehabilitation as evidenced by the following:

Verbalizes awareness of memory deficit

> Provide opportunities for patient to discuss concerns about impaired memory. *There is a positive relationship between awareness and treatment outcome.*

> Assure patient that memory impairment is not unusual following neurological trauma. *Cognitive difficulty is frequently noted as a residual symptom following brain injury.*

Maintain ability to attend to environmental routine as evidenced by the following:

Participates in the memory rehabilitation process.

> Collaborate with family and significant others to identify previous organizational styles and methods. *Information is better learned and retained when it is related to previously learned skills and knowledge.*

> Collaborate with other disciplines to determine appropriate therapeutic techniques and approaches. *A multidisciplinary treatment approach is required from a few weeks to 2 years following brain injury.*

> Include family members in the process of evaluation and rehabilitation. *Individuals with disabilities can set health goals and achieve them; family*

Memory, impaired

members are often actively engaged in assisting with therapy and rehabilitation.

Assist with selection of a recording system that is meaningful to the patient, such as a daily calendar, note cards, or memory book. *Adaptation and adjustment to disabilities are major areas of focus on the course of recovery. Interventions that focus on purposeful activity often improves cognitive function.*

Demonstrate method of recording meaningful information in memory book.

Assist patient to record data in memory book.

Reinforce use of memory book for reference to attend therapy sessions. *There is a feeling of success when a person can practice and master a task.*

Proceed from simple to complex instruction. *Consistent technique applied to multiple contexts facilitates transfer to information.*

Be consistent in using memory training techniques. *Consistent technique applied to multiple contexts facilitates transfer of information.*

Provide feedback and validation as patient gains independence in use of recorded information. *Perceived ability to complete health practice increases the likelihood of maintaining behavior.*

REFERENCES

Becker H and others: Self-rated abilities for health practices: A health self-efficacy measure, *Health Val* 17(5):42-50, 1993.

Harrington DE and others: Current perceptions of rehabilitation professionals towards mild traumatic brain injury. *Arch Phys Med Rehabil* 74(6):579-586, 1993.

McDowell I and others: Late rehabilitation for late head injury: Clinical psychologists' interventions, *Clin Rehabil* 9:150-156, 1995.

Paulanka BJ, Griffin LS: Behavioral responses to memory impaired clients to selected nursing interventions. *Phys Occupa Ther Geriatr* 12(1):65-78, 1993.

Rosenthal M: Mild traumatic brain injury syndrome. *Ann Emer Med* 22(6):1048-1051.

Stuifbergen AK, Becker HA: Predictors of health promoting lifestyles in persons with disabilities, *Res Nurs Health* 17:3-13, 1994.

Mobility, impaired physical

CLINICAL CONDITION/ MEDICAL DIAGNOSIS	RELATED FACTORS
Systematic lupus erythematosus (SLE)	Acute and chronic joint pain, fatigue

> **Patient goals**
> **Expected outcomes**
> > Associated nursing/collaborative interventions *and scientific rationale*

Improve pain management as evidenced by the following:

Rates pain as a 3 or less on a scale of 0 to 10 over a 48-hour period (0, no pain; 10, worst pain)

Teach patient how to use a numerical pain scale.

Apply warm moist heat to affected joints.

Provide warm showers as needed and at bedtime to promote comfort. Avoid excessively hot water *because this might increase fatigue.*

Teach patient how to use progressive relaxation as an adjunct to analgesics as needed and at bedtime. *Pain control is a major component in maintaining optimal muscle and joint mobility.*

Self-administers prescribed antiinflammatory and/or analgesic medications consistently and on schedule

Teach appropriate use of antiinflammatory medications and analgesics, *which are most effective when administered on a consistent and fixed schedule to maintain adequate serum levels.*

Reports a minimum of 7 hours of uninterrupted sleep for 3 consecutive days

Provide egg-crate mattress or similar joint-cushioning material for patient's bed to increase comfort.

Suggest back massage at bedtime to promote sleep.

Counsel patient to limit naps to no more than two a day. *Excessive napping during the day can interfere with normal sleep patterns.*

Monitor patient's emotional response to disease process, *because emotional state may have an impact on patient's ability to manage pain.*

Protect currently affected (acute) joints while maintaining function of joints affected by chronic lupus symptoms as evidenced by the following:

Maintains full range of motion in chronically affected joints

Coach patient through passive ROM before initiating active ROM twice daily to all but acutely affected joints *to ensure safety and efficiency.*

Rests and supports acutely affected joints

Provide rest and support to acutely affected joints *to stabilize and reduce stress on the joint and aid in muscle relaxation.*

Splint inflamed wrists and hands. *By immobilizing the joint, splinting can decrease pain and prevent contractures from forming in nonfunctional positions.*

Maintains daily exercise regimen as prescribed by physician and/or physical therapist

Balance rest therapy with active physical exercise program *to promote strength and function and to minimize fatigue related to activity level.*

Achieve optimal level of physical mobility as evidenced by the following:

Provides own daily self-care within limits of any existing physical disabilities

Assist patient with task analysis of daily activities.

Teach patient how to use a walker and other assistive devices correctly.

Performs activities of daily living (ADLs) in a manner that promotes joint conservation and protection

Provide information about task simplification, assistive devices, and other energy-conserving techniques.

Identify resources within patient's social support systems and in wider community that may aid in meeting ADLs outside the bounds of patient's current physical abilities (e.g., assistance with housework and transportation).

REFERENCES

Creason NS: Toward a model of clinical validation of nursing diagnoses: developing conceptual and operational definitions of impaired physical mobility. In Carroll-Johnson RM, ed: *Classification of nursing diagnoses: proceedings of the ninth conference,* Philadelphia, 1991, JB Lippincott.

Halverson PB, Holmes SB: Systemic lupus erythematosus: medical and nursing treatments, *Orthopaed Nurs* 11(6):17, 1992.

Kasper CE and others: Alterations in skeletal muscle related to impaired physical mobility: an empirical model, *Res Nurs Health* 16(4):265-273, 1993.

Kraft LS, Maas M, Haroy MA: Diagnostic content validity of impaired physical mobility in the older adult, ed 2, In Carroll-Johnson RM: *Classification of nursing diagnoses: proceeding of the tenth conference,* Philadelphia, 1992, JB Lippincott.

Krupp LS and others: A study of fatigue in SLE, *J Rheumatol* 17(11):1450, 1990.

McCloskey JC, Bulechek GM: Exercise therapy: joint mobility. In *Nursing interventions classification (NIC),* ed 2, St Louis, 1996, Mosby.

Mehmert PA, Delaney CW: Validating impaired physical mobility, *Nurs Diagn* 2(4):143, 1991.

Metzler DJ, Harr J: Positioning your patient properly, *AJN* 96(3):33-37, 1996.

Mobily PR, Skemp Kelly IS: Introgenesis in the elderly: factors of immobility, *J Gerontolog Nurs* 17(9):5-28, 1991.

Morse JM, Bottorff, Hutchinson S: The paradox of comfort, *Nurs Res* 44(1):14-19, 1995.

Quellet LL, Rush KL: A synthesis of selected literature on mobility: a basis for understanding impaired mobility, *Nurs Diagn* 3(2):72, 1992.

Mobility, impaired physical—cont'd

Noncompliance (therapeutic regimen)

CLINICAL CONDITION/ MEDICAL DIAGNOSIS	RELATED FACTORS
Degenerative joint disease (older adult)	Complexity of exercise regimen Side effects of medication

Patient goals
Expected outcomes
> Associated nursing/collaborative interventions *and scientific rationale*

Integrate exercise prescription into activities of daily living as evidenced by the following:

Records in exercise log time and distance walked
> Collaborate with patient/significant other to develop and implement a weekly exercise (activity/rest) plan.

> Teach patient/significant other how to use exercise log.

Records joint pain on scale of 0 to 10 (0, no pain; 10, worst pain) before and after exercise and adjusts time and distance walked as appropriate

Modifies activities that consistently increase pain
> Teach patient/significant other use of visual analog scale to record joint pain. *Logging exercise and rest may increase compliance with activity/rest prescription.*

> Discuss pain log with patient/significant other and suggest ways to modify activity/rest plan.

Adhere to schedule for taking medications as evidenced by the following:

Takes nonsteroidal antiinflammatory drugs (NSAIDs) with food

Records medications taken and missed and any side effects
> Collaborate with patient/significant other to implement plan for taking medications. *Active participation in decision-making about therapeutic regimen may increase compliance.*

Noncompliance (therapeutic regimen)

NANDA-Approved Nursing Diagnoses

Disuse syndrome, risk for
Diversional activity deficit
Dysreflexia
Energy field disturbance
Environmental interpretation syndrome, impaired
Family processes, altered: alcoholism
Family processes, altered
Fatigue
Fear
Fluid volume deficit
Fluid volume deficit, risk for
Fluid volume excess
Gas exchange, impaired
Grieving, anticipatory
Grieving, dysfunctional
Growth and development, altered
Health maintenance, altered
Health-seeking behaviors (specify)
Home maintenance management, impaired
Hopelessness
Hyperthermia
Hypothermia
Incontinence, functional
Incontinence, reflex
Incontinence, stress
Incontinence, total
Incontinence, urge
Infant behavior, disorganized
Infant behavior, disorganized: risk for
Infant behavior, organized: potential for enhanced
Infant feeding pattern, ineffective
Injection, risk for

Injury, risk for
Knowledge deficit (specify)
Loneliness, risk for
Management of therapeutic regimen, community: ineffective
Management of therapeutic regimen, families: ineffective
Management of therapeutic regimen, individual: effective
Management of therapeutic regimen, individuals: ineffective
Memory, impaired
Mobility, impaired physical
Noncompliance (specify)
Nutrition, altered: less than body requirements
Nutrition, altered: more than body requirements
Nutrition, altered: risk for more than body requirements
Oral mucous membrane, altered
Pain
Pain, chronic
Parent/infant/child attachment, altered: risk for
Parental role conflict
Parenting, altered
Parenting, altered, risk for
Peripheral neurovascular dysfunction, risk for
Personal identity disturbance
Poisoning, risk for
Post-trauma response
Powerlessness
Protection, altered
Rape-trauma syndrome
Rape-trauma syndrome: compound reaction
Rape-trauma syndrome: silent reaction
Relocation stress syndrome
Role performance, altered

NANDA-Approved Nursing Diagnoses

Activity intolerance
Activity intolerance, risk for
Adaptive capacity, decreased: intracranial
Adjustment, impaired
Airway clearance, ineffective
Anxiety
Aspiration, risk for
Body image disturbance
Body temperature, altered, risk for
Bowel incontinence
Breastfeeding, effective
Breastfeeding, ineffective
Breastfeeding, interrupted
Breathing pattern, ineffective
Cardiac output, decreased
Caregiver role strain
Caregiver role strain, risk for
Communication, impaired verbal
Community coping, potential for enhanced
Community coping, ineffective
Confusion, acute
Confusion, chronic
Constipation
Constipation, colonic
Constipation, perceived
Coping, defensive
Coping, family: potential for growth
Coping; ineffective family: compromised
Coping; ineffective family: disabling
Coping, ineffective individual
Decisional conflict (specify)
Denial, ineffective

------------------------------ FOLD HERE ------------------------------

Self-care deficit, feeding
Self-care deficit, toileting
Self-esteem disturbance
Self-esteem, chronic low
Self-esteem, situational low
Sel-mutilation, risk for
Sensory/perceptual alterations (specify) (visual, auditory, kinesthetic, gustatory, tactile, olfactory)
Sexual dysfuncition
Sexuality patterns, altered
Skin integrity, impaired
Skin integrity, impaired, risk for
Sleep pattern disturbance
Social interaction, impaired
Social isolation
Spiritual distress (distress of the human spirit)
Spiritual well-being, potential for enhanced
Suffocation, risk for
Swallowing, impaired
Thermoregulation, ineffective
Thought processes, altered
Tissue integrity, impaired
Tissue perfusion, altered (specify type) (renal, cerebral, cardiopulmonary, gastrointestinal, peripheral)
Trauma, risk for
Unilateral neglect
Urinary elimination, altered
Urinary retention
Ventilation, inability to sustain spontaneous
Ventilatory weaning reponse, dysfunction (DVWR)
Violence risk for: self-directed or directed at others

Review side effects of medications (e.g., gastrointestinal irritation from NSAIDs).

Teach patient/significant other to record in pain log medication taken and missed.

Discourage patient from discontinuing medications without consulting physician.

Makes and keeps appointment to evaluate compliance with regimen

Make appointment to interview patient and conduct "pill count" to evaluate compliance with medication regimen. *Patient interview is the most accurate measure of compliance.*

REFERENCES

Conn VS, Taylor SG, Kelley S: Medication regimen complexity and adherence among older adults, *Image J Nurs Schol* 23(4):231-235, 1991.

Hegyvary ST: Patient care outcomes related to management of symptoms, *Annu Rev Nurs Res* 11:145-68, 1993.

Keeling A and others: Noncompliance revisited: a disciplinary perspective of a nursing diagnosis, *Nurs Diagn* 4(3):91-98, 1993.

Kison C: Health beliefs and compliance of cardiac patients, *Appl Nurs Res* 5(4):181-185, 1992.

McCloskey JC, Bulechek GM: Self-modification assistance. In *Nurs interventions classification (NIC)*, St Louis, 1996, Mosby.

Miller P, Wikoff R, Hiatt A: Fishbein's model of reasoned action and compliance behavior of hypertensive patients, *Nurs Res* 41(2):104-109, 1991.

Reodeker NS: Health beliefs and adherence to chronic illness, *Image J Nurs Schol* 20(1):31-35, 1988.

Roberson MHB: The meaning of compliance: patient perspective, *Qual Health Res* 2(1):7-26, 1992.

Rogers A, Caruso CC, Aldrich MS: Reliability of sleep diaries for assessment of sleep/wake patterns, *Nurs Res* 42(6):368-372, 1993.

Wewers ME, Lowe NK: A critical review of visual analogue scales in the measurement of clinical phenomena, *Res Nurs Health* 13:227, 1990.

Simons MR: Interventions related to compliance. In Bulechek GM, McCloskey JC, eds: Symposium on nursing interventions *Nurs Clin North Am* 27(2):477-494, 1992.

Noncompliance (therapeutic regimen)—cont'd

Nutrition, altered: less than body requirements

CLINICAL CONDITION/ MEDICAL DIAGNOSIS	RELATED FACTORS
Chronic obstructive lung disease; oxygen dependent	Inadequate intake of nutrients
	Gastric distress

Patient goals
Expected outcomes
    Associated nursing/collaborative interventions *and scientific rationale*

Consume a well-balanced, high-calorie diet (2400 calories) as evidenced by:

Weight remains plus or minus three pounds from current and increases by one to two pounds per month

Teach use of food diary *to facilitate self-monitoring.*

Analyze with patient and wife the food diary weekly. *Documenting oral intake and patient's progress facilitates early detection of inadequate intake and serves as a teaching tool.*

Help patient to identify food preferences including foods high in complex carbohydrates and protein. *Several small additions, such as adding margarine or butter to hot cereal, will increase the caloric intake.*

Teach importance of oral hygiene before meals *to enhance taste.*

Encourage a pattern of four to six small meals per day after rest periods. *Several small meals and snacks are less fatiguing than three large meals.*

Schedule bronchodilators and steroids with food/ milk products *to reduce the gastric irritation.*

Establish a dietary prescription in collaboration with a dietician.

Establish a pattern of rest and activity as evidenced by:

Participates in activities of enjoyment and necessity

Teach pacing of ADLs.

Teach appropriate use of oxygen to increase ability to engage in exercise. *Independence in self-care will maximize the patient's self-esteem.*

Teach/monitor inspiratory muscle-training exercises as appropriate. *Increasing inspiratory muscle strength can help reduce shortness of breath.*

Teach patient self-care practices to prevent respiratory infection. If bronchitis develops, consult physician for antibiotic prescription as appropriate. *Infection increases the work of breathing.*

Facilitate patient's enrollment in an outpatient pulmonary rehabilitation program. *Group interactions provide reinforcement and support and an opportunity for socialization.*

Explain/review use of exercise log. *Exercise log reinforces positive behavior and promotes motivation.*

REFERENCES

Birchenall J, Streight M: *Care of the older adult,* ed 3, Philadelphia, 1993, JB Lippincott.

Bodkin NI, Hansen BC: Nutritional studies in nursing, *Ann Rev Nurs Res* 9:203-220, 1991.

Chiang L, Ku N, Lo CK: Clinical validation of the etiologies and defining characteristics of altered nutrition: less than body requirements in patients with cancer. In Carroll-Johnson RM, ed: *Classification of nursing diagnoses: proceedings of the tenth conference,* Philadelphia, 1992, JB Lippincott.

Rankin S, Stallings K: *Patient education—issues, principles, practices,* ed 3, Philadelphia, 1996, JB Lippincott.

Stoller J, Aboussouan L: Chronic obstructive lung diseases: emphysema, chronic bronchitis, bronchiectasis, and cystic fibrosis. In George R and others, eds: *Chest medicine,* ed 3, Baltimore, 1995, Williams and Wilkins.

Townsend C: *Nutrition and diet therapy,* ed 6, Albany, NY, 1994, Delmar.

Nutrition, altered: more than body requirements

CLINICAL CONDITION/ MEDICAL DIAGNOSIS	RELATED FACTORS
Obesity	Long-established overeating habits; no regular pattern of exercise

Patient goals
Expected outcomes
> Associated nursing/collaborative interventions *and scientific rationale*

Verbalize need to lose weight

Demonstrates commitment to lose weight

> Assist patient to identify relationship between current health problems and excess weight.
>
> Explore motivation to lose weight.
>
> Reinforce commitment to lose weight. *Motivation occurs when the patient identifies a significant need.*
>
> Establish written contract with patient to use techniques to modify eating behaviors. *Provides patient and nurse with clear expectations about the agreed-on goals and responsibilities each has in moving toward weight loss.*

Eat a well-balanced diet as evidenced by:

Choose foods from the food pyramid groups

> Teach use of food diary *to facilitate self-monitoring.*
>
> Analyze food diary with patient weekly. Include food eaten, time of day, surroundings, circumstances, and where eating occurs.
>
> Suggest techniques to change diet and eating behaviors.
>
> Identify low-calorie food preferences. *Identifying food preferences increases likelihood of compliance.*
>
> Encourage water consumption to eight glasses a day. *This provides adequate hydration necessary for body metabolism.*

Participate in activities to increase metabolic rate as evidenced by the following:

Increases use of energy utilization techniques

Explore current level of activity.

Discuss with patient methods to increase energy utilization techniques such as parking the car well away from an entrance, using stairs instead of elevators, and walking to work or shopping instead of driving. *Initially, increasing energy utilization techniques is easier to accomplish than a formal exercise program and provides positive reinforcement.*

Encourage patient to commit to using at least one energy utilization technique. *Commitment increases likelihood of follow-through.*

Praise patient accomplishments. *This provides positive reinforcement.*

Engages in regular exercise for 20 minutes at least three times a week

Explain relationship between exercise, weight loss, and hypertension. *Knowledge increases likelihood of compliance.*

Offer pamphlets/samples of exercise.

Encourage patient to decide on exercise regimen. *Patient involvement increases adherence to exercise program.*

Review use of exercise log. *Exercise log reinforces positive behavior and promotes motivation.*

Review health precautions to take when exercising (e.g., check pulse, stop exercising if experiencing muscle or chest pain).

Achieve gradual weight loss to 20% to 30% over ideal weight as evidenced by:

Loses 1 to 2 pounds per week

Monitor weight weekly or twice weekly *to provide feedback/reinforcement.*

REFERENCES

Bodkin NI, Hansen BC: Nutritional studies in Nursing, *Annu Rev Nurs Res* 9:203-220, 1991.

Gabello W: Dietary counseling, *Patient Care* 27(5):168, 1993.

Nutrition, altered: more than body requirements—cont'd

Hanson MJS: Modifiable risk factors for coronary heart disease in women, *Am J Crit Care* (3):177-184.

Olson A: Women and weight control. In McElmurry BJ and Parker RS, editors: *Annual review of women's health,* 1993.

Rankin S, Stallings K: *Patient education—issues, principles, practices,* ed 3, Philadelphia, 1996, JB Lippincott.

Robison J and others: Redefining success in obesity intervention: the new paradigm, *J Am Diet Assoc* 95(4):422, 1995.

Townsend C: *Nutrition and diet therapy,* ed 6, Albany, NY, 1994, Delmar.

Vickers MJ: Understanding obesity in women, *J Obstet Gynecol Neonatal Nurs* 22(1):17, 1993.

Wadden TA and others: Relationship of dieting history to resting metabolic rate, body condition, eating behavior and subsequent weight loss, *Am J Clin Nutr* 56:2035-2085, 1992.

Nutrition, altered: risk for more than body requirements

CLINICAL CONDITION/ MEDICAL DIAGNOSIS	RISK FACTORS
Obesity	Disruption of significant relationship
	Dysfunctional pattern of intake

Patient goals
Expected outcomes
   Associated nursing/collaborative interventions *and*
      scientific rationale

Alter pattern of intake as evidenced by the following:

Holds present weight for 1 week followed by loss of 1 to 2 lb per week until desired weight is achieved

Verbalizes the relationship between experience of loss and pattern of intake

   Develop a method for patient to keep a daily
      record of intake and cues associated with intake.
   Analyze weekly log to determine relationship of
      patient's feelings to pattern of intake.
   Have patient identify desired weight.
   Contract with patient for desired weekly weight
      loss.
   Develop with patient a diet prescription.
   Evaluate patterns of intake.
Limits alcohol intake to one drink, containing no more than 1 oz of alcohol, per week
   Alert patient to dangers of using alcohol as a
      coping strategy.
   Have patient log alcohol intake along with food
      intake.

Increase energy expenditure as evidenced by the following:

Translates awareness of need for increased physical activity into common energy-expending activities (e.g., uses stairs, walks to grocery store)

325

Participates in energy-expending diversional activities for 30 minutes daily

Help patient to identify, select, and participate in one or more energy-expending activities on a daily basis. Record activity, type, and length.

Monitor involvement in selected activities.

Patients need help incorporating exercise into their daily lives. Planning to exercise three times a week is more difficult to implement than exercising daily, that is, making a lifestyle change.

Engage in relationships that facilitate positive coping as evidenced by the following:

Seeks support and assistance from selected relationships

Assist patient in identifying pattern of social relationships.

Help patient to verbalize his/her responses to efforts to increase or strengthen social network.

Maintain an atmosphere of genuineness, empathy, and unconditional positive regard.

Monitor influence of social interaction on food intake.

REFERENCES

Allan JD: Exercise program. In Bulechek GM, McClosky JC, eds: *Nursing interventions—essential nursing treatments,* ed 2, Philadelphia, 1992, WB Saunders.

Bodkin WL, Hansen BC: Nutritional studies in nursing, *Annu Rev Nurs Res* 9:203, 1991.

Crist JK: Weight management. In Bulechek GM, McCloskey JC, eds: *Nursing interventions—essential nursing treatments,* ed. 2, Philadelphia, 1992, WB Saunders.

Miller KD: Compulsive overeating, *Nurs Clin North Am* 26(3):677-697, 1991.

Riley EA: Codependency and the eating disorder client, *Nurs Clin North Am* 26(3):765, 1991.

Wadden TA and others: Relationship of dieting history to resting metabolic rate, body composition, eating behavior and subsequent weight loss, *Am J Clin Nutr* 56:2035-2085, 1992.

Oral mucous membrane, altered

CLINICAL CONDITION/ MEDICAL DIAGNOSIS	RELATED FACTORS
Cancer	Trauma associated with chemotherapy

Patient goals
Expected outcomes
    Associated nursing/collaborative interventions *and scientific rationale*

Maintain a comfortable and functional oral cavity

Demonstrates knowledge of a routine oral hygiene regimen

Provide verbal and written information on how to prevent, recognize and treat stomatitis. *Patients who received education materials have a lower incidence of severe stomatitis.*

Demonstrates absence from oral inflammation and infection

Examine oral cavity daily for inflammation, infection, or ulceration. *White or yellow patches may indicate* Candida albicans.

Establish a mouth care regimen before and after meals and at bedtime *to prevent infection.*

Increase mouth care to every 2 hours and twice at night for severe stomatitis. *Omission of oral hygiene for periods of 2 to 6 hours nullifies past benefits.*

Remove dentures. Brush, soak, and cleanse thoroughly. In case of severe stomatitis instruct patient to remove dentures for at least 8 hours daily. *Dentures will irritate inflamed mucosa and cause necrotic ulceration, bleeding, pain when eating or talking.*

Select a small soft toothbrush for removal of dental debris. To soften toothbrush, soak in hot water before brushing, and rinse in hot water during brushing. Rinse well after use and store in a cool dry place. *Toothbrushes may be contraindicated in severe stomatitis, thrombocytopenia, and neutropenia.* Use a finger wrapped in gauze to help remove dental debris.

Oral mucous membrane, altered

Use toothpaste designed for fragile, sensitive mucosa.

Use toothettes or disposable foam swabs *to stimulate gums and clean oral cavity.* Avoid use of lemon-glycerin swabs, *which irritate the oral mucosa and contribute to tooth decalcification.*

Encourage flossing between teeth twice a day with unwaxed dental floss if platelet levels are above 50,000/mm. *Unwaxed fiber strands separate when pressed against the flat tooth surface, permitting cleansing of a larger surface area.* Alternatives to unwaxed floss include waxed dental tape or a double strand of waxed floss.

Encourage frequent rinsing of mouth with mouthwashes and gargles *to cleanse the mouth, reduce microscopic flora, and soothe and relieve local discomfort.*

Chlorhexidine gluconate is an antimicrobial mouthwash that can be used prophylactically *to reduce the incidence and severity of mucositis. Solutions stronger than 0.5% may cause mucosal burning and browning of teeth.*

Sodium bicarbonate helps remove thick mucus. Mix 1 quart of lukewarm water, ½ tsp baking soda, and ½ tsp salt. Change solution daily.

Warm saline is a nonirritating and efficient way to apply heat and cleanse inflamed mucous membranes. *It is economical, readily available, isotonic, and it facilitates the granulation process.* Saline may not be effective in removing hardened crusts or debris.

Avoid the use of hydrogen peroxide solutions. *Peroxide may promote bacterial growth and destroy newly granulating cells.*

Administer oral antibacterial or antifungal agents as prescribed. *Candida albicans* can be treated with a nystatin mouth rinse or troche. Nonspecific stomatitis can be treated with a mixture of 60 ml tetracycline 125 mg, 120 ml of diphenhydramine 25 mg/10 ml, and 60 ml of kaolin-pectin.

Oral mucous membrane, altered—cont'd

Maintains symptomatic relief of mucosal dryness with moistening agents and/or agents that increase the flow of saliva

Instruct patient to avoid tobacco, alcohol, and commercial mouthwashes, *which dry the oral mucosa.* Avoid hot, coarse, spicy foods and citrus juices, *which irritate the mouth.*

Encourage patient to take frequent sips of fluids. Have a fluid available throughout the night.

Encourage the use of synthetic saliva products when mouth feels dry.

Provide hard, sour, sugarless gum or candy *to stimulate saliva production. Caution patient that the chronic use of oral lozenges and candy can lead to oral mucosal damage caused by pressure and changes in oral osmolarity.*

Provide adequate room humidification.

Apply vitamin A & D ointment in a lanolin-petrolatum–based lip balm *to keep lips moist and to promote healing of cracked lips.*

Administer sialogogues (products that increase the flow of saliva) as prescribed.

Reports oral comfort in swallowing and talking

Modify diet to include soft or pureed foods. *Foods with high water content or those served in cream sauces or gravy are easy to swallow even without normal amounts of saliva.*

Apply topical analgesics such as viscous lidocaine or administer systemic analgesics as prescribed.

REFERENCES

Graham KM and others: Reducing the incidence of stomatitis using a quality assessment and improvement approach, *Cancer Nurs* 16:2, 1993.

Hill C and others: Oral care, *Oncol Nurs Forum* 19:6, 1992.

Holmes S: The oral complications of specific anticancer therapy, *Int J Nurs Stud* 28:4, 1991.

Kenny SA: Effect of two oral care protocols on the incidence of stomatitis in hematology patients, *Cancer Nurs* 13:6, 1990.

Miaskowski C, Rostad M: Implementing the ANA/ONS Standards of Oncology Nursing Practice, *J Nurs Qual Assur* 4:3, 1990.

Weimart TA: Common ENT emergencies: the acute nose and throat, Part 2, *Emerg Med* 30:24-26, 1992.

Zebra MG and others: Relationships between oral mucositis and treatment variables in bone marrow transplant patients, *Cancer Nurs* 15:3, 1992.

Pain (acute)

CLINICAL CONDITION/ MEDICAL DIAGNOSIS	RELATED FACTORS
Inoperable cancer (2 days postoperative)	Inadequate pain relief from as needed analgesic
	Reluctance to take pain medication

Patient goals
Expected outcomes
>   Associated nursing/collaborative interventions *and*
>   *scientific rationale*

Obtain pain relief in hospital and at home as evidenced by the following:

Verbalizes comfort and pain relief after taking analgesic
Reports 3 to 4 hours of uninterrupted sleep at night

>   Collaborate with physician to establish a regular schedule for administration of parenteral and/or oral narcotics.
>
>   Collaborate with physician to provide upward adjustment of dose when substituting oral for parenteral narcotic.
>
>   Use a flow sheet to monitor pain in terms of quality, intensity, duration, and effects of narcotics and comfort measures *to determine adequacy of pain medication.*
>
>   Teach patient/significant other to continue scheduled narcotic use at home to maximize pain relief.
>
>   Find ways to overcome reluctance to taking pain medication.
>
>   Provide patient/significant other with verbal and/or written, accurate information about narcotic analgesics.
>
>   Teach concept of "rescue" dose when using extended-release oral morphine. *"Rescue" dose of immediate-release oral morphine will relieve breakthrough pain.*

Pain (acute)

Assist patient/significant other with downward adjustment of narcotic (if indicated) after completion of chemotherapy. *Collaboration with physician and patient/significant other provides opportunity for joint evaluation of analgesic regimen.*

Augment narcotic-induced pain relief as evidenced by the following:

Uses music tapes, television, and radio for diversion
Learns/uses progressive muscle relaxation
Collaborates with nurse to test/evaluate selected cognitive and physical measures to augment comfort and pain control

Teach patient use of selected strategies to augment pain relief (relaxation, guided imagery, diversion). *Diversion through use of auditory stimulation (music) may augment pain relief by release of endorphins.*

Evaluate use of physical measures, (massage, heat, etc.) to increase patient comfort.

Teach patient/significant other to use daily log of pain and activities to determine what precipitates/relieves pain.

Teach family members to use back massage and other comfort-inducing measures. *Use of comfort measures such as back rub, massage, or clean sheets may facilitate restful night's sleep and increase ability to cope with pain.*

REFERENCES

Acute Pain Management Guideline Panel: *Acute pain management: operative or medical procedures and trauma. Clinical practice guidelines,* AHCPR Pub. No. 92-0032. Rockville, Md, 1992, Agency for Health Care Policy and Research, Public Health Service, US Department of Health and Human Services.

Davis GC: The meaning of pain management: a concept analysis, *Adv Nurs Sci* 15(1):77-86, 1992.

Fortin JD, Schwartz-Barcott D, Rossi S: The postoperative pain experience, *Clin Nurs Res* 1(3):292-304, 1992.

Good M: A comparison of the effects of jaw relaxation and music on postoperative pain, *Nurs Res* 44(1):52-57, 1995.

Greipp ME: Undermedication for pain: an ethical model, *Adv Nurs Sci* 15(1):44-53, 1992.

Herr KA, Mobily PR: Comparison of selected pain assessment tools for use with elderly, *Appl Nurs Res* 6(1):39-46, 1993.

Hegyvary ST: Patient care outcomes related to management of symptoms, *Annu Rev Nurs Res* 11:145-168, 1993.

Pain (acute)—cont'd

Kolcaba KY: Holistic comfort: operationalizing the construct as a nurse-sensitive outcome, *Adv Nurs Sci* 15(1):1-10, 1992.

McCaffery M, Ferral BR: How to use the new AHCPR guidelines, *AJN* 94(7):42-47, 1994.

McCloskey JC, Bulechek GM: Pain management. In *Nursing interventions classification (NIC)*, ed 2, St Louis, 1996, Mosby.

McDonald DH: Gender and ethnic stereotyping and narcotic analgesic administration, *Res Nurs Health* 17:45-49, 1994.

Morse JM, Bottorff JL, Hutchinson S: The paradox of comfort, *Nurs Res* 44(1):14-19, 1995.

Passero CL: How to calculate a rescue dose, *AJN* 41:65-66, 1996.

Scandrett-Hibdon S, Uecker S: Relaxation training. In Bulechek GM, McCloskey JC, eds: *Nursing interventions—essential nursing treatments*, ed 2, Philadelphia, 1992, WB Saunders.

Sieggreen M and others: Pain: report of a work group. In Rantz MJ, LeMone P: *Classification of nursing diagnoses: proceedings of the eleventh conference*, Glendale, Calif, 1995, CINAHL.

Simon JM, Nolan L, Bauman MA: Validation of the nursing diagnoses acute pain and chronic pain. In Rantz MJ, LeMone P, eds: *Classification of nursing diagnoses: proceedings of the eleventh conference*, Glendale, Calif, 1995, CINAHL.

Taylor G: Pain, *Annu Rev Nurs Res* 5:23, 1987.

Whipple B, Glynn NJ: Quantification of the effects of listening to music as a noninvasive method of pain control, *Schol Inq Nurs Pract* 6(1):43-58, 1992.

Villarruel AM: Mexican-American cultural meanings, expressions, self-care and dependent-care actions associated with experiences of pain, *Res Nurs Health* 18(5):427-436, 1995.

Pain (acute)—cont'd

Pain, chronic

CLINICAL CONDITION/ MEDICAL DIAGNOSIS	RELATED FACTORS
Laminectomy	Inadequate knowledge of chronic pain management

Patient goals
Expected outcomes
> Associated nursing/collaborative interventions *and scientific rationale*

Take an active role in pain management as evidenced by the following:

Identifies measures that have helped relieve pain in the past

Verbalizes desire to gain control over pain

> Elicit patient's ideas about measures to control pain.
>
> Pay attention to language used to describe pain and its severity.
>
> Teach early intervention in the pain experience.
>
> Elicit patient's knowledge of analgesics and nonsteroidal antiinflammatory drugs (NSAIDs) used to control pain.

Records pain episodes, measures used to control pain, and pain relief

> Teach and monitor use of pain log to record type of pain, measures used to control pain, and pain relief obtained. *Recording pain experiences and measures used to relieve pain increases patient's perception of control.*
>
> Teach and monitor use of pain log to record all medications patient is taking. *Combinations of prescription and over-the-counter drugs place individuals at risk for adverse drug reactions.*
>
> Teach patient to self-monitor for side effects of medications, such as gastrointestinal irritation. *Long-term users of NSAIDs may require a medication to inhibit gastric acid secretion, such as ranitidine (Zantac).*

Pain, chronic—cont'd

Implement a mutually established pain management program as evidenced by the following:

Collaborates with physician and pharmacist in selection of cost-effective analgesic/NSAID

Expresses willingness to try new strategies to augment pain relief

Practices and records relaxation with music sessions in pain log

Uses heat and rest to augment pain relief

Discuss importance of trying a pain-control technique more than one time. *Pain relief obtained from a pain control measure may differ from day to day; measure may not be effective the first time used.*

Coach and monitor relaxation practice sessions. Instruct in safe use of heating pad; use moist heat (e.g., Thermophore, a heating pad with special cover). *Moist heat helps to relieve pain and promotes relaxation/rest.*

REFERENCES

Hegyvary ST: Patient care outcomes related to management and symptoms, *Ann Rev Nurs* 11:145-168, 1993.

Jacox A: Pain control. In Bulechek GM, McCloskey JC: *Nursing interventions: essential nursing treatments,* Philadelphia, 1992, WB Saunders.

Kolcaba KY: Holistic comfort: operationalizing the construct as a nurse-sensitive outcome, *Adv Nurs Sci* 15(1):1-10, 1992.

Mahon SM: Concept analysis of pain: implications related to nursing diagnosis, *Nurs Diagn* 5(1):14-25, 1994.

McCaffery M, Ferral BR: How to use the new AHCPR guidelines, *AJN* 94(7):42-47, 1994.

McCloskey JC, Bulechek GM: Pain management. *Nursing interventions classification (NIC),* ed 2, St Louis, 1996, Mosby.

McDonald DH: Gender and ethnic stereotyping and narcotic analgesic administration, *Res Nurs Health* 17(1):45-49, 1994.

Moran KJ: The effects of self-guided imagery and other-guided imagery on chronic low back pain. In Funk SG and others, eds: *Key aspects of comfort,* New York, 1989, Springer.

Pain Management Guideline Panel: *Acute pain management: Operative or medical procedures and trauma. Clinical practice guidelines.* AHCPR Pub. No. 92-0032. Rockville, Md, 1992, Agency for Health Care Policy and Research, Public Health Service, US Department of Health and Human Services.

Pollow RL and others: Drug combinations and potential for risk of adverse drug reaction among community-dwelling elderly, *Nurs Res* 43(1):44-49, 1994.

Pain, chronic—cont'd

Schoor JA: Music and pattern change in chronic pain, *Adv Nurs Sci* 15(4):27-36, 1993.

Simon JM, Nolan L, Bauman MA: Validation of the nursing diagnoses acute pain and chronic pain. In Rantz MJ, LeMone P, eds: *Classification of nursing diagnoses: proceedings of the eleventh conference,* Glendale, Calif, 1995, CINAHL.

Sieggreen M, and others: Pain. Report of a work group. In Rantz MJ, LeMone P. *Classification of nursing diagnoses: proceedings of the eleventh conference,* Glendale, Calif, 1995, CINAHL.

Vallerand AH: Gender differences in pain, *Image: J Nurs Scholar* 7(3):235-237, 1995.

Whipple B: Methods of pain control: review of research and literature, *Image: J Nurs Scholar* 19(3):142, 1987.

Wild LR: Caveat emptor: a critical analysis of the costs of drugs used for pain management, *Adv Nurs Sci* 16(1):52-61, 1993.

Parent/infant/child attachment, altered: risk for

CLINICAL CONDITION/ MEDICAL DIAGNOSIS	RISK FACTORS
Prematurity	Separation

Patient goals
Expected outcomes
> Associated nursing/collaborative interventions *and scientific rationale*

Share feelings about altered parental role as evidenced by:

Verbalize experience of pregnancy and delivery

Provide an opportunity for parents to discuss their feelings about their high-risk pregnancy and premature delivery. *Parents are often unprepared for the premature birth and have unresolved pregnancy and childbirth issues in the immediate postpartum period.*

Help parents examine reasons for their infant's premature birth. *Feeling guilty is a common response after a premature birth. Self-blame may offer some parents a sense of control over the future.*

Express feelings about having a hospitalized premature infant

Create a caring environment so that parents will feel comfortable sharing their feelings.

Validate the emotional reactions of parents by informing them about the common responses about premature infants. *Parents of premature infants express feelings of disappointment, helplessness, isolation, uncertainty about the infant's survival and prognosis, and loss of the role as primary caregiver for their infant.*

Monitor parents' response to having a preterm infant, accepting individual and gender differences in coping styles. *There is variability in parents' adaptation to the premature birth. There are no prescribed stages of parental adjustment to a premature birth.*

Accept parents' need to ask questions about other infants in the unit. *Parents cope by comparing their infant's condition to that of other infants in the unit.*

Refer parents to parent support groups or other parents of premature infants.

Refer parents to appropriate religious support. *Seeking religious explanations for the premature birth is a coping strategy for some parents.*

Utilize support systems

Assist parents to share information with family, friends, and other parents. *Assisting parents to provide information may enhance the support they receive from others.*

Refer to social services as needed.

Parents will acquire adequate information as evidenced by the following:

Become familiar with the hospital unit environment

Acquaint parents with the environment of the hospital unit. *The sights and sounds of the hospital unit are stressors for parents.*

Introduce parents to the personnel of the unit and explain each staff member's role and any rotating patterns of staffing.

Use written and audiovisual materials to educate and reinforce parent teaching.

Learn about the infant's condition

Provide parents with complete and honest information, and arrange periodic patient care conferences with the parents. *Information should be provided in a respectful, unbiased, and caring manner that allows parents to communicate their feelings, ideas, and questions.*

Provide consistent information between health care members, avoiding any criticism of each other's care.

Acquaint parents with the infant's physical appearance and behaviors by performing a physical examination of the infant in the presence of the parents. *The infant's physical appearance and behaviors are stressors for parents.*

Emphasize the individual behavioral responses of the infant, including those infant cues that signal appropriate stimulation. *Parents usually elicit positive behaviors in their infants, such as smiling, which promote parent-infant attachment. However, some parents may not be able to elicit positive behaviors due to a lack of knowledge about appropriate infant stimulation and therefore, need education.*

Participate in the care of their infant as evidenced by the following:

Express desired level of participation in the care of their infant

Ask parents how often they wish to call and visit.

Identify any circumstances that may affect the parent's ability to call or visit. *Other life stressors or inadequate child care for other children may make it difficult for parents to visit their infant frequently.*

Monitor parents' desired level of participation in care and decision making, including when the parents want to be notified of changes in the condition or treatment of their infant. *Parents desire different levels of involvement in the care of their hospitalized infant.*

Participate in setting visitation rights and limits to their infant

Support parents' need for unrestricted visitation.

Arrange unit activities, such as patient care rounds or unit meetings, so that parents do not have to leave their infant's bedside during the activity.

Ask parents to identify those other individuals who have the parents' permission to visit their infant. *Parents, not unit personnel, should identify appropriate visitors for the infant.*

Have adequate resources for visiting and caring for their infant

Assess any financial concerns. *Parents may lack the financial resources to travel to the hospital or care for their infant after discharge.*

Refer to appropriate resources.

Demonstrate attachment behaviors to the infant

Allow the parents to visit the infant soon after the

infant's admission to the unit and to hold the infant when the infant is stabilized. *Attachment behaviors include maintaining close proximity to the infant.*

Remove mechanical barriers such as non–life-sustaining equipment and phototherapy lights.

Provide photographs of the infant.

Visit the mother in her hospital room if she is unable to visit her infant, and transport the infant to her room when the infant's condition permits.

Call the parents if they are unable to call or visit their infant.

Encourage parents to name their infant, and refer to the infant by his or her name.

Participate in infant caregiving from the beginning of the infant's hospitalization

Encourage parents to participate in caregiving to the infant. *Caregiving is one component of the parental role, and an alteration in the parental role is a stressor for parents of premature infants.*

Offer parents the opportunity to participate in infant caregiving during the acute and convalescent stages of hospitalization. *Mastery of the new parental role cannot be achieved without direct participation in caregiving.*

Schedule appointments for parents to learn or participate in infant caregiving.

Plan infant caregiving, such as bathing and feeding, at the time of the parents' visits.

Encourage parents to participate in caregiving that is exclusively within the domain of the parents, such as skin-to-skin contact and breastfeeding. *Mothers of premature infants have commented that breastfeeding is the one activity that only they can do for their infant.*

Reinforce parents' success in infant caregiving. *Positive feedback enhances self-esteem and competence, and increased competence facilitates attachment.*

Document parent caretaking so that the parents' ability to provide care to their infant is consistently supported by the hospital staff. *Parents should have adequate opportunity to master those infant caregiving activities required after discharge.*

Parents view themselves as the primary nurturer and caregiver for the infant as evidenced by the following:

View the nurse as a professional rather than as a substitute parent for their infant

> Establish "milestone" caregiving activities for which the parents want to be a participant, such as the first tub bath. *Parents mourn the loss of the anticipated role as primary caregiver, and have blurred boundaries between themselves and the nurse.*
>
> Request parents' permission before photographing their infant for special holidays, such as Christmas.
>
> Provide only those clothes and toys that parents have purchased or approved for the infant.
>
> Maintain a professional relationship with the infant and family.

REFERENCES

Affleck G, Tennen H: The effect of newborn intensive care on parents' psychological well-being, *Child Health Care* 20(1):6, 1991.

Affonso DD, Hurst I, Mayberry LJ, Haller L, Yost K, Lynch ME: Stressors reported by mothers of hospitalized premature infants, *Neonatal Netw* 11(6):63, 1992.

Affonso D, Bosque E, Wahlberg V, Brady JP: Reconciliation and healing for mothers through skin-to-skin contact provided in an American tertiary level intensive care nursery, *Neonatal Netw* 12(3):25, 1993.

Brady-Fryer B: Becoming the mother of a preterm baby. In Field PA, Marck PB, eds: *Uncertain motherhood: negotiating the risks of the childbearing years,* Thousand Oaks, Calif, 1994, Sage.

Griffin T: Nurse barriers to parenting in the special care nursery, *J Perinatal Neonatal Nurs* 4(2):56, 1990.

Harrison H: The principles of family-centered neonatal care, *Pediatrics* 92(5):643, 1993.

Hayes N, Stainton MC, McNeil D: Caring for a chronically ill infant: a paradigm case of maternal rehearsal in the neonatal intensive care unit, *J Pediat Nurs* 8(6):355, 1993.

McNeil D: Uncertainty, waiting, and possibilities: Experiences of becoming a mother with an infant in the NICU, *Neonatal Netw* 11(7):78, 1992.

Mercer RT, Ferketich SL: Predictors of parental attachment during early parenthood, *J Adv Nurs* 15:268, 1990.

Miles MS, Funk SG, Kasper MA: The stress response of mothers and fathers of preterm infants, *Res Nurs Health* 15:261, 1992.

Miller DB, Holditch-Davis D: Interactions of parents and nurses with high-risk preterm infants, *Res Nurs Health* 15:187, 1992.

Sharp MC, Strauss RP, Lorch SC: Communicating medical bad news: parents' experiences and preferences, *J Pediatr* 121:539, 1992.

Parent/infant/child attachment, altered: risk for—cont'd

DONNA M. DIXON, KAREN KAVANAUGH, AND ALICE M. TSE

Parental role conflict

CLINICAL CONDITION/ MEDICAL DIAGNOSIS	RELATED FACTORS
Childhood chronic illness	Home care of a child with special technologic needs

Patient goals
Expected outcomes
> Associated nursing/collaborative interventions *and scientific rationale*

Participate in technology-related care as evidenced by the following:

Maintains desired levels of participation with health professionals

Participates in routine and complex caretaking activities

Makes independent, safe decisions related to acute episodes of the illness, equipment malfunction, or need for professional assistance

Adapts information for the development of a personal style of performing skills

> Monitor parents' desired level of participation in care and decision making.
>
> Provide consistent contact with health professionals for information gathering and follow-up.
>
> Determine style of parental relationship with health professionals, for example, silent in care, recipients of care, monitors of care, and managers of care, *because they differ according to the level of trust in professionals, information gathering style, and decision-making patterns.*
>
> Monitor knowledge base and competency related to equipment and required technical care.
>
> Assess level of anxiety related to skill performance.
>
> Teach equipment operation, maintenance, safety, and necessary backup.
>
> Teach CPR as necessary.
>
> Provide opportunities to master required home health-care skills when the child is hospitalized.

Parental role conflict

Teach factors that increase frequency of complications, such as exposure to infections and immobility.

Review management of acute episodes.

Evaluate parents' understanding of special care and provide clarification as needed. *Learning is a complex process that requires time for integration into the family's current lifestyle. Continual assessment of barriers to learning, anxiety and competency enhance the process.*

Develop plans for ordering supplies and contacting vendors.

Express feelings and concerns about parental role demands as evidenced by the following:

Verbalizes feelings and perceptions of self, role change, fears, and level of stress

Maintains roles of primary caretaker, educator, protector, and disciplinarian

Has adequate financial resources

Has minimal health problems related to stress

Maintains desired level of contact with significant others for emotional and caretaking support

Monitor parents' perception of current situation as they compare with previous parenting patterns.

Help parents to verbalize any fears, expectations for the future, and feelings of isolation and overwhelming responsibility.

Determine extended family and friends' positive and negative reactions to child's situation.

Assist the parents to involve the child in age-appropriate self-care and home responsibilities.

Discuss ways to maintain appropriate parent-child relationship without overprotectiveness, guilt, or anger.

Assess financial status and concerns and refer to appropriate resources.

Counsel parents to develop strategies for the future to facilitate expression of feelings and concerns.

Refer to support groups and parents in similar situations as available and desired by the parents.

Assess involvement in community religious groups.

Teach parents about specific strategies used by families in difficult situations, such as acquiring social support, reframing, seeking social support, mobilizing of family to acquire and accept support and passive appraisal. *Families of technology-assisted children often lack financial resources, feel isolated, receive unwanted advice from others, and expend tremendous energy mobilizing community assistance and support.*

Incorporate technology in family life as evidenced by the following:

Evaluates family boundaries, goals, patterns of interaction, and values in relation to the health of the child

Develops adjustment strategies and problem-solving and adaptive coping skills

Integrates new patterns of behavior and responsibility into individual, family, and school routines

Assist family to identify stressors and strains related to incorporation of the technology, specific strengths related to the stage of development/ career, and resources. *Long-term effects of pediatric home care vary over time and warrant continual reevaluation.*

Assist family to determine their accord about competencies as a family, such as quality of marital communication, shared orientation to childrearing and illness management, and satisfaction with quality of life. *Adaptability is the ability of the family to reorganize its power structure, roles, and rules. Emotional bonding, boundaries, supports, and time for recreation influence family cohesion.*

Help parents incorporate necessary lifestyle changes.

Provide anticipatory guidance regarding schooling and/or child care.

Help family to plan and implement necessary social and environmental adaptations at home and school.

Assist parents to involve siblings in the care of the child and home responsibilities.

Assist parents to involve the child in age-appropriate self-care and home responsibilities. *A family management style develops when a family incorporates the care of a chronically ill child.*

REFERENCES

Christian BJ: Quality of life and family relationships in families coping with their child's chronic illness. In Funk SG and others: *Key aspects of caring for the chronically ill: hospital and home,* New York, 1994, Springer.

Cohen MH: The unknown and the unknowable—managing sustained uncertainty, *West J Nurs Res* 15(10):77-96, 1993.

Copeland LG: Caring for children with chronic conditions: model of critical times. *Holistic Nurs Prac* 8(1):45-55, 1993.

Gibson CH: The process of empowerment in mothers of chronically ill children, *J Adv Nurs* 21:1201-1210, 1995.

Jerret MD: Parents' experience of coming to know the care of a chronically ill child, *J Adv Nurs* 19:1050-1056, 1994.

Knafl KA, Cavallari KA, Dixon DM: *Pediatric hospitalization: family and nurse perspectives,* Glenview, Ill, 1988, Scott Foresman.

LaMontagne LL, Johnson BD, Hepworth JT: Evolution of parental stress and coping processes: a framework for critical care practice, *J Ped Nurs* 10(4):212-221, 1995.

Miles MS, Frauman AC: Nurses' and parents' negotiation of caregiving roles for medically fragile infants: barriers and bridges. In Funk SG and others: *Key aspects of caring for the chronically ill: hospital and home,* New York, 1994, Springer.

Ray LD, Ritchie JA: Caring for chronically ill children at home: factors that influence parents' coping, *J Ped Nurs* 8(4):217-225, 1993.

Thorne SE: *Negotiating health care: the social context of chronic illness,* Newbury Park, Calif, 1993, Sage.

Parental role conflict—cont'd

Parenting, altered

CLINICAL CONDITION/ MEDICAL DIAGNOSIS	RELATED FACTORS
Mother experiencing major depression	Inadequate role identity; unrealistic expectations

Patient goals
Expected outcomes
> Associated nursing/collaborative interventions *and scientific rationale*

Provide safe environment for child as evidenced by the following:

Remains physically and psychologically safe

Provide physically and psychologically safe environment for the child, which is the basic function of a parent.

Assess degree of risk to child's physical and psychological safety.

Contact other family members or appropriate authorities if child's safety seems jeopardized. *Deficiencies in this area may range from routinely ignoring a child's diet or personal hygiene to homes with multiple safety hazards to severe physical abuse.*

Provide interventions that are designed to focus the parent's awareness of the child's needs. In situations where the parent(s) cannot provide for the minimum safety and physiologic needs of the child, mechanisms designed by the community must be engaged to remove the child to a safer environment.

Achieve role identity as parent as evidenced by the following:

Identifies socially expected parenting behaviors

Identify major components and priorities within role identity (i.e., child of one's parents, spouse, career identity).

Identify source of verbalized "ideal" parenting behavior.

Parenting, altered

Identify perception of specific parenting behaviors.

Encourage patient to verbalize presence or absence of effective role models.

Encourage patient to verbalize incongruence between "ideal" parenting behaviors and actual behaviors.

Incorporates concept of "parent" as integral part of role identity

Observe parent-child interactions for congruence between verbalized "ideal" of parent behavior and actual behavior.

Provide opportunity for parent to explore role identity through individual counseling or group interaction.

Provide learning opportunities for additional parenting behavior.

Provide opportunity for parents to observe or experience effective parenting behaviors.

Provide opportunity for parent to implement alternative parenting behaviors.

Give positive reinforcement for additional parenting behavior that will support incorporation of concept or "parent" into role identity. *Parenting is a learned behavior. In many communities the opportunity for observing parenting behavior is limited, and persons rely on their perception of how they were parented. Interventions that provide information about alternative parenting behaviors and opportunity to discuss the changes in life-style required as a parent broaden the perspective of the parent and aid in internalizing the parenting role.*

Acquire realistic expectations of self, spouse, and infant or child within family as evidenced by the following:

Develops realistic expectations of self, spouse and infant or child

Assist patient to identify present expectations of self, spouse and infant or child.

Assist patient to identify areas of failure to meet expectations of self.

Assist patient to identify areas where others fail to meet expectations.

Provide opportunity for patient to express feelings about unmet expectations.

Encourage patient to speculate on reasons for expectations being unmet.

Encourage patient to acknowledge own responsibility for attempting to meet expectations as well as realistic limits of self and others.

Help patient to develop realistic expectations as result of increased knowledge of normal development and basic needs.

Develops strategies that increase the possibility that expectations will be met

Help patient to develop alternative strategies to increase possibility of having expectations met (e.g., discussing expectations with spouse, identifying steps that must occur in order to meet expectations). *Many parents have unrealistic expectation of their role and abilities as a parent, of their spouse's role and abilities, and the role and ability of the child in the relationship. This may lead to increased frustration and anxiety as the expected behaviors are not manifested. Since anxiety is frequently transformed into anger or depression, the potential for disruption of parenting function is great. Helping the parent to identify the source of the anger and develop more realistic expectations diffuses the anxiety and offers opportunity to develop alternative behaviors.*

REFERENCES

Denehy JA: Interventions related to parent-infant attachment, *Nurs Clin North Am* 27(2):4225, 1992.

Gross D: At risk: children of the mentally ill, *J Psychosoc Nurs* 28(8):14, 1989.

Hall LA and others: Psychosocial predictors of maternal depressive symptoms, parenting attitudes, and child behavior in single-parent families, *Nurs Res* 40(4):214, 1991.

Karl D: The consequences of maternal depression for early mother-infant interaction: a nursing issue, *J Ped Nurs* 6(6):384, 1991.

Martel LK: Postpartum depression as a family problem, *MCN* 15(2):90, 1990.

McCloskey JC, Bulechek GM, eds: *Nursing interventions classification (NIC),* ed 2, St Louis, 1996, Mosby.

Parenting, altered—cont'd

Mrazek DA, Mrazek P, Kinnert M: Clinical assessment of parenting, *J Am Acad Child Adolesc Psychiatry* 34:272, 1995.

Norris DM, Hoyer PJ: Dynamism in practice: parenting within King's framework, *Nurs Sci Quart* 6(2):79, 1993.

Olshansky EF: Parenting, altered. In McFarland GK and Thomas MD: *Psychiatric mental health nursing: application of the nursing process,* New York, 1991, JB Lippincott.

Senner A: Munchausen syndrome by proxy, *Comp Ped Nurs* 12(5):345, 1989.

Parenting, altered—cont'd

Parenting, altered, risk for

CLINICAL CONDITION/ MEDICAL DIAGNOSIS	RISK FACTORS
Growing preterm infant (6 months of age)	Inadequate knowledge

Patient goals
Expected outcomes
    Associated nursing/collaborative interventions *and scientific rationale*

Acquire adequate knowledge base for effective parenting as evidenced by the following:

Verbalizes desired knowledge about specific aspects of parenting

Assist parent(s) to identify knowledge deficits related to caring for a growing preterm infant.

Identify learning readiness and learning capability of parent(s).

Provide information related to normal growth and development as well as specific information for growing preterm infant.

Teach parent(s) skills and behaviors related to caring for a growing preterm infant.

Demonstrates more effective parenting behavior, such as providing for child's physical, psychological, emotional, and social needs

Provide opportunity for parent(s) to test out new information.

Encourage age-appropriate play activities between parent(s) and child.

Encourage age-appropriate caretaking activities by parent(s). *Lack of information, lack of role models, lack of external resources, and ineffective coping skills may all be decreased through appropriate patient-education methods.*

Parenting, altered, risk for

Experience emotional, social and physical support as evidenced by the following:

Recognizes realistic limitations of self and support systems

Assist parent(s) to identify specific areas of needed emotional, social, or physical support.

Assist parent(s) to identify specific strengths of parent(s) and support systems.

Encourage parent(s) to express feelings about areas of need.

Activates additional support systems as needed

Provide information about additional resources available to meet areas of need.

Assist parent(s) to select appropriate resources to supplement self and support system.

Act as liaison or advocate as needed in obtaining help from appropriate resources. *Many of the defining characteristics of Altered Parenting are the result of insufficient emotional, social, or physical support. Persons whose own basic needs for safety, nutrition, or love have not been met will be unable to meet the needs of another. Once specific areas of deficiencies have been identified, the nurse may offer information about services available to provide the support needed.*

REFERENCES

Denehy JA: Interventions related to parent-infant attachment, *Nurs Clin North Am* 27(2):4225, 1992.

Griffin T: Nurse barriers to parenting in the special care nursery, *J Peri Neo Nurs* 4(2):56, 1990.

McCain GC: Parenting growing preterm infants, *Ped Nurs* 16(5):467, 1990.

McCloskey JC, Bulechek GM, eds: *Nursing interventions classification (NIC)*, ed 2, St Louis, 1996, Mosby.

Mrazek DA, Mrazek P, Kinnert M: Clinical assessment of parenting, *J Am Acad Child Adolesc Psychiatry* 34:272, 1995.

Younger JB: A model of parenting stress, *Res Nurs Health* 14(3):197, 1991.

Peripheral neurovascular dysfunction, risk for

CLINICAL CONDITION/ MEDICAL DIAGNOSIS	RISK FACTORS
Bone fractures of upper or lower extremity	Mechanical compression (e.g., tourniquet, cast)

Patient goals
Expected outcomes
> Associated nursing/collaborative interventions *and scientific rationale*

Maintain neurovascular integrity to the extremity as evidenced by the following:

Experiences absence of pain, pallor or cyanosis, pulse-lessness, paresthesia, and paralysis ("five P's")

> Perform neurovascular assessment every hour for first 24 hours; then every 2 hours for 8 hours; then every 4 hours. Continue as long as mechanical compression is present (extremity cast, check involved distal extremity; spica or body cast, check all 4 extremities; halo cast, check cranial nerves).

> Observe capillary filling after compression of arteries of extremity. *Failure of circulatory return to extremity when pressure is released indicates arterial injury.*

> Feel and compare temperature of both extremities.

> Observe color of skin of both extremities.

> Observe for presence and amount of edema (e.g., insert fingers under cast or measure circumference of extremities). *As swelling within muscle compartment increases, neurovascular compromise occurs.*

> Palpate and compare pulses of both extremities at least every 2 hours. Report absent or diminished pulses (1 or less on 4+ scale).

> Monitor oxygen saturation by pulse oximetry. *Oxygen saturation may be compromised even in presence of palpable peripheral pulses.*

Peripheral neurovascular dysfunction, risk for

Monitor for evidence of paresthesia, and decreased or absent sensation including 2-point discrimination. *Two-point discrimination is best check of sensitivity.*

Assess mobility of involved extremity (flexion, extension, abduction, and adduction) of fingers and toes. Bring tips of thumb and fingers together to form circle. *Impossible to perform circle maneuver if radial, ulnar, and median nerves are not intact to intrinsic muscles.*

Assess for pain out of proportion to injury. *The primary concern of neurovascular dysfunction is impairment of nerves or blood vessels distal to the area of the cast, splint, or traction. Early detection of neurovascular compromise can avoid irreversible and permanent damage.*

Progresses through cast, splint, or brace therapy without experiencing complications

Document and report immediately and persistently, if necessary, any evidence of neurovascular compromise. *Permanent and irreversible damage resulting in paresis, paralysis, or amputation can occur rapidly, within 4 to 12 hours.*

Elevate extremity to level of heart until edema is controlled. Avoid elevating above person's central venous pressure (normal CVP = 6-13 cm H₂O pressure; 2.5 cm = 1 inch). *Elevating extremity aids venous return to decrease edema. Elevating above person's CVP impedes arterial flow and increases rather than decreases edema.*

Apply icebags to lateral surfaces of cast or traction for 24 to 48 hours—avoid placing over arterial areas. *Cold decreases edema; applying over artery could impede arterial flow.*

Avoid pressure over peroneal nerve.

Observe for paresthesia at anterior surface of affected leg, dorsum of foot, and great toe and inability to dorsiflex foot or extend toes. *Pressure on peroneal nerve can result in permanent foot drop.*

Split cast down one or both sides and rewrap splint cast with elastic bandage if necessary; remove traction or splint and reapply more loosely.

Irreversible and permanent damage can result in 6 hours if pressure is not relieved.

Notifies nurse or physician of signs and symptoms of peripheral neurovascular compromise while in the hospital and after discharge

Instruct client and significant other about signs and symptoms of peripheral neurovascular compromise.

Emphasize importance of notifying nurse or physician immediately of numbness or tingling, increasing pain, increased swelling, or change in color. *Complications from cast, splint, or traction therapy can occur at any time. Changes in body weight, edema loss, and softening of the cast can create changes in neurovascular status.*

Prevent compartment syndrome and Volkmann's ischemic fracture resulting from compression or severance of an artery as evidenced by the following:

Normal compartment pressure (< 10 mm Hg), adequate tissue perfusion as noted by brisk (< 3 sec) capillary refill, and normal range of motion in all extremities

Assess for increasing and progressive pain on passive motion every 1 to 2 hours. *Pain on passive motion is earliest and most significant sign of compartment syndrome.*

Assess for evidence of pallor or cyanosis. *Tissue damage results when oxygen is reduced because of lack of blood supply; hypoxia resulting from entrapment of vessels or nerves can result in ischemic contracture or ischemic myositis.*

Immobilize traumatized extremity. *Movement of arm or leg can result in further injury to nerves and blood vessels.*

Perform and document tissue pressure readings. *Normal tissue pressure is 0 to 10 mm Hg. Increase in pressure recordings denotes impending compartment syndrome.*

Report immediately tissue pressure readings of 30 mm Hg or above. *Pressures of 30 mm Hg or above*

Peripheral neurovascular dysfunction, risk for—cont'd

can result in irreversible damage if not relieved within 6 hours; 30 mm Hg is criterion used for surgical decompression. If pressure in compartment equals diastolic blood pressure, microcirculation ceases.

REFERENCES

Anglen J, Banovetz J: Compartment syndrome in the well leg resulting from fracture—table positioning, *Clin Orthop Related Res* 301:239-242, 1994.

Harris IE: Supracondylar fractures of the humerus in children, *Orthopedics* 15:811-817, 1992.

Hawkins BJ, Bays PN: Catastrophic complication of simple cast treatment—Case report, *J Trauma* 34:760-762, 1993.

Mohler LR and others: Pressure generation beneath a new thermoplastic cast, *Clin Orthop Related Res* 322:262-267, 1996.

Myerson M, Manoli A: Compartment syndromes of the foot after calcaneal fractures, *Clin Orthop Related Res* 290:142-150, 1993.

Simpson NS, Jupiter JB: Delayed onset of forearm compartment syndrome—a complication of distal radius fracture in young adults, *J Orthop Trauma* 9:411, 1995.

Weiner G, Styf J, Nakhostine M, Gershuni DH: Effect of ankle position and a plaster cast on intramuscular pressure in human leg, *J Bone Joint Surg Am* 76A:1476-1481, 1994.

Zavotsky KE, Banavage A: Management of the patient with complex orthopedic fractures, *Orthop Nurs* 14(5):53-57, 1995.

Peripheral neurovascular dysfunction, risk for—cont'd

Personal identity disturbance

CLINICAL CONDITION/ MEDICAL DIAGNOSIS	RELATED FACTORS
Borderline personality disorder (BPD)	History of severe, traumatic interpersonal experiences

> **Patient goals**
> **Expected outcomes**
>   Associated nursing/collaborative interventions *and scientific rationale*

Maintain a positive concept of personal identity over time as evidenced by the following:

Distinguishes between self and non-self and responds to others as separate from self

Develop a trusting, accepting relationship with patient.

Support the patient's independence and autonomous ventures *to reinforce establishment of separate, differentiated relationships with others in the environment and support existing ego strengths.*

Maintain personal boundaries and clarify expectations about the nurse-patient relationship *to decrease ambivalence and anxiety.*

Encourage independent decision making, providing nonjudgmental feedback.

Integrates thoughts, emotions, and behaviors into an organized cohesive, continuing self

Show empathy and awareness of the patient's vulnerability to feelings of abandonment and aloneness. *These internal states may trigger anger, anxiety, and acting-out by the patient.*

Modify environment stressors *to decrease a sense of threat, disorganization, and overstimulation for the patient.*

Teach patient stress management strategies.

Teach patient to record thoughts and feelings *to reinforce a continuous sense of self and decrease fragmentation.*

Personal identity disturbance

Assess patient's ability to differentiate between internal and external stimuli *to evaluate reality-testing.*

Monitor mental status *to identify presence of organic causes of symptoms and reality-testing difficulties.*

Demonstrates positive acceptance and identification of self

Encourage patient to discuss personal values, beliefs, and goals for the future.

Encourage patient to discuss relationships and experiences that have influenced self-concept in order *to assess impact of events on development of self.*

Support positive self-designations and self-affirmation statements *to reinforce positive self-image and competencies.*

REFERENCES

Buck MH: The personal self. In Roy SC, Andres A, eds: *The Roy adaptation model,* Norwalk, Conn, 1991, Appleton & Lange.

Goldstein WN: The borderline patient: update on the diagnosis, theory, and treatment from a psychodynamic perspective, *Am J Psychother* 49(3):317, 1995.

Kerr NJ: Ego competency: a framework for formulating nursing care, *Perspect Psychiatr Care* 26(4):30, 1990.

Hauser ST and others: Paths of adolescent ego development: links with family life and individual adjustment, *Psychiatr Clin North Am* 13(3):489, 1990.

Kroll J: *PTSD/borderlines in therapy,* New York, Norton, 1993.

Lego S: The fear of moving beyond one's parents, *Perspect Psychiatr Care* 26(1):28, 1990.

LeMone P: Analysis of a human phenomenon: self-concept, *Nurs Diagn* 2(3):126, 1991.

Ricci MS: Aloneness in tenuous self-states, *Perspect Psychiatr Care* 27(2):7, 1991.

Sayre J: Psychodynamics revisited: an object-relations framework for psychiatric nursing, *Perspect Psychiatr Care* 26(1):7, 1990.

Sebastian L: Promoting object constancy—writing as a nursing intervention, *J Psychosoc Nurs* 29(1):21, 1991.

Poisoning, risk for

CLINICAL CONDITION/
MEDICAL DIAGNOSIS

RISK FACTORS

Elderly woman with
reduced vision and
hearing

Large stock of medications stored in
an inappropriate place; poor lighting

Patient goals
Expected outcomes
Associated nursing/collaborative interventions *and*
scientific rationale

**Adapt home environment to reduce risk of
accidental poisoning as evidenced by the following:**

Selects an appropriate storage area for medications
**Permanently removes all cleaning supplies from
bathroom**
**Discards outdated prescription and over-the-counter
drugs**
Collaborate with patient to establish a separate
storage area for medications.
Evaluate with patient contents of medicine cabinet
and discard outdated medications.
**Replaces 25- and 60-watt bulbs with 100-watt bulbs
where appropriate**
**Keeps hall and bathroom lights on during evening
and night**
**Keeps a flashlight at bedside, in kitchen, and next to
favorite chair in living room**
Teach patient to keep environment well lighted.
Assist patient with selection of places to keep flash-
lights in case of power failure.
Place list of emergency telephone numbers near
telephone.
Provide patient with information about life-line
services available from local hospital.

**Establish a safe method for taking medications as
evidenced by the following:**

**Uses magnifying glass to check contents of each bot-
tle of medication**

Poisoning, risk for

357

Sets up medications for 24-hour period in well-lighted area
Demonstrates agreed-on method to set up medications
Counts with nurse amount of medication remaining in containers

Help patient to develop a way to identify medications accurately.

Discuss and demonstrate way to set up medications for 24 hours. *Setting up medication for 24-hour period decreases risk of missing a dose or taking an extra dose.*

Monitor medication taking. *Omission of doses is the most common error in self administration of medications by elderly.*

Seek medical evaluation of reduced vision as evidenced by the following:

Schedules an appointment for visit from social worker
Makes and keeps appointment to see ophthalmologist
Family members agree to assist with transportation to keep appointments

Provide patient with list of medical and financial resources in community.

Help patient to make appointments.

Develop plan with patient and family for medical evaluation.

REFERENCES

Janken JK, Cullinan CL: Auditory sensory/perceptual alteration: suggested revision of defining characteristics, *Nurs Diagn* 1(4):147-154, 1990.

Kanak MF: Interventions related to safety, *Nurs Clin North Am* 27(2):371-396, 1992.

McCloskey JC, Bulechek GM: Surveillance: safety. In *Nursing interventions classification (NIC)*, St Louis, 1996, Mosby.

Neill KM: The need for safety. In Yura H, Walsh MB, eds: *Human needs and the nursing process,* Norwalk, Conn, 1983, Appleton-Century-Crofts.

Nelson MA: Economic impoverishment as a health risk: methodologic and conceptual issues, *Adv Nurs Sci* 16(3):1-12, 1994.

Williams MA: The physical environment and patient care, *Annu Rev Nurs Res* 6:61-84, 1988.

Poisoning, risk for—cont'd

Post-trauma response

CLINICAL CONDITION/ MEDICAL DIAGNOSIS	RELATED FACTORS
Multiple injuries	Overwhelming guilt about auto accident: temporary loss of mobility

Patient goals
Expected outcomes
    Associated nursing/collaborative interventions *and scientific rationale*

Use new coping strategies to deal with excessive feelings of guilt as evidenced by the following:

Decreases excessive verbalization of details of accident

Schedules regular visits with minister or psychologist

Develops an objective appraisal of the event

Explore guilt feelings with patient. Pace intervention to readiness for assistance. *Free expression of feelings is more productive after initial period of denial.*

Support the use of appropriate defense mechanisms.

Provide consultation or referral to deal with excessive feelings of guilt.

Maintains relationship with significant other

Contact family of significant other to obtain information about injury of significant other.

Arrange for telephone and personal visits with significant other.

Allow for privacy during interactions with significant other. *This will enable patient to deal with feelings of guilt.*

Maintain relationship with family and friends as evidenced by the following:

Accepts assistance of parents and siblings to deal with outside obligations

Asks parents to manage insurance and legal aspects of accident

Initiates telephone visits with friends and personal visits with close friends

Provide family members with information about patient's physical status.

Instruct family members about importance of frequent, short visits from family members and close friends.

Request family members to bring meaningful personal items for patient's use.

Discuss with family an interim-interaction approach; answer patient's questions about accident but avoid excessive details, including pictures. *The preceding actions help patient, family, and significant other to express and accept feelings and reactions to the traumatic event.*

Maintain structural and physiological integrity of body systems as evidenced by the following:

Retains muscle strength in unaffected limbs
Retains full range of motion (ROM) in affected limbs
Skin remains intact with no redness, abrasions
Circulation and sensory and motor functions remain intact in affected limbs

Instruct and assist with active ROM in unaffected limbs.

Assist with passive ROM in affected limbs (within limits imposed by injuries).

Make small changes in body position every 2 hours.

Monitor and massage pressure-prone areas of skin.

Monitor warmth, sensation, and movement of fingers and toes in casted extremities. *Providing ROM and proper position assists in maintaining structural integrity of body systems.*

Maintains pretrauma pattern of urine and bowel elimination

Monitor adequate fluid and fiber intake to prevent bladder and bowel elimination problems.

Provide for adequate intake of fluids and foods high in fiber.

Use assistive devices to enhance self-care ability as evidenced by the following:

Transfers from bed to wheelchair with assistance of one person
Attends physical therapy sessions twice a day to gain muscle strength and learn crutch walking
Practices crutch walking with nursing assistance
Resumes responsibility for activities of daily living (ADLs) gradually within limits of injuries

Guide patient in learning transfer techniques.
Arrange for physical therapy.
Praise patient for small gains in ADLs.
Monitor for side effects of increased activity (e.g., increased discomfort or pain in affected limbs).
Focus on taking more responsibility for ADLs helps patient to control intrusive thoughts about accident.

REFERENCES

Komnenich P, Feller C: Disaster nursing, *Annu Rev Nurs Res* 9:123-134, 1991.
McCloskey JC, Bulechek GM: Coping enhancement. In *Nursing interventions classification (NIC)*, ed 2, St Louis, 1996, Mosby.
McCloskey JC, Bulechek GM: Support system enhancement. In *Nursing interventions classification (NIC)*, ed 2, St Louis, 1996, Mosby.
Norman EM, Getek DM, Griffin CC: Post-traumatic stress disorder in an urban trauma population, *Appl Nurs Res* 4(4):171-176, 1991.
Murphy SA: Human responses to catastrophe, *Annu Rev Nurs Res* 9:57-76, 1991.
Oberst MT: Response to coping amid uncertainty: an illness trajectory perspective, *Schol Inq Nurs Pract* 7(1):33-35, 1993.
Thompson JM and others: Posttrauma response. In *Mosby's clinical nursing*, ed 3, St Louis, 1993, Mosby.
Wiener CL, Dodd MJ: Coping amid uncertainty: an illness trajectory perspective, *Schol Inq Nurs Pract* 7(1):17-31, 1993.

Post-trauma response—cont'd

Powerlessness

CLINICAL CONDITION/ MEDICAL DIAGNOSIS	RELATED FACTORS
Cancer requiring frequent hospitalizations; undifferentiated schizophrenia	Controlling or authoritative health care environment; lifestyle of helplessness

---

Patient goals
Expected outcomes
    Associated nursing/collaborative interventions *and scientific rationale*

Experience an increased sense of control over life situation and own activities along with a decrease in a lifestyle of helplessness as evidenced by the following:

Verbalizes positive feelings about own ability to achieve tasks and control of activities

Assist patient to identify preferences, needs, values, and attitudes that may affect task achievement and self-control of activities.

Mutually explore with the patient readiness to initiate and sustain health-promotion behaviors.

Discuss with the patient desirable health behaviors.

Identify with the patient undesirable health behaviors and assist patient to formulate specific plans to avoid such behaviors.

Identify with the patient situations in which powerlessness is experienced. *Personal power is very important to one's own sense of self.*

Explore reality perceptions and clarify if necessary by providing or correcting misinformation. *Verbalizing and exploring feelings increases understanding of individual coping styles and defense mechanisms.*

Modify the environment and organization if needed to facilitate the patient's active involvement in self-care. *Many factors can contribute to a sense of powerlessness including organizational and environmental factors.*

Encourage a sense of partnership with the health care team and reinforce the patient's right to ask questions. *Active patient involvement in decision making and active participation in care can help patient feel in control and prevent a sense of powerlessness.*

Provide procedural and sensory information related to specific treatment interventions for cancer; consider using peer models who demonstrate successful mastery *because such role models can promote mastery and reduce anxiety.*

Engage in problem-solving behaviors

Help the patient develop awareness of care aspects that are patient-controlled.

Eliminate unpredictability of events by informing and involving patient in scheduling.

Alleviate pain and any physical discomfort that diminishes energy reserve and/or make patients feel helpless. *Chronic pain can contribute to a sense of helplessness and powerlessness.*

Provide positive reinforcement for increasing involvement in self-care.

Provide relevant learning material about clinical condition, that is, cancer and schizophrenia.

Assist the patient to maintain realistic expectations through strategies such as proximal goal setting.

Involve the patient in role play to strengthen ability to express concerns.

Teach coping skills (e.g., relaxation, distraction, visual imagery, comforting and positive self-talk, self monitoring). *Focused coping strategies enhance potential for mastery over specific aspects of care.*

Integrates therapeutic regimen into lifestyle

Provide opportunity for the expression of positive emotions (e.g., hope, faith, sense of purpose).

Help the patient identify strength and improvements in condition and mastery of self-care and coping resources.

Involve the family or significant others in reinforcing and supporting health-enhancing behaviors. *Maintaining optimal health is important in keeping inpatient hospital stay to a minimum and in reducing the potential for powerlessness to increase or recur.*

Facilitate continuity of significant activities and roles patient fills in everyday life or help the patient find alternative activities or roles, interests and use of talents.

Assist the patient in planning things that may deplete energy so that support systems are available.

Support involvement in self-help groups or self-help education when indicated. *Social support systems provide ongoing reinforcement of health-desirable behaviors and enhance compliance.*

REFERENCES

Braden CJ: A test of the self-help model: learned response to chronic illness experience, *Nurs Res* 39(1):42, 1990.

Clements S, Cummings S: Helplessness and powerlessness: caring for clients in pain, *Holistic Nurs Pract* 6(1):76-85, 1991.

Fleury JD: Empowering potential: a theory of wellness motivation, *Nurs Res* 40(5):286, 1991.

Mack JE: Power, powerlessness, and empower in psychotherapy, *Psychiatry* 57:178-198, 1994.

McFarland GK, McFarlane EA: *Nursing diagnosis and intervention: planning for patient care,* ed 3, St Louis, 1997, Mosby.

Miller JF: *Coping with chronic illness: overcoming powerlessness,* ed 2, St Louis, 1993, Mosby.

Nystrom AEM, Segesten KM: On sources of powerlessness in nursing home life, *J Nursing* 19:124-133.

Richmond TS and others: Powerlessness in acute spinal cord injury patients: a descriptive study, *J Neurosci Nurs* 24(3):146-152, 1992.

Swearingen PL: *Manual of medical surgical nursing care: nursing interventions and collaborative management,* ed 3, St Louis, 1994, Mosby.

Thompson JM, McFarland GK, Hirsch JE and Tucker SM: *Mosby's clinical nursing,* ed 4, St Louis, 1997, Mosby.

Walding MF: Pain, anxiety, and powerlessness, *J Adv Nurs* 16:388-397, 1991.

Powerlessness—cont'd

Protection, altered

CLINICAL CONDITION/ MEDICAL DIAGNOSIS	RELATED FACTORS
Hematologic cancer	Altered immune and hematopoietic function

Patient goals
Expected outcomes
  Associated nursing/collaborative interventions *and scientific rationale*

Maintain protective defenses as evidenced by the following:

Establishes a pattern of personal hygiene consistent with other demands of daily living

Teach strategies to promote personal and environmental cleanliness.

Assist with daily shower and oral hygiene. *Skin and mucous membranes are the frontline of defense and cleanliness decreases exposure to microbes.*

Monitor vital signs. *Early report of abnormal vital signs (e.g., fever) can reduce complications.*

Incorporates safety measures, prevent infection, bleeding

Teach and demonstrate safety precautions to patient and family.

Re-orient and assist patient during periods of confusion. *Injury from falls and trauma have a high risk of complications due to deficient protective mechanisms.*

Restore protective defenses as evidenced by the following:

Maintains normal body weight and fluid balance

Establish diet plan in collaboration with patient and dietician.

Weigh patient daily.

Offer small frequent meals.

Prescribe dietary supplement as needed.

Encourage fluid intake.

Monitor intake and output. *Nausea, vomiting, anorexia, diarrhea, and stomatitis are associated with therapy and impact nutritional status and fluid balance.*

Incorporates period of rest before or after activities

Teach measures to conserve energy (e.g., pacing of ADLs).

Symptoms resolve in response to therapy

Provide comfort for symptoms (e.g., chills, fever, myalgias). *Flu-like symptoms cause distress and may lead to stress and decreased quality of life.*

Promote protective defenses as evidenced by the following:

Reports increased sense of well-being

Initiate stress management.

Teach relaxation exercises.

Teach alternate coping strategies.

Assist with communication between patient and family.

Provide supportive nurse interactions. *Psychoneuroimmunology provides rationale for mind-body interaction, stress and immunodepression, and justifies interventions of touching, listening, and caring attitudes of the nurse.*

REFERENCES

American Nurses Association, Oncology Nursing Society: *Standards of oncology nursing practice,* Kansas City, 1987, American Nurses Association.

Bauer SM: Psychoneuroimmunology and cancer: an integrated review, *J Adv Nurs* 19:1114-1120, 1994.

Sheppard KC: Altered protection: A nursing diagnosis. In R Carroll-Johnson R, editor: *Classification of nursing diagnoses: proceedings of the ninth conference,* Philadelphia, 1991, JB Lippincott.

Tomaszewski JG and others: Overview of biotherapy, *Cancer Nurs* 18(5):397-414, 1995.

Volker D: Neoplasia. In Beare PG and Myers JL: *Principles and practice of adult health nursing,* ed 2, St Louis, 1994, Mosby.

Protection, altered—cont'd

Rape-trauma syndrome (acute)

CLINICAL CONDITION/ MEDICAL DIAGNOSIS	RELATED FACTORS
Raped by acquaintance	Fear of reprisal; anxiety about acquired immunodeficiency syndrome (AIDS)

> **Patient goals**
> **Expected outcomes**
>   Associated nursing/collaborative interventions *and scientific rationale*

Obtain relief from emotional responses to rape experience as evidenced by the following:

Accepts immediate and ongoing counseling from rape-crisis center staff

Acknowledge appropriateness and support of patient responses to victimization.

Provide empathetic support during physician and police interviews.

Provide for continuity of support throughout entire emergency room experience.

Identifies individuals in family and peer group who would provide support

Verbalizes decrease in fears, anxieties, and concerns

Help patient identify, select, and contact individual with whom rape experience could be discussed. *Women who receive crisis support recover more quickly than those who do not.*

Assist with identifying and avoiding individuals who are upsetting.

Assist significant other to focus on subjective experience of rape rather than on whether rape occurred. *A nonjudgmental attitude helps to alleviate feelings of guilt and self blame.*

Assume decision-making role as evidenced by the following:

Asks questions that enable her to make decisions about health care

Offer information about medical and legal options to facilitate making choices.

Rape-trauma syndrome (acute)

Identify decisions that can be postponed.

- *Rape challenges an individual's sense of power, autonomy, and control; making own decisions can maintain power, sense of control, and feeling of responsibility.*

Verbalizes concern of exposure to human immunodeficiency virus (HIV) or AIDS infection

Makes appointment to discuss HIV testing and accepts written information about ethical issues surrounding HIV testing

Help patient identify fears related to rape, pregnancy, HIV transmission. *Patient's verbalization of concern of AIDS will enable her to seek and accept help toward recovery.*

Discuss benefit of periodic HIV testing, 5-year window of infection, and right to know assailant's HIV status versus right to privacy and informed consent.

Provide written information about ethical issues related to HIV testing and potential loss of employment and access to health insurance if seropositive.

- *Individual has the right to know benefits and risks of HIV testing and status of debate about ethical and legal issues.*

Cope with concern for personal safety as evidenced by the following:

Asks family member/peer to stay with her for a few days

Set goal of returning to usual activities by a specified date

Collaborate with patient to identify safety measures to decrease vulnerability.

Provide a list of immediate and long-term responses to rape experience such as nightmares, flashbacks; emphasize that reactions are not unusual.

REFERENCES

Blair T, Warner CG: Sexual assault, *Topics Emerg Med* 14(4):58, 1992.

Burgess AW, Baker T: AIDS and victims of sexual assault, *Commun Psychiatry* 43(5):447, 1992.

Rape-trauma syndrome (acute)—cont'd

Burgess AW and others: HIV testing of sexual assault populations: ethical and legal issues, *J Emerg Nurs* 16(5):331, 1990.

Larson E, Ropka ME: An update on nursing research and HIV infection, *Image: J Nurs Scholar* 23:4-12, 1991.

Marden MO, Rice MJ: The use of hope as a coping mechanism in abused women, *J Holistic Nurs* 13(1):70-82, 1995.

McArthur MJ: Reality therapy with rape victim, *Arch Psychiatr Nurs* 6:360, 1990.

McCloskey JC, Bulechek GM: Crisis intervention. In *Nursing interventions classification (NIC)*, ed 2, St Louis, 1996, Mosby.

McCloskey JC, Bulechek GM: Rape-trauma treatment. In *Nursing interventions classification (NIC)*, ed 2, St Louis, 1996, Mosby.

Norwood SL: The social support APGAR: instrument development and testing, *Res Nurs Health* 19(2):143-152, 1996.

Turner JG: AIDS-related knowledge, attitudes, and risk for HIV infection among nurses, *Annu Rev Nurs Res* 11:205-224, 1993.

Visser E: AIDS as a result of incest, *AIDS Patient Care* 6(3):113, 1992.

Rape-trauma syndrome: compound reaction

CLINICAL CONDITION/ MEDICAL DIAGNOSIS	RELATED FACTORS
Did not seek medical/ psychological help to deal with trauma	Inadequate support system; inability to resolve rape-trauma experience

---

Patient goals
Expected outcomes
   Associated nursing/collaborative interventions *and scientific rationale*

Develop significant other or family support as evidenced by the following:

Verbalizes that significant other has begun to express warmth and concern

   Assist significant other or family to focus on the subjective experience of rape.

   Help patient identify individuals with whom the rape experience could be discussed.

Accepts and keeps appointment with counselor at rape-crisis center

   Refer patient and significant other to rape counseling center.

   Assist patient and significant other with seeking individual and group counseling. *Group counseling assists members with changing negative attitudes and behaviors.*

   Determine need for family members to seek counseling. *Failure of significant other or family to provide support leads to feelings of guilt and self-blame; feelings require resolution before current physical and emotional problems can be successfully treated.*

Make realistic decisions about actual or potential health problems as evidenced by the following:

Keeps follow-up medical appointments
Takes medication in keeping with prescribed regimen

Makes appointment to discuss HIV testing and accepts written information about ethical and legal issues surrounding HIV testing

Teach importance of medication regimen.

Monitor adherence to medical regimen.

Discuss benefit of periodic HIV testing, 5-year window of infection, and right to know assailant's HIV status versus right to privacy and informed consent.

Provide written information about ethical issues related to HIV testing and potential loss of employment and access to health insurance if seropositive. *Individual has the right to know benefits and risks of HIV testing and status of the debate about ethical and legal issues.*

Cope with cognitive and emotional responses to rape and other stressors as evidenced by the following:

Verbalizes anger and resolves self-blame
Keeps and discusses feelings recorded in separate journal

Teach and monitor use of journal to express anger and related feelings. *Discussing anger and related feelings enables couple to support one another.*

Provide and discuss written list of long-term responses to rape experience; emphasize that reactions are not unusual.

Monitor resolution of symptoms with Rape-Trauma Symptom Rating Scale.

Practices relaxation and cognitive coping strategies
Participates in rape support group

Teach relaxation strategies.

Teach use of cognitive coping strategies such as thought stopping, desensitization, guided imagery, and refuting irrational ideas.

Resume a satisfying lifestyle as evidenced by the following:

Reestablishes intimate relationship with significant other
Reports feeling more secure

Maintains contact with legal system

Collaborate with patient in pacing social activities.
Select strategies to protect from future assaults.
Monitor and support patient's experiences with
legal system.

REFERENCES

Blair T, Warner CG: Sexual assault, *Topics Emerg Med* 14(4):58, 1992.
Burgess AW, Baker T: AIDS and victims of sexual assault, *Hosp Commun Psychiatry* 43(5):447, 1992.
Burgess AW and others: HIV testing of sexual assault population: ethical and legal issues, *J Emerg Nurs* 16(5):331, 1990.
Larson E, Ropka ME: An update on nursing research and HIV infection, *Image: J Nurs Scholar* 23:4-12, 1991.
McCloskey JC, Bulechek GM: Crisis intervention. In *Nursing interventions classification (NIC)*, ed 2, St Louis, 1996, Mosby.
McCloskey JC, Bulechek GM: Rape-trauma treatment. In *Nursing interventions classification (NIC)*, ed 2, St Louis, 1996, Mosby.
Visser E: AIDS as a result of incest. *AIDS Patient Care* 6(3):113, 1992.

Rape-trauma syndrome: compound reaction—cont'd

Rape-trauma syndrome: silent reaction

CLINICAL CONDITION/ MEDICAL DIAGNOSIS	RELATED FACTORS
Concern for personal safety	Anxiety, denial

Patient goals
Expected outcomes
   Associated nursing/collaborative interventions *and scientific rationale*

Cope with personal safety concern as evidenced by the following:

Verbalizes feeling of insecurity
   Establish a trusting relationship with patient.
   Actively listen to patient's perceptions of increased vulnerability.
   Collaborate with patient to identify safety measures to decrease vulnerability.

Makes some progress in relating anxiety about safety to the rape event
   Assist patient to identify source of anxiety about personal safety.
   Provide opportunity to discuss safety concerns with a female police officer. *Establishing a trusting relationship and providing direct assistance with safety measures may reduce anxiety enough to enable patient to deal with the unidentified problem of rape.*

Decrease reliance on denial to maintain sense of well-being as evidenced by the following:

Begins to verbalize feelings of anger and shame related to rape
Verbalizes fear of male friends and relatives since rape
   During routine interview, ask patient if anyone has ever attempted to assault her or hurt her in any way.
   Avoid direct questioning; allow patient to continue at own pace to reveal details of the rape event.

Rape-trauma syndrome: silent reaction

Determine readiness for referral to rape counselor. *Avoiding direct confrontation of denial may enable patient to begin to deal with fears and anxieties associated with the rape.*

Reveals some details of rape experience

Help patient identify specific concerns related to rape experience such as concern about pregnancy and sexually transmitted diseases (STDs).

Assume decision-making about health-care needs as evidenced by the following:

Asks questions about health care resources

Offer information about medical and legal options to facilitate making choices.

Identify decisions that should be made soon and those that can be postponed.

Verbalizes fear of human immunodeficiency virus (HIV) and acquired immunodeficiency syndrome (AIDS)

Does not return to full denial during discussion of HIV testing

Offer information about HIV testing. Discuss benefit of periodic HIV testing, 5-year window of infection, and right to know assailant's HIV status versus right of privacy and informed consent.

Provide written information about ethical issues related to HIV testing and potential loss of employment and access to health insurance if seropositive. *Individual has the right to know benefits and risks of HIV testing and status of debate about ethical and legal issues.*

Cope with cognitive and emotional responses to rape experience as evidenced by the following:

Verbalizes anger and resolves self-blame
Practices cognitive coping strategies
Participates in rape support group

Teach use of cognitive coping strategies such as thought stopping, desensitization, guided imagery, and refuting irrational ideas.

Provide information about support-group opportunities and benefits.

Teach and monitor use of journal to express anger and related feelings. *Discussion of fear, anger, and related feelings enables individual to obtain support from group.*

REFERENCES

Blair T, Warner CG: Sexual assault, *Topics Emerg Med* 14(4):58, 1992.

Burgess AW, Baker T: AIDS and victims of sexual assault, *Hosp Commun Psychiatry* 43(5):447, 1992.

Burgess AW and others: HIV testing of sexual assault populations: ethical and legal issues, *J Emerg Nurs* 16(5):331, 1990.

McCloskey JC, Bulechek GM: Crisis intervention. In *Nursing interventions classification (NIC)*, ed 2, St Louis, 1996, Mosby.

McCloskey JC, Bulechek GM: Rape-trauma treatment. In *Nursing interventions classification (NIC)*, ed 2, St Louis, 1996, Mosby.

Turner JG: Acquired immunodeficiency syndrome, *Annu Rev Nurs Res* 8:195-210, 1990.

Turner JG: AIDS-related knowledge, attitudes, and risk for HIV infection among nurses, *Annu Rev Nurs Res* 11:205-224, 1993.

Visser E: AIDS as a result of incest, *AIDS Patient Care* 6(3):113, 1992.

Relocation stress syndrome

CLINICAL CONDITION/ MEDICAL DIAGNOSIS	RELATED FACTORS
Pelvic fracture (Indochinese refugee)	Sudden environmental change within context of recent migration

Patient goals
Expected outcomes
   Associated nursing/collaborative interventions *and scientific rationale*

Adapt to sudden change associated with hospitalization and migration as evidenced by the following:

Demonstrates reduced levels of fear and anxiety

Establish a supportive relationship with patients *to build trust and a sense of security.*

Orient patient to new surroundings and routines *to decrease unfamiliarity, uncertainty, and a sense of disruption.*

Assess patient's current level of stressors (e.g., resettlement and acculturation stress, developmental crises, family roles, impact of changed health status) *to determine patient's appraisal of relocation events and level of loss and vulnerability.*

Provide structure and consistent caregivers whenever possible *to minimize further changes for the patient and establish predictable relationships.*

Communicates about changes and losses associated with relocation (e.g., loss of culture, status, roles, social network) and describes impact on coping with changed health status

Provide opportunities for patient to verbalize feelings about perceived or actual changes and losses associated with relocation *to acknowledge distress, facilitate grieving, and promote problem-solving.*

Use consultants when appropriate (e.g., language translators, volunteers from culture-specific community programs) *to maximize communication between the patient and care providers.*

Relocation stress syndrome

Acknowledge patient's positive statements about new environment and acceptance of changed surroundings.

Assess for dysfunctional grieving responses (e.g., explore somatic complaints) and make psychiatric referrals if indicated.

Maintains a sense of self-worth and positive personal identity during transition to new setting

Acknowledge patient's cultural preferences whenever possible (e.g., diet, family involvement, communication patterns) and incorporate into care.

Protect patient's privacy and encourage participation in decision making about care *to decrease powerlessness, uncertainty, and feelings of marginality.*

Assess sources of support for patient (e.g., family, friends, ethnic community, religious organizations) and facilitate contact.

Accepts support from appropriate resources during adjustment period to hospitalization as evidenced by the following:

Verbalizes acceptance of referrals to community agencies and health care providers before discharge

Initiate early discharge planning for culturally relevant follow-up in the community.

Initiate early patient predischarge teaching, working with language translators and others in the patient's support system.

Refer patient to relevant self-help support groups (e.g., resettlement classes, ethnic clinics, church groups) *to rebuild disrupted social network, promote feelings of universality, decrease isolation, and increase support during the adjustment period and convalescence.*

REFERENCES

Aroian KJ: A model of psychological adaptation to migration and re-settlement, *Nurs Res* 39(1):5, 1990.

Aroian KJ: Mental health risks and problems encountered by illegal immigrants, *Issues Ment Health Nurs* 14:379, 1993.

Beiser M, Edward RG: Mental health of immigrants and refugees, *New Direct Ment Health Serv* 20(61):73, 1994.

Relocation stress syndrome—cont'd

377

Cravener P: Establishing therapeutic alliance across cultural barriers, *J Psychosoc Ment Health Nurs* 14:379, 1993.

Frye BA, D'Avanzo C: Themes in managing culturally defined illness in the Cambodian refugee family, *J Commun Health Nurs* 11(2):89-98, 1994.

Hertz DG: Bio-psycho-social consequences of migration stress: a multidimensional approach, *Isr J Psychiatry Relat Sci* 30(4):204, 1993.

Kinzie JD, Boehnlein JK: Psychotherapy of the victims of massive violence: countertransference and ethical issues, *Am J Psychother* 47(1):90-102, 1993.

Moore LJ, Boehnlein JK: Posttraumatic stress disorder, depression, and somatic symptoms in 65 mien patients, *J Nerv Ment Dis* 179(12):728, 1991.

Sack WH, Clark GN, Seeley J: Post-traumatic stress disorder across two generations of Cambodian refugees, *J Am Acad Child Adololesc Psychiatr* 34(9):1160, 1995.

Relocation stress syndrome—cont'd

Role performance, altered

CLINICAL CONDITION/ MEDICAL DIAGNOSIS	RELATED FACTORS
Chronic obstructive pulmonary disease (COPD)	Inadequate role performance; decline in strength and endurance

Patient goals
Expected outcomes
    Associated nursing/collaborative interventions *and*
      scientific rationale

Engage in functional role performance within limitation of health status changes as evidenced by the following:

Describes realistic expectations for self and behaviors necessary for fulfilling modified role expectations

    Encourage patient to express concerns and feelings about chronic illness, physical limitations, and other losses.

Determines nature of role performance disturbance and limitations (e.g., role stress, role strain, role overload, role failure, role loss, interpersonal role conflict, or role insufficiency) to plan strategies to cope with role changes

    Assess scope and nature of situational transition experienced by patient *to determine degree of actual role disturbance and limitations, as well as patient's perceptions regarding the impact of these changes.*

    Determine role of the patient within family and social contexts *to identify responsibilities and expectations held by patient and others. Major situational events that families are confronted with can affect the functioning of roles within the family and the family as a unit.*

    Determine cultural factors influencing role expectations and performance.

    Encourage patient to clarify role expectations with family or partner and discuss potential impact

Role performance, altered

379

of changed role performance. *To cope, patient may use a cognitive redefinition coping strategy by reevaluating the importance of a previously valued role.*

Uses constructive strategies to cope with situational transition related to changes in health status

Assist patient in identifying strengths and resources, including positive role models and opportunities for decision-making regarding role performance *to increase and reinforce functional role performance.*

Assist patient and family or partner in identifying previous coping strategies and resources to apply to current situation.

Discuss impact of role changes with family or partner *to assess degree of support available to patient and to increase collaborative problem-solving. Reducing altered role performance can contribute to lowered feelings of distress.*

Teach patient specific strategies to cope with physical disability (e.g., problem-focused strategies of positioning and breathing techniques; emotion-focused strategies of relaxation exercises).

Use role playing *to teach new behaviors, provide opportunities for role rehearsal, and reinforce desired changes.*

Provide patient with positive feedback for initiating and practicing new behaviors *to reinforce changes and build self-esteem related to role transition.*

Seeks assistance from appropriate resources within the health care system and community

Initiate early discharge planning and collaborate with patient and family or partner in planning rehabilitation care *to maximize a sense of control and decrease anxiety. Social support can reduce stress related to role performance.*

Provide patient with referrals to relevant self-help support groups in the community *to facilitate reference group interaction, information-sharing, and advocacy.*

Provide supportive family counseling or referral for such *since an optimally functional family can be helpful to patient coping.*

REFERENCES

Andrews HA: Overview of the role function mode. In Roy SR, Andrews A, eds: *The Roy adaptation model,* Norwalk, Conn, 1991, Appleton & Lange.

Doyle DL, Stern PA: Negotiating self-care in rehabilitation nursing, *Rehabil Nurs* 17(6):319, 1992.

Evans RL and others: Poststroke family function: an evaluation of the family's role in rehabilitation, *Rehabil Nurs* 17(3):127-132, 1992.

Gift AG, Austin DJ: The effects of a program of systematic movement on COPD patients, *Rehabil Nurs* 17(1):6, 1992.

Kersten L: Changes in self-concept during pulmonary rehabilitation, Part I, *Heart Lung* 19(5):456, 1990.

Kersten L: Changes in self-concept during pulmonary rehabilitation, Part II, *Heart Lung* 19(5):463, 1990.

Krause N: Stressors in salient social roles and well-being in later life. *J Gerontology* 49(3):137-148, 1994.

Lancee WJ and others: The impact of pain and impaired role performance on distress in persons with cancer, *Can J Psychiatry* 39(10):617-622, 1994.

Sexton DL, Munro BH: Living with a chronic illness—the experience of women with chronic obstructive pulmonary disease (COPD), *West J Nurs Res* 10(1):26, 1988.

Spitze G and others: Middle generation roles and the well-being of men and women, *J Gerontology* 49(3):S107-S116, 1994.

Temple A, Fawdry K: King's theory of goal attainment-resolving filial caregiver role strain. *J Gerontolog Nurs* 8(B):11-15, 1992.

Warda M: The family and chronic sorrow: role theory approach, *J Pediatr Nurs* 7(3):205-210, 1992.

Self-care deficit (bathing/hygiene; dressing/grooming; feeding; toileting)

CLINICAL CONDITION/ MEDICAL DIAGNOSIS	RELATED FACTORS
Cerebrovascular accident (CVA)	Disability requiring modified lifestyle

Patient goals
Expected outcomes
> Associated nursing/collaborative interventions *and scientific rationale*

Modify lifestyle to maximize self-care ability and increase independence within limitations

Recognizing that self-care practices are necessary for managing activities of daily living (ADLs) and overcoming limitations

> Provide opportunity for expression of feelings related to CVA and physical limitations (e.g., denial, anxiety, or depression).

> Encourage patient to identify motivations to engage in self-care behaviors.

> Assist patient to identify factors that support or hinder self-care activity.

> Provide factual and/or technical information relevant to meet self-care requisites. *Adequate information will allow the patient to be as independent as possible, to make intelligent decisions about his/her care, and to decrease anxiety.*

> Discuss with patient a means of negotiating and instilling a sense of responsibility or commitment to self-care (i.e., contract learning). *A sense of responsibility gives a patient some form of control during a time of uncertainty and powerlessness.*

> Consistently convey value of patient's knowledge and competence necessary to engage in health promoting self-care activities.

Demonstrates self-care activities as much as possible within limitations

> Assist patient to set short, realistic, and attainable goals.

Assist patient to make free choices of self-care activity and methods of assistance. *A chance of free choice will give patient a sense of control and self-esteem.*

Allow patient to make own schedule for ADLs.

Provide sufficient time and personal care supplies necessary for self-care.

Provide patient and family support and knowledge to empower them to manage self-care limits more effectively. *Education and support reinforce positive psychological and social outcomes, and reduce fear and anxiety related to physical limitations.*

Avoid emphasis on self-care limitations that could heighten self-criticism and lowered physical self-concept.

Assist patient to select self-care practices that enhance adjustment to disability (e.g., maintaining balanced exercise/rest regimen).

Encourage patient to engage in ADLs for herself/himself as much as possible.

Explore the use of self-help devices/assistive devices to help patient become more self-sufficient.

Provide assistance, supervision, and teaching as necessary to improve self-care practices.

Provide opportunity for building self-care confidence by frequent reinforcement of positive feedback. *Positive reinforcement emphasizes the need for continuing self-care behaviors.*

Allow patient to explore feelings associated with positive changes.

Uses strengths and weaknesses to engage in self-care activities within limitations

Assist patient to identify and utilize own strengths, intact roles, and resources to maximize sense of ability for regaining control.

Assist patient to identify past self-care abilities and present limitations. *Self-care abilities and perceived self-efficacy have an effect on self-care behavior.*

Facilitate discussion by patient and family of topics that are not related to disability (e.g., current events, hobbies, recreational interests, family activities).

Encourage patient to maintain previously learned self-care activities.

Assist patient to identify previous coping behaviors and support system for problem solving to generate a sense of hope and self-control. *Patients using problem-focused coping strategies appear to have less psychosocial difficulty with post-CVA adjustment.*

Reassess goals periodically and set new goals as possible.

Reinforce patient's progress, no matter how small, with positive feedback.

Utilizes available support system and community resources

Assess the family's willingness to support patient's self-care limitations, changed lifestyle, and patient's ability to increase independence.

Actively include family and significant others in entire stroke rehabilitation process. *The perceived beliefs of significant others are important for patient's adherence to medical regimen.*

Teach the family the role of supervision rather than the role of activity maintenance. *The pessimistic attitude of family member impedes the patient from doing what he/she is capable of doing and leads to regression and low self-esteem.*

Assist patient and family to use available resources such as Medicare, Social Security, and disability insurance.

Encourage patient and family to use community resources such as stroke support group, interest group, senior citizen center, or adult day care for diversional activity.

Keep patient's significant others who can influence patient, informed of patient's progress, so they can give patient positive feedback. *Family could provide validation of worth to the patient in the family within the patient's ability to function.*

REFERENCES

Barron M: Life after stroke, *Nurs Times* 88(10):32, 1992.

Borgman MF, Passarella P: Nursing care of the stroke patient using Bobath principles: an approach to altered movement, *Nurs Clin North Am* 26(4):1019, 1991.

Brandriet LM, Lyons M, Bently J: Perceived needs of poststroke elders following termination of home health services, *Nurs Health Care* 15(10):514-520, 1994.

Bronstein KS: Psychosocial components in stroke: implication for adaptation, *Nurs Clin North Am* 26(4):1007, 1991.

Farzan DT: Reintegration for stroke survivors: home and community consideration, *Nurs Clin North Am* 26(4):1019, 1991.

Gibbon B: Stroke nursing care and management in the community: a survey of district nurses' perceived contribution in one health district in England, *J Adv Nurs* 20(3):469-476, 1994.

Palmer S: Primary nursing care of patients who have had a stroke, *Br J Nurs* 4(1):8-14, 1995.

Sutton P: Positive progress, *Nurs Times* 88(5):38, 1992.

Walkins M: Can you tread this emotional high wire? *Prof Nurse* 8(9):604, 1993.

Self-esteem disturbance

CLINICAL CONDITION/ MEDICAL DIAGNOSIS	RELATED FACTORS
Rheumatoid arthritis (elderly patient)	Reduced self-care ability; limited coping mechanisms

> **Patient goals**
> **Expected outcomes**
> > Associated nursing/collaborative interventions *and scientific rationale*

Experience and maintain self-esteem as evidenced by the following:

Identifies strategies for coping with negative feelings about self

Help patient to describe effects of illness on self-appraisal, daily activities, family, and friends. *Rheumatoid arthritis accompanied by functional incapacities may be associated with decreased levels of self-esteem.*

Convey respect and acceptance of the patient as a unique individual. *Creating an atmosphere of acceptance and interest is important so that the patient can begin to explore presenting problems and the significance of current experiences.*

Encourage discussion of illness *to facilitate acceptance of reality of illness. Patients who accept the reality of a disease and integrate this reality into their own self-concept experience higher levels of self-esteem.*

Discourage the use of palliative coping responses (e.g., wishful thinking, ruminating on past problems and failures) *because these coping behaviors are associated with ongoing lowered self-esteem.*

Inspire hope by describing situations in which other patients have managed similar difficulties.

Help patient set initial goals that can be achieved within a short period.

Encourage patient to evaluate goal achievement and reflect on small accomplishments *because self-esteem may be augmented through experience of small successes.*

Encourage decision-making in planning and directing own care *to promote patient autonomy and to decrease avoidance of constructive problem-solving.*

Teach meditation and relaxation skills *to provide the patient with the ability to successfully cope with stressors and to improve his/her self-esteem and life satisfactions.*

Facilitate participation in treatment modalities that emphasize support, acceptance, and belonging.

Encourage development of a health-promoting activity such as an exercise program, to extent possible. *Participation in a regular exercise program increases self-esteem.*

Achieves goals within family and social environment that reflects awareness of personal talents and limitations

Encourage identification and description of existing strengths and potentials.

Acknowledge recognition of patient's expertise or knowledge *to reinforce patient's recognition of existing strengths and competencies.*

Encourage patient to initiate realistic activities in which success can be anticipated *because failure and negative feedback from others can influence patient's self-confidence.*

Help patient strengthen desired coping skills and become involved in actions to meet goals within the patient's functional capacity. *Strengthening a positive coping response lessens the patient's tendency to avoid problems or stressors.*

Monitor extent to which patient's family influences patient's perception of self.

Teach family members to recognize the influence of their interactive style on patient's perceptions of self.

Encourage participation in volunteer programs (e.g., programs sponsored by church affiliation or community-based programs) *to reinforce perception to self and others of ability to make positive contributions to others.*

Teach patient to create and maintain relationships that provide successful social interaction.

Maintains self-care skills necessary for functioning in society as evidenced by the following:

Engages in daily activities to meet personal needs (e.g., personal hygiene practices, good grooming, meal preparation, home maintenance, planning leisure time) to extent possible

Monitor ongoing pain levels as well as patient's expectations of pain control. *Acute and chronic arthritic pain affects an individual's ability to maintain routine self-care skills.*

Monitor patient's ability to identify and accurately report symptoms.

Compare subjective descriptions with objective measurements *to determine possible discrepancies between the patient's ability and willingness to participate in self-care skills.*

Encourage participation in treatment modalities such as an ADLs group that focuses on learning or relearning how to live independently in a community and achieving highest level of functional capacity.

Emphasize the importance of participating in activities that maximize the patient's ability to maintain optimal health, personal hygiene, and independent living (e.g., meal planning and preparation, money management and leisure time). *Maintaining optimal level of health and functioning aids in maintaining self-esteem, as well as optimal social functioning.*

REFERENCES

Bednar RL, Wells MG, Peterson SR: *Self-esteem: paradoxes and innovations in clinical theory and practice,* Washington, DC, 1989, American Psychological Association.

Bonheur B, Young SW: Exercise as a health-promoting lifestyle choice, *Applied Nurs Res* 4(1):2, 1991.

Borelli MD, DeLucas E: Physical health promotion, *Psychosocial Nursing* 31(3):15-18, 1993.

Cornwell CJ, Schmitt MH: Perceived health status, self-esteem and body image in women with rheumatoid arthritis or systemic lupus erythematosus, *Res Nurs Health* 13:99, 1990.

Self-esteem disturbance—cont'd

Greenblatt F: Maintaining self-esteem, *J Long Term Care Admin* 20(4):7, 1992.

McFarland GK, Wasli EL, Gerety EK: *Nursing diagnoses and process in psychiatric mental health nursing,* ed 3, Philadelphia, 1997, JB Lippincott.

Norris J: Nursing intervention for self-esteem disturbances, *Nurs Diagn* 3(2):48, 1992.

O'Brien M: Multiple sclerosis: the relationship among self-esteem, social support, and coping behavior, *Appl Nurs Res* 6(2):54, 1993.

Pigg JS, Schroeder PM: Frequently occurring problems of patients with rheumatic diseases: the ANA outcome standards for rheumatology nursing practice, *Nurs Clin North Am* 19(4):697, 1984.

Rugel RP: *Dealing with the problem of low self-esteem,* Springfield, Ill, 1995, Charles C. Thomas.

Walsh A, Walsh PA: Love, self-esteem, and multiple sclerosis, *Soc Sci Med* 29(7):793, 1989.

White NE, Richter JM, Fry C: Coping, social support, and adaptation to chronic illness, *West J Nurs Res* 14(2):211, 1992.

Self-esteem disturbance—cont'd

Self-esteem, chronic low

CLINICAL CONDITION/
MEDICAL DIAGNOSIS

Eczematous
dermatitis (young
female adult)

RELATED FACTORS

Repeated negative and stressful
interpersonal relationships

Patient goals
Expected outcomes
    Associated nursing/collaborative interventions *and*
        scientific rationale

**Develop more positive self-evaluations as evidenced
by the following:**

**Increase in positive statements about self and own
capabilities**

Explore with patient nature of feelings about self
and extent of existence and change over time *to
help the patient begin to understand the associations
between repeated negative interpersonal statements
and current state of low self-esteem.*

Demonstrate empathy.

Help patient describe experiences that make her
feel worthwhile and good about herself.

Convey genuine interest in and concern for patient
to reinforce sense of self-worth.

Teach patient to recognize negative and distorted
thoughts about self *so that she can begin to learn
techniques for interrupting or stopping self-defeating
thoughts.*

Support patient's endeavors to practice techniques
to stop and replace negative and self-defeating
thoughts about self.

Encourage identification and description of realistic and positive self-assessments.

Share techniques for improving self-esteem based
on self-awareness and self-talk, such as self affir-
mations and positive messages *to help the patient
identify actions to change behaviors that negatively
impact self-esteem.*

Self-esteem, chronic low

Engage in constructive interpersonal relationships as evidenced by the following:

Develops positive interpersonal relationships

Teach patient to observe pattern of interactions with mother, significant other, employer, and friends.

Help patient to identify and describe problems in relating to these people.

Suggest that patient keep journal *to assist in problem solving and obtaining feedback.*

Teach patient strategies for building self-confidence (e.g., improving communications skills, making constructive use of defenses, developing hobbies and interests, and developing personal opinions about issues).

Evaluates self as able to deal with interpersonal relationships

Acknowledge to patient that she does have choices in life.

Discourage rumination about past failures.

Assist patient in setting realistic goals for improving interpersonal relationships.

Role play a variety of ordinary interpersonal encounters *to help patient become aware of strengths and difficulties in interactions with mother, significant other, employer, and friends.*

Evaluate need for referral to specific additional treatment modalities (e.g., brief psychotherapy, social skills training, women's issues group therapy, or women's support group). *These modalities can serve as additional resources for helping the patient learn new skills in establishing and maintaining constructive interpersonal relationships.*

Develop more healthful physical lifestyle as evidenced by the following:

Participates in planning to make lifestyle changes to enhance physical health and well-being

Assess patient's current physical health status.

Teach patient to recognize relationship between physical health and positive feelings about self.

Assist patient in identifying ways to promote health and well-being.

Reinforce health-promoting practices such as exercise, relaxation, and diversional activity.

REFERENCES

Antonucci TC, Peggs JF, Marquez JT: The relationship between self-esteem and physical health in a family practice population, *Fam Pract Res J* 9(1):65, 1989.

Bonheur B, Yong SW: Exercise as a health-promoting lifestyle choice, *Appl Nurs Res* 4(1):2, 1991.

Crouch MA, Straub V: Enhancement of self-esteem in adults, *Fam Commun Health* 6(2):65, 1983.

Decarlo JJ, Mann WC: The effectiveness of verbal versus activity groups in improving self-perceptions of interpersonal communication skills, *Am J Occup Ther* 39(1):20, 1985.

Kinney CK, Mannetter R, Carpenter MA: Support groups. In Bulechek GM, McCloskey JC: *Nursing interventions: essential nursing treatments,* ed 2, Philadelphia, 1992, WB Saunders.

Maynard C: Psychoeducational approach to depression in women, *J Psychosoc Nurs* 31(12):9-14, 1993.

Norris J: Nursing intervention for self-esteem disturbances, *Nursing Diagn* 3(2):48, 1992.

Prehn RA, Thomas P: Does it make a difference? The effect of a women's issues group on female psychiatric inpatients, *Psychosoc Nurs Ment Health Serv* 28(11):34, 1990.

Rugel RP: Dealing with the problem of low self-esteem, Springfield, Ill, 1995, Charles C. Thomas.

Stanwyck DJ: Self-esteem through the life span, *Fam Commun Health* 6(2):11, 1983.

JOAN M. CALEY, ELIZABETH KELCHNER GERETY, AND GERTRUDE K. MCFARLAND

Self-esteem, situational low

CLINICAL CONDITION/
MEDICAL DIAGNOSIS

Adjustment disorder
with work inhibition
(Female administrator
in complex health
care organization that
is undergoing
restructuring)

RELATED FACTORS

Organizational instability; impending
job loss

Patient goals
Expected outcomes
- Associated nursing/collaborative interventions *and
  scientific rationale*

Regain former realistic positive self-esteem as evidenced by the following:

Increases confidence in handling job situation

Encourage identification and description of
changes in feelings about self.

Discuss self-care strategies and their relationship to
feelings about self; *to feel good about self, person
must be able to take care of self.*

Assist patient in clearly describing previous state of
positive self-evaluation.

Assess patient's perception of the current situation,
availability of supportive resources, and current
coping strategies *to obtain information about
patient's education, counseling, support, and
referral needs.*

Explore with patient current employment environment in organization (e.g., degree of organizational instability, level of interpersonal conflict,
extent of personal involvement, impending
threat to current job).

Help patient to assess realistic options for self
within current organization and other potential
employment opportunities, short-term and
long-term, *to assist patient in identifying and mobilizing own resources and strengths.*

Self-esteem, situational low

393

Engage patient in problem solving (e.g., assess realities of situation, examine personal assets and strengths, identify incremental goals, develop action plan to meet goals). *These actions promote awareness of positive relationship between self-esteem and effective problem solving.*

Increases ability to problem solve, set goals, and take action

Help patient to explore community groups and resources that could help with problem solving and decision making about transitions.

Offer patient reading materials that might assist in problem solving.

Teach conflict-resolution skills.

Teach patient constructive defenses against attacks from others *to help patient regain sense of competency and control.*

Assist patient to identify available resources for exploring job opportunities.

Increases understanding of situational factors and self-behaviors that have an impact on current situation

Assist patient in describing current level of on-the-job performance; perceptions of feeling valued, needed, or important in relation to the overall organization; and impact of current situation on other aspects of daily living.

Help patient identify previous problem-solving strategies and strengths, limitations, and potentials.

Offer hope that situation can be handled, by describing others who have overcome similar job instabilities.

Suggest that patient keep journal *to assist in problem solving and obtaining feedback.*

Support patient's decision-making efforts. *These actions create a supportive reality-based environment for effective problem solving and feedback.*

Maintain physical health as evidenced by the following:

Improves balance between physical and mental health states

Assess patient's current physical health status.

Teach patient awareness of potential harmful effects of negative self-talk.

Teach patient about relationship between physical health and positive feelings about self *to promote awareness of positive relationship between self-esteem and physical health.*

Assist patient in identifying ways to promote health and well-being.

Reinforce health-promoting practices, such as exercise program, use of relaxation techniques, and diversional activity. *These types of activities serve to reduce anxiety, and they facilitate exploration of constructive problem solving.*

REFERENCES

Antonucci TC, Peggs JF, Marquez JT: The relationship between self-esteem and physical health in a family practice population, *Fam Pract Res J* 9(1):65, 1989.

Bonheur B, Young SW: Exercise as a health-promoting lifestyle choice, *Appl Nurs Res* 4(1):2, 1991.

Bunkers SJ: A strategy for staff development: self-care and self-esteem as necessary partners, *Clin Nurse Specialist* 6(3):154-162, 1992.

Crouch MA, Straub V: Enhancement of self-esteem in adults, *Fam Commun Health* 6(2):65, 1983.

DeCarlo JJ, Mann WC: The effectiveness of verbal versus activity groups in improving self-perceptions of interpersonal communication skills, *Am J Occup Ther* 39(1):20, 1985.

Gilberts R: The evaluation of self-esteem, *Fam Commun Health* 6(2):29, 1983.

Hagerty BM and others: Sense of belonging: a vital mental health concept, *Arch Psychiatric Nurs* 6(3):172, 1992.

LeMone P: Analysis of a human phenomenon: self-concept, *Nurs Diagn* 2(3):126, 1991.

Norris J: Nursing intervention for self-esteem disturbances, *Nurs Diagn* 3(2):48, 1992.

Rugel RP: *Dealing with the problem of low self-esteem,* Springfield, 1995, Charles Thomas.

Self-esteem, situational low—cont'd

Self-mutilation, risk for

CLINICAL CONDITION/ MEDICAL DIAGNOSIS	RISK FACTORS
Borderline personality	Psychosis; history of physical, emotional, or sexual abuse

Patient goals
Expected outcomes
   Associated nursing/collaborative interventions *and scientific rationale*

Experience fewer episodes of self-mutilation as evidenced by the following:

Identifies and manages anxiety

Develop trusting relationship with patient.

Assist patient in recognition of anxiety and situations in which he/she becomes anxious. *This step is necessary before plans for reducing anxiety can be developed.*

Explore with patient approaches to reduce anxiety (e.g., music, physical activity).

Constructively uses resources to deal with stressors

Create nonthreatening environment *because an increase in stressors can lead to self-mutilation.*

Assist patient to identify perceived stressors.

Explore with patient past successes in reducing stress *to capitalize use of patient's strengths.*

Collaborate with patient to develop a plan to cope with stressors.

Have patient demonstrate use of stress-reduction techniques.

Demonstrate self-differentiation

Engage patient in values clarification, self-appraisal, and identification of ideal self *to develop clearer sense of self-identity.*

Provide opportunities in which patient can maximize use of his/her strengths *to enhance self-esteem.*

Offer unconditional positive regard when interacting with patient *to enhance feelings of self-esteem.*

Displays positive family interactions

Determine to what extent the patient's self-perception is affected by his or her dysfunctional family.

Discuss alternative strategies with patient to enhance family interaction (e.g., family therapy) *so as to decrease any stress or threat to self.*

REFERENCES

Favazza A: *Bodies under siege: self-mutilation in culture and psychiatry,* Baltimore, 1993, Johns Hopkins Press.

Naschinski C: High risk for self-mutilation. In Thompson JM, McFarland GK, Hirsch JE and Tucker SM: *Mosby's clinical nursing,* ed 4, St Louis, 1997, Mosby.

Russ M and others: Subtypes of self-injurious patients with borderline personality disorder, *Am J Psychiatr* 150:1869-1871, 1993.

Sabo A and others: Changes in self-destructiveness of borderline patients in psychotherapy, *J Nerv Ment Dis* 183(6):370-375, 1995.

Sansone R, Sansone L, Wiederman M: The prevalence of trauma and its relationship to borderline personality symptoms and self-destructive behaviors in a primary care setting, *Arch Fam Med* 4:439-442, 1995.

Shearer S: Phenomenology of self-injury among inpatient women with borderline personality disorder, *J Nerv Ment Dis* 182(9):524-526, 1994.

Sensory/perceptual alterations

CLINICAL CONDITION/ MEDICAL DIAGNOSIS	RELATED FACTORS
Schizophrenia, undifferentiated type	Poor symptom management

> **Patient goals**
> **Expected outcomes**
>> Associated nursing/collaborative interventions *and scientific rationale*

Experience reduction in hallucinations and/or distress they cause as evidenced by:

Recognizes that auditory hallucinations can be self-managed

Use empathy and listening in the relationship with patient. *Schizophrenic patients are sensitive to the clinical relationship, which can produce feelings of safety and understanding, or helplessness and being controlled.*

Identify common tasks in process of self-management, such as recognizing symptoms, use of medication, handling acute episodes, maintaining a social network, etc. *Knowing specific tasks assists the patient in understanding and participating in the treatment process.*

Discuss common coping styles: seeking help, isolating self, looking for escape, distracting.

Identify denial as a way to deal with anxiety. *Often daily life events are overestimated or negatively perceived, increasing anxiety and sense of helplessness and contributing to relapse.*

Identifies actions to be taken which are specific and meaningful to self

Teach patient to recognize early signs of relapse in self, that is, rejecting or alienating others, forgetting to take medicine, not keeping appointments. *Knowing the signs of relapse will assist patient in taking preventive action for self.*

Sensory/perceptual alterations

Teach what factors will assist the patient in evaluating progress toward self-management, such as: Do I need reminders to bathe, to eat? Am I being asked to do things with others? Have I been in any arguments this week? Am I keeping appointments and taking medications?

Develop cognitive and behavioral coping strategies to deal with hallucinations as evidenced by:

Reports fewer hallucinations and/or feelings of distress as he/she goes about daily routines

Teach strategies to deal with traumatic emotional event such as appraising correctly daily life events or stopping automatic behavior responses.

Teach strategies to deal with social contexts in which hallucinations are experienced.

Demonstrates ways to handle hallucinations and to share with others

Teach use of self-talk, talking to another, television or radio, other diversional activity. *Providing a number of strategies for the patient to try will encourage further development of techniques to manage self.*

Provide opportunity to exchange experiences with others *as a way to further enhance the patient's social support system.*

Verbalizes knowledge of hallucinations as a neurophysiological malfunction and/or expression of levels of anxiety

Listen and validate patient's experience of anxiety, anger, lack of self-worth, powerlessness, sexuality, *thereby assisting him/her to understand the experience and achieve success in learning to manage the voices.*

Listen and validate the experience of having drug- and/or alcohol-related hallucinations, *thereby assisting patient to understand the experience and take appropriate action for self to avoid their use.*

Sensory/perceptual alterations—cont'd

REFERENCES

Buccheri R and others: Auditory hallucinations in schizophrenia: Group experience in examining symptom management and behavioral strategies, *J Psychosoc Nurs Ment Health Serv* 34(2):12-25, 1996.

Carter DM, MacKinnon A, Copolov DL: Patient's strategies for coping with auditory hallucinations, *J Nerv Ment Dis* 184(3):159-164, 1996.

Frederick J, Cotanch P: Self-help techniques for auditory hallucinations in schizophrenia, *Issues Ment Health Nurs* 16(3):213-224, 1995.

Murphy MF, Moller MD: Relapse management in neurobiological disorders: The Moller-Murphy Symptom Management Assessment Tool, *Arch Psychiatr Nurs* 7(4):226-235, 1993.

O'Connor FW: A vulnerability-stress framework for evaluating clinical interventions in schizophrenia, *Image J Nurs Schol* 26(3):231-236, 1994.

Pollack LE: Inpatient self-management of bipolar disorder, *Appl Nurs Res* 9(2):71-79, 1996.

San Blise ML: Everything I learned, I learned from patients: Radical positive reframing, *J Psychosoc Nurs Ment Health Serv* 33(12):18-25, 1995.

Sensory/perceptual alterations—cont'd

Sexual dysfunction

CLINICAL CONDITION/ MEDICAL DIAGNOSIS	RELATED FACTORS
Generalized anxiety disorder	Misinformation and/or inadequate knowledge; conflicting values.

Patient goals
Expected outcomes
    Associated nursing/collaborative interventions *and*
       scientific rationale

Verbalize increased knowledge about sexual concerns as evidenced by the following:

Identifies personal sexual concerns

Assist patient in identifying possible factors that may contribute to sexual dysfunction. *Medications, alcohol or drug abuse or clinical conditions can affect sexual functioning.*

Encourage patient to describe current sexual interactions and behavior patterns (e.g., compatibility with sexual partner; comfort with sexual interactions or frequency of sexual interactions). *Patients need reassurance from authoritative source that it is permissible to think, read, talk, and fantasize about sex.*

Provide privacy when discussing sexual matters. Provide climate in which patient can openly discuss concerns. Use nonjudgmental attitude. *Comfort factors show respect to client and promote expression of feeling.*

Acknowledge patient's feelings of anxiety about discussing sexual concerns *to establish rapport and create an internal state of trust for patient.*

Verbalizes knowledge about human sexuality

Explore patient's knowledge deficit about sexuality. *Patients with sexual dysfunctions often lack sex education.*

Dispel any myths or misinformation patient may have about sexual activities (e.g., that masturbating will make you crazy). *Patients need to have*

Sexual dysfunction

myths dispelled and be provided with accurate information about sexual functioning.

Use terminology that patient understands.

Offer information about specific needs, assigning books to read or to discuss.

Clarify with patient any uncertainties about terminology being used (slang or street terminology can have a variety of meanings). *Because the same words may have different meaning for different people, the nurse must be constantly prepared to define or clarify the meaning of a word or phrase.*

Identify and discuss personal sexual beliefs and values as evidenced by the following:

Selects socially acceptable behaviors consistent with personal beliefs and values

Explore with patient beliefs and values regarding sexuality, without placing your personal beliefs and values on the patient. For example, how do factors such as patient's early childhood beliefs, religious beliefs, and perceptions of parental attitudes toward sex affect present beliefs and values?

Offer suggestions to patient about alternative sexual behaviors or outlets within own scope of knowledge and level of comfort.

Allow patient the opportunity to discuss suggestions. *Make facts available whenever patient needs or asks for them since this builds trust, orients, enables decision making, and decreases anxiety, frustration, or other distressing feelings that hinder realistic action, thereby helping the patient focus on deeper concerns.*

Listen to what the patient has to say without jumping to conclusions or interpreting behavior prematurely.

Provide specific facts that address expressed needs. *Careful listening conveys respect and promotes self-esteem and a sense of security and safety.*

Attend closely to verbal and nonverbal signals suggesting anxiety or indications that a problem is more extensive than originally presented. *Nonverbal behavior often conveys more directly the feelings and is often the key to the message.*

Assist the patient in describing behavior rather than labeling (e.g., "I have difficulty becoming sexually aroused" instead of "I am frigid").

Help the patient determine whether behavior is helpful or useful in reaching goals, instead of labeling behavior as good or bad. *Patients need help in arriving at their own answers and determining what is right or wrong; do not judge for the patient what is right or wrong, normal and abnormal.*

Withhold personal opinions. *Patients must decide what is normal for themselves.*

Focus on changing nonsexual behavior that contributes to sexual problems by assigning assertiveness training, communication training, stress-reduction exercises, problem-solving techniques. *Skills training provides the patient with the behavioral repertoire needed to successfully interact with others.*

Encourage communication between partners.

Recommend a self-help program or refer to individual or group counseling, as appropriate.

REFERENCES

Annon JS: The plissit model: a proposed conceptual scheme for behavioral treatment of sexual problems, *J Sex Educa Ther* 2(1):1-15, 1976.

Donohue J, Gebhard P: The Kinsey Institute/Indiana University report on sexuality and spinal cord injury, *Sexual Disabil* 13(1):7, 1995.

Golding JM: Sexual assault history and limitations in physical functioning in two general population samples, *Res Nurs Health* 19(1):33, 1996.

Sbrocco T, Weisberg RB, Barlow DH: Sexual dysfunction in the older adult: assessment of psychosocial factors, *Sexual Disabil* 13(3):201, 1995.

Visser AP, Pascalle B: Effectiveness of sex education provided to adolescents *Patient Educ Counsel* 23(1):147, 1994.

Wilson HS, Kneisl CR: Clients with gender identity and sexual disorders. In *Psychiatric nursing*, Redwood City, Calif, 1996, Addison-Wesley.

Sexual dysfunction—cont'd

Sexuality patterns, altered

CLINICAL CONDITION/ MEDICAL DIAGNOSIS	RELATED FACTORS
Myocardial infarction (MI)	Knowledge/skill deficit about alternative responses to health-related transitions

Patient goals
Expected outcomes
  Associated nursing/collaborative interventions *and scientific rationale*

Attain satisfying level of sexual activity compatible with functional capacity as evidenced by the following:

Verbalizes knowledge related to the resumption of sexual activity

  Encourage patient and partner to ask questions about sexuality or sexual functioning in relation to their medical condition. Actively listen to patient's and partner's fears and concerns about altered self-image and sexual functioning. This will *promote open and therapeutic communication.*

  Assess level of comfort in discussing topic alone or with partner. Provide opportunity for both. *Individual counseling allows discussion of issues that may cause discomfort if discussed with partner present.*

  Provide specific information to patient and partner about limitations; correct myths and misinformation; address issues with sensitivity to customs and cultural issues. *Misinformation and myths may create unrealistic expectations about sexuality and sexual experiences. Patients who receive education and counseling report improved sexual satisfaction and performance because of decreased anxiety.*

  Use information obtained through sexual history about sexual activity before MI as basis for teaching and counseling; assess for long-standing sexual dysfunction, which can be caused by a psychogenic problem. *Assessment of patterns of sexual activity provides basis for individualized counseling and can help identify previous patterns associated with physiologic and psychologic stress.*

Examine concerns about sexuality and adequacy of sexual function. *Issues that may influence resumption of sexual activity are fear of sudden death or precipitation of symptoms such as angina, dyspnea, and palpitations; perceived change in body image; depression, which can affect ability to invest emotionally and be a factor in sexual dysfunction; forced dependency; changes in feelings of self-worth; and attractiveness to sexual partner.*

Address stress, fears, and sexual concerns of partner and examine relationship with sexual partner. *Partner should be included in the counseling process; if not, he or she may become overprotective and seek to limit those activities that are seen as potentially harmful to patient.*

Teach patient about possible side effects of drugs such as digitalis, hypnotics, tranquilizers, and diuretics. *Commonly prescribed medications may decrease libido and cause orgasmic and/or erectile dysfunction.*

Assess physical status that indicates when sexual activity can be resumed, patient's general health, tolerance for physical activity before MI, extent of myocardial damage, frequency and severity of angina or arrhythmias, and patient's ability to tolerate progression of activity. *Base advice to patient on consultation with physician. Depending on individual case, patient may resume sexual intercourse 5 to 8 weeks after postinfarction based on Index of Sexual Readiness (ability to take a brisk walk or climb two flights of stairs without chest pain). The O_2 demand of intercourse is in the 4-to-5 (metabolic equivalent) MET range. The ability to exercise at 5 or 6 METs and attain a heart rate of 115 to 120 beats per minute without such symptoms as ischemic changes or significant arrhythmias signifies that resumption of sexual activity will be safe.*

Explain alternative means/forms of expressing intimacy and/or sexual expression such as touching and positions that conserve energy.

Resumes sexual activity at or near level before MI

Assist patient in developing individualized plan of progressive physical and sexual activity based on physiologic limitations. *Sexual activity should be resumed gradually. Similar to any physical activity, sexual intercourse places increased demands on the cardiovascular system.*

Instruct about potential for angina during sexual intercourse and how to respond (if angina is experienced, stop intercourse and take nitroglycerin; may resume after relief is obtained). *If couple is advised that angina may occur, they know what to do, and they may be better able to cope. If they do encounter this problem, additional medication may be needed to prevent angina.*

Advise patient to avoid sexual activity for 2 or more hours after eating. *Angina may occur because of increased blood flow to gastrointestinal organs and increase demands caused by sexual activity. This results in decreased blood flow to myocardium.*

Advise patient to avoid sexual activity after excessive alcohol intake. *Alcohol causes decreased cardiac output, which may decrease the amount of exercise that can be performed without provoking angina.*

Teach patient warning signs that must be reported to physician: rapid pulse or respiratory rate that persists 4 to 5 minutes after orgasm, feeling of extreme fatigue after sexual activity. Anginal symptoms during or after sexual activity. *Potentially significant dysrhythmias and arrhythmias can be precipitated by sexual activity. Cardiovascular symptoms that occur during sexual activity may require further evaluation, use of medication, and physical conditioning, which would allow the patient to exercise in greater comfort.*

REFERENCES

Fridlund D and others: Recovery after myocardial infarction: effects of a caring rehabilitation programe, *Scandinav J Caring Sci* 5(1), 1991.

Glick DF: Home care of patients with cardiac disease. In Kinney MR and others: *Comprehensive cardiac care,* St Louis, 1991, Mosby.

Hamilton GA, Seldman RN: A comparison of the recovery period for women and men after an acute myocardial infarction, *Heart Lung* 22(4), 1993.

Jones C: Sexual activity after myocardial infarction, *Nurs Standard* 6(48), 1992.

Miller NH: Cardiac rehabilitation. In Kinney MR and others: *Comprehesive cardiac care,* St Louis, 1991, Mosby.

Piper KM: When can I do "it" again nurse? Sexual counseling after a heart attack, *Prof Nurse* 8(3), 1992.

Seidl A, and others: Understanding the effects of a myocardial infarction and sexual functioning: a basis for sexual counseling, *Rehabil Nurs* 16(5), 1991.

Steinke EE, Patterson-Midgley P: Sexual counseling of MI patients: nurses' comfort, responsibility, and practice, *Dimen Crit Care Nurs* 15(4):216-223, 1996.

Tardif GS: Sexual activity after a myocardial infarction, *Arch Phys Med Rehabil* 70:763-766, 1989.

Sexuality patterns, altered—cont'd

Skin integrity, impaired

CLINICAL CONDITION/ MEDICAL DIAGNOSIS	
Pressure ulcer	RELATED FACTORS
	Physical immobilization
	Altered circulation

Patient goals
Expected outcomes
 Associated nursing/collaborative interventions *and scientific rationale*

Manifest intact skin in area of disruption as evidenced by the following:

Skin lesion clean and healing

Discuss treatment options with patient and family.

Perform assessment of wound (Stage 1-4) and surrounding skin as a baseline and document daily or when dressing is changed, at least weekly.

Provide wound treatment based on stage and drainage, using AHCPR* guidelines; if using hydrocolloid, place triangle dressings narrow point down.

Debride and clean wound using AHCPR guidelines.

Ambulate patient if possible.

When patient is in bed, turn every 1 to 2 hours; use all four sides (lateral, prone, dorsal) unless contraindicated.

Position patient off pressure ulcer.

Select support surface according to AHCPR guidelines.

Keep pressure off skeletal prominences by positioning patient with pillow and/or foam devices.

Do not position directly on trochanter *because higher interface pressures and lower transcutaneous O_2 tension occurs.*

Use lifting devices and/or sheets to position patients.

Do not drag patient *because dragging causes shear.*

*Agency for Health Care Policy Research

Skin integrity, impaired

Use static devices (filled with foam or water, air, or gel) as necessary.

Do not massage skin; *rubbing may cause additional trauma.*

Prevent head of bed elevation of more than 30 degrees for long periods *because shearing forces are generated on sacrum, causing mechanical stress.*

Use underpads or briefs that absorb moisture and leave a quick-drying surface toward the skin if skin is continuously moist (incontinence, perspiration, drainage). *Excessive moisture reduces the resistance of skin to ulceration and increases risk of pressure sore formation fivefold.*

Avoid use of doughnuts and rubber rings because these increase pressure and damage tissue.

Have patient do active or passive range of motion (ROM) exercises every 2 hours *to promote circulation to skin and to alter weight-bearing.*

Elevate legs to prevent edema. *Edema slows oxygen diffusion and metabolic transport from capillary to cell.*

Teach patient to change position if possible.

Provide the following:

- Increased calories and protein 30 to 35 calories per day and 1.25 to 1.50 gms protein per day *because tissues are more vulnerable to necrosis with smaller amounts of pressure if the diet is deficient in these.*
- Increased fluid intake to prevent dehydration (2600 mL/day if possible).
- Supplement iron and vitamin C as needed. *Vitamin C is important for wound healing, fosters collagen synthesis and capillary function; iron improves oxygen-carrying capacity of blood.*

Assess and treat pain related to pressure ulcer and treatment according to AHCPR guidelines for acute pain management.

Monitor laboratory values that have an impact on skin and report abnormalities: Hct/Hbg *because low levels compromise oxygen delivery to tissues;* BUN *because elevated levels may indicate renal disease, which may affect albumin;* albumin *because low amounts cause interstitial edema, which impedes exchange of nutrients and waste products;* bilirubin *because levels may indicate liver disease, which may affect albumin;* arterial blood gases *because they indicate oxygen available for tissues.*

Patient/significant other demonstrates proper skin care

Teach patient/significant other above interventions.

Teach to call physician regarding signs and symptoms of infection or worsening of ulcer.

REFERENCES

Acute Pain Management Guideline Panel: *Acute pain management: operative or medical procedures and trauma.* Clinical Practice Guideline, No 1, AHCPR Publication No. 92-0032, Rockville, Md, 1992, Agency for Health Care Policy and Research, Public Health Service, US Department of Health and Human Services.

Barnes S: Patient/family education for the patient with pressure necrosis, *Nurs Clin North Am,* 22(2):463, 1987.

Day A: Managing sacral pressure ulcers with hydrocolloid dressings: results of a controlled clinical study, *Ostomy/Wound Manage* 41(2):52, 1995.

Gosnell D: Assessment and evaluation of pressure sores, *Nurs Clin North Am,* 22(2):399, 1987.

Robel L: Nutritional implications in the patient with pressure sores, *Nurs Clin North Am,* 22(2):379, 1987.

Treatment of Pressure Ulcers Guideline Panel: *Treatment of pressure ulcers,* AHCPR Publication No. 95-0652, Rockville, Md, 1994, Agency for Health Care Policy and Research, Public Health Service, US Department of Health and Human Services.

Skin integrity, impaired—cont'd

Skin integrity, impaired, risk for

CLINICAL CONDITION/ MEDICAL DIAGNOSIS	RELATED FACTORS
Acute CVA	Prolonged bedrest

Patient goals
Expected outcomes
Associated nursing/collaborative interventions *and scientific rationale*

Maintain intact skin tissue as evidenced by the following:

No reddened areas, no broken skin

Assess patient for the following risk factors or use a risk assessment scale: incontinence, immobility, inactivity, poor nutrition, edema, diminished sensation, decreased mental status.

Inspect skin for redness, cyanosis, blistering temperature, and pulses daily.

Keep skin clean and dry after washing.

Prevent extremes in environmental temperature and humidity.

Lubricate dry skin *because dry skin results in reduced pliability, fissuring, and cracking.*

Keep pressure off skeletal prominences by positioning patient with pillows or foam devices.

Ambulate patient if possible.

Use all four sides (lateral, prone, dorsal) unless contraindicated. When patient is in bed, turn every 1 to 2 hours.

Do not position directly on trochanter *because higher interface pressures and lower transcutaneous O_2 tension occurs.*

Do not drag patient; *dragging causes shear.* Use lifting devices/sheets to position patient.

Teach patient to change position if possible.

Use static devices (filled with foam or water; air or gel) as necessary.

Do not massage skin; *rubbing may cause additional trauma.*

revent head of bed elevation of more than 30
degrees for long periods. *Shearing forces are
generated on sacrum, causing mechanical stress.*
Use underpads or briefs that absorb moisture and
leave a quick-drying surface toward the skin if
skin is continuously moist (incontinence, perspiration, drainage). *Excessive moisture reduces
the resistance of skin to ulceration and increases
risk of pressure sore formation fivefold.*
Avoid use of doughnuts and rubber rings *because
these increase pressure and damage tissue.*
Provide adequate nutrition, including the following: sufficient calories and protein because *tissues are more vulnerable to necrosis with small
amounts of pressure if the diet is deficient in calories
and protein;* fluid intake adequate to prevent dehydration (2600 mL/day if possible).
Have patient do active or passive range of motion
(ROM) exercises every 2 hours to *promote
circulation to skin and to alter weight-bearing.*
Elevate legs to prevent edema. *Edema slows oxygen
diffusion and metabolic transport from capillary
to cell.*
Monitor blood chemistry levels that have an impact on skin and report abnormalities when
present: Hct/Hbg *because low levels compromise
oxygen delivery to the tissue;* BUN *because elevated
levels may indicate renal disease, which may affect
albumin;* albumin *because low amounts cause interstitial edema, which impedes exchange of nutrients and waste products;* bilirubin *because elevated
levels may indicate liver disease, which may affect
albumin;* arterial blood gases *because of indication
of oxygen available for tissues.*
Returns demonstration of proper skin care.
Provide *Preventing Pressure Ulcers: Patient Guide,* and
AHCPR publication, or other patient education
materials.
Teach patient/partner above interventions.
Teach to call physician if symptoms worsen.

REFERENCES

Barnes S: Patient/family education for the patient with pressure necrosis, *Nurs Clin North Am* 22(2):463, 1987.

Bergstrom N, et al: The Braden scale for predicting pressure sore risk, *Nurs Res* 36(4):205, 1987.

Bobel L: Nutritional implications in the patient with pressure sores, *Nurs Clin North Am* 22(2):379, 1987.

Maklebust J: Pressure ulcers: etiology and prevention, *Nurs Clin North Am* 22(2):359, 1987.

Panel for the Prediction and Prevention of Pressure Ulcers in Adults: *Pressure ulcers in adults: prediction and prevention,* Clinical Practice Guideline, No 3, AHCPR Publication No. 92-0047, Rockville, Md, 1992, Agency for Health Care Policy and Research, Public Health Service, US Department of Health and Human Services.

Skin integrity, impaired, risk for—cont'd

Sleep pattern disturbance

CLINICAL CONDITION/ MEDICAL DIAGNOSIS	RELATED FACTORS
Major medical illness	Disruptions in life-style or usual sleep habits

Patient goals
Expected outcomes
> Associated nursing/collaborative interventions *and scientific rationale*

Understand factors contributing to sleep pattern disturbances as evidenced by the following:

Participates in determining potential or actual causes for inadequate sleep

> Compare patient's current sleep pattern with usual sleep habits before hospitalization or current episode of sleep disturbance.
>
> Monitor and discuss possible causes for disturbed sleep (e.g., patient's worries, concerns, pain).
>
> Encourage expression of concerns if and when patient is unable to sleep.
>
> Confer with family or significant others about potential causes of sleep disturbance.
>
> Evaluate effects of patient's medications (e.g., steriods, diuretics) that may interfere with sleep. *Emotional problems may occur when corticosteriods are used, including mood swings, insomnia, etc.*
>
> Observe and monitor patient's daytime habits and activities.

Verbalizes understanding of specific plan to manage or correct causes of inadequate sleep

> Plan daytime activities to assure adequate physical and mental activity.
>
> Discourage daytime napping *only* if daytime naps negatively affect nighttime sleep. *Unsynchronized circadian sleep-wake cycles result from short naps dispersed over a 24-hour period.*

Sleep pattern disturbance

Monitor patient to avoid excessive time in bed (if medically appropriate).

Sleep through the night or at least for increased lengths of uninterrupted periods as evidenced by the following:

Falls asleep within 30 minutes of going to bed

Determine patient's usual nighttime habits and provide for routine as closely as possible (e.g., provide warm milk if allowed on medical regimen and if no nighttime voiding problem exists). Explain reasons for any necessary modifications in usual routine. *Changing a person's usual pattern of food intake in the evening has been found to impair subsequent sleep.*

Decrease fluid intake before bedtime (if wakening for frequent voiding occurs).

Have patient empty bladder at bedtime.

Avoid caffeine for 8 hours before sleep (if fluids are needed, substitute decaffeinated drinks).

Promote relaxation at bedtime: select interventions approved by the patient (e.g., provide soft music, back massage, security objects; suggest guided imagery techniques; teach muscle-relaxation techniques).

Provide patient with comfortable environment to promote sleep or rest (e.g., turn off lights; provide adequate room ventilation; provide warmth or coolness as needed; avoid noise disturbances). *Cortical inhibition on reticular formation is eliminated during sleep, enhancing autonomic responses; thus, cardiovascular responses to noise are greater during sleep.*

Avoid strenuous physical or mental activity just before bedtime.

Minimal number of essential interruptions occur

Sleeps during longer intervals between nursing care functions

Verbalizes feeling of being rested or refreshed after nighttime sleeping

Schedule assessments or interventions to allow for longer sleep periods (e.g., check vital signs and turn patient at same time). *Sleep deprivation occurs with frequent interruption of sleep and may impair recovery because of psychologic and physiologic disturbances. Patient's own circadian rhythm is disturbed by interruptions.*

Explain to patient the need for essential interruptions.

Help patient to maintain a normal day/night pattern to facilitate night sleeping.

Provide sedation as prescribed only if necessary, temporarily, and preferably on an intermittent, not nightly, basis.

Determine effectiveness of sedative prescribed (i.e., optimal dosage, no rebound effects).

Monitor level of daytime alertness and daytime functioning.

REFERENCES

Edwards GB, Schuring LM: Pilot study: validating nurses' observations of sleep and wake states among critically ill patients, using polysomnography, *Am J Crit Care* 2(2):125-131, 1993.

Floyd JA: Another look at napping in older adults, *Geriatr Nurs* 16(3):136-138, 1995.

Halfens R, Cox K, Kuppen-Van Merwijk A: Effect of the use of sleep medication in Dutch hospitals on the use of sleep medication at home, *J Adv Nurs* 19:66-70, 1994.

Jensen DP, Herr KA: Sleeplessness, *Adv Clin Nurs Res* 28(2):385-403, 1993.

Sheely LC: Sleep disturbances in hospitalized patients with cancer, *Oncol Nurs Forum* 23(1):109-111, 1996.

Spenceley SM: Sleeping inquiry: A look with fresh eyes, *Image* 25(3):249-256, 1993.

Sleep pattern disturbance—cont'd

Social interaction, impaired

CLINICAL CONDITION/ MEDICAL DIAGNOSIS	RELATED FACTORS
Chronic undifferentiated schizophrenia	Knowledge/skill deficit about enhancing mutuality
	Absence of available significant other

Patient goals
Expected outcomes
  Associated nursing/collaborative interventions *and scientific rationale*

Improve social competence in interpersonal interactions and enhance social network as evidenced by the following:

Identifies strengths and limitations in current patterns of social interaction

  Establish trusting one-on-one nurse-patient relationship

  Assess with the patient the strengths and limitations of current social interaction style.

  Assess family relationships and patterns of relating to family members

  Observe and assist the patient to identify nonverbal behaviors of which he or she may not be aware.

  Review the patient patterns of relating with peers.

  Encourage the patient to express feelings and perceptions of social skills. *Self-perceptions can be altered to promote adaptive changes and growth.*

  Explore with the patient feelings that are associated with discomfort in social situations.

  Help patient identify situations in which others are alienated because of patient's behavior.

Uses enhanced social skills in both familiar and new interpersonal situations in order to enhance to mutuality

  Provide opportunities for meaningful task performance within the milieu.

Social interaction, impaired

417

Facilitate conversation between patient and peers or significant others to enhance mutuality.

Help patient identify others with whom he or she feels comfortable and encourage interaction and activities with them.

Provide feedback about observed interactions; consider use of videotaping to review learning.

Structure milieu to provide opportunities for socialization (small areas for reading, games, refreshments).

Use social skill training to assist patient to identify strategies and role play more effective behavior, obtain social reinforcement, and practice the behavior in a real situation.

Modeling, structuring, and providing feedback promote learning and awareness of positive actions and problem areas.

Increase interactions with others as evidenced by the following:

Resumes or adds to socialization and activities with expressed satisfaction in interpersonal relationships

Help patient identify opportunities for increased social interaction.

Encourage visits and involvement of family or significant others.

Use creative activities and group interaction to provide opportunities for self-expression and demonstration of abilities.

Encourage attendance at activities, resumption of hobbies or involvement in support groups or volunteer work to expand social networks.

Provide positive reinforcement for demonstration of more effective social skills.

These actions provide increased opportunity for positive social reinforcement and repetition of successful social behaviors.

REFERENCES

Eastland LS: Recovery as an interactive process: explanation and empowerment in 12-step programs, *Qual Health Res* 5(3):292, 1995.

Social interaction, impaired—cont'd

Hayes RL, Halford WK, Varghese FT: Social skills training with chronic schizophrenic patients: effects on negative symptoms and community functioning, *Behav Therapy* 26(3):433-449, 1995.

Hughes I and others: Developing a family intervention service for serious mental illness: clinical observations and experiences, *J Ment Health* 5(2):145-159, 1996.

Liberman RP, DeRisi WJ, Mueser KT: *Social skills training for psychiatric patients,* New York, 1989, Pergamon Press.

Manderino M, Bzdek V: Social skill building with chronic patients, *J Psychosoc Nurs Ment Health Serv* 25(9):18-23, 1987.

McFarland GK, McFarlane EA: *Nursing diagnosis and intervention: planning for patient care,* ed 3, St Louis, 1997, Mosby.

Simmons A: Social networks: their relevance to mental health nursing, *J Adv Nurs* 19:281, 1994.

Topf M, Dambacher B: Teaching interpersonal skills: a model for facilitating optimal interpersonal relations, *Psychosoc Nurs* 19:29-33, 1981.

Social interaction, impaired—cont'd

Social isolation

CLINICAL CONDITION/ MEDICAL DIAGNOSIS	RELATED FACTORS
Third degree burns	Loss of significant relationship and of work role
Facial disfigurement	Inability to engage in or sustain satisfying relationships

Patient goals
Expected outcomes
> Associated nursing/collaborative interventions *and scientific rationale*

Develop a trusting relationship as evidenced by the following:

Expresses feelings of aloneness, absence of supportive significant others, and feelings of rejection

Facilitate and explore expressions of feelings.

Explore dynamics of past relationships: process and outcome.

Engage in active listening.

Alert patient to negative self-talk and discuss inaccuracies of perception.

Assess social skills through varied behavioral observation. Incorporate findings into personalized strategies for successful socialization.

Assess situational and chronic low self-esteem. Assess need for referral.

Help patient to recognize bodily reactions to cognitions. *Awareness is a first step in gaining control over thoughts, feelings, and behaviors.*

Reduce degree of social isolation as evidenced by the following:

Regularly participates in a pertinent, therapeutic group meeting
Invites at least one person to visit home at regular intervals

Selects and participates in at least one leisure group activity every 2 weeks

Structure with patient a self-modification program using self-selected strategies.

Provide information about available pertinent groups (e.g., social skills training, cognitive reappraisal, social support).

Provide positive reinforcement for even the slightest movement toward involvement with others.

Develop one or two meaningful relationships as evidenced by the following:

Identifies one or two individuals who are important and why they are important
Interacts with these individuals regularly, such as one phone call per week

Identify barriers to forming meaningful relationships.

Discuss relationships of personal responsibility and social isolation.

Discuss and analyze at each visit positive and negative aspects of interpersonal interactions that occurred in previous week.

Discuss reality and risks and benefits of opening oneself to others.

Develop interest in volunteering to assist someone or an organization as evidenced by the following:

Makes at least one phone call per week for 3 weeks, inquiring about volunteer service

Discuss satisfaction that can be experienced through helping others.

Provide patient with information about volunteer possibilities in immediate vicinity. *Engaging in volunteer activities provides recognition and allows patient to experience satisfying personal relationships.*

Contract with patient for at least one phone call to a volunteer service per week. Elicit feelings about the phone call at next session.

Expand and engage in new interest as evidenced by the following:

Engages in one satisfying leisure activity appropriate to developmental stage with another individual(s) on a regularly planned basis.

Negotiate with patient to complete a leisure assessment.

Discuss findings of leisure assessment; elicit feelings regarding assessment and finding.

Explore with patient obstacles to involvement in one leisure activity identified as interesting.

Help patient to engage in strategies to overcome obstacles.

REFERENCES

Donohue B and others: Social skills training for depressed, visually impaired older adults. A treatment manual, *Behav Modif* 19(4):379-424, 1995.

Elsen J, Blegen M: Social isolation. In Maas M, Buckwalter KC, Hardy M, eds: *Nursing diagnoses and interventions for the elderly,* Philadelphia, 1991, WB Saunders.

Kell JH, Frisch NC: A transcultural concept analysis of social isolation. In Carroll-Johnson RM, ed: *Classification of nursing diagnoses: proceedings of the tenth conference,* Philadelphia, 1992, JB Lippincott.

Kinney CK, Mannettu R, Carpenter MA: Support groups. In Bulechek GM, McCloskey JC, eds: *Nursing interventions: essential nursing treatments,* ed 2, Philadelphia, 1992, WB Saunders.

Lien-Greschen Validation of social isolation related to maturational age: elderly, *Nurs Diagn* 4(1):37, 1993.

Luggen AS, Rini AG: Assessment of social networks and isolation in community-based elderly men and women, *Geriatr Nurs* 16(4):179-181, 1995.

McCloskey JC, Bulecheck GM, editors: Socialization enhancement. *Nursing interventions classification (NIC),* ed 2, St Louis, 1996, Mosby.

Pender NJ: Self-modification. In Bulechek GM, McCloskey J, editors: *Nursing interventions treatment for nursing diagnosis,* Philadelphia, 1985, WB Saunders.

Porter EJ: Older widows' experience of living alone at home, *Image* 26(1):19-24, 1994.

Russel D: The measurement of loneliness. In Peplau LA, Perlman D, eds: *Loneliness,* New York, 1982, John Wiley & Sons.

Scandrett-Hibdon S: Cognitive reappraisal. In Bulecheck GM, McCloskey JC, eds: *Nursing interventions: essential nursing treatments,* ed 2, Philadelphia, 1992, WB Saunders.

Stevens SR: Post-trauma response. In Thompson JM and others: *Mosby's clinical nursing,* ed 3, St Louis, 1993, Mosby.

Whalen P: Tu, solou (you, alone): alienation and resocialization of the elderly, *J Gerontol Nurs,* 6,348, 1980.

Spiritual distress (distress of the human spirit)

CLINICAL CONDITION/ MEDICAL DIAGNOSIS	RELATED FACTORS
Human immunodeficiency virus/acquired immunodeficiency syndrome (HIV/AIDS)	Fear, hopelessness, guilt, and sense of alienation

---

Patient goals
Expected outcomes
  Associated nursing/collaborative interventions *and scientific rationale*

Improve personal harmony and serenity as evidenced by the following:

Makes positive statements about self and life
Achieves high Existential Well-Being score (40 to 60) on the Spiritual Well-Being Index
Expresses a sense of hope, forgiveness, and loss of guilt
Expresses a sense of meaning in illness and purpose in life

  Encourage expression of feeling through presence, active listening, and being nonjudgmental. *Presence and active listening will help to build trust and positive regard.*

  Encourage storytelling by encouraging patient to review life story; share stories of others who have found meaning in diversity. *Storytelling will help the nurse to develop a better understanding of the patient and help the patient find meaning in life.*

  Monitor hope and existential well-being with the Spiritual Well-Being Index and the Hopelessness Scale. *There is a positive relationship between spiritual well-being and hope in persons with AIDS.*

  Inspire hope by referring to AIDS as a chronic illness; inform patient that newer treatments can prolong life for many years.

Spiritual distress (distress of the human spirit)

423

Improve personal harmony and connections with friends, family, members of personal faith and culture, and other support systems as evidenced by the following:

Initiates and maintains ongoing relationship with other individual

Explores, discusses, and maintains ongoing relationships with family, culture, and faith system

Participates in AIDS support group and systems

Encourage patient to continue relationships with significant others; realize that many of patient's significant others may be ill or have died from AIDS. *Helping patients cope with and express grief over losses will help them cope with own personal loss of future.*

Encourage patient to contact and communicate with family members and members of faith system. *Support system and spiritual heritage are important for persons coping with chronic illness; they help prevent alienation and are often helpful for finding meaning and purpose in life.*

Help the patient deal with the hurtful and destructive elements from family and spiritual heritage; be compassionate and open to nontraditional (blood and surrogate) families that seek reentry to faith system.

Provide information on AIDS support systems in community; collaborate with social worker in seeking out and encouraging participation in the support systems.

Familiarize self with African-American and Hispanic-American family systems. *African-American and Hispanic-American cultures have strong family systems and beliefs, and are statistically in a high-risk group for HIV/AIDS.*

Improve harmony with God, Supreme Being, or Power beyond self as evidenced by the following:

Scores high on the Spiritual Well-Being Scale; acknowledges that there is a loving and forgiving God

Expresses sense of being loved by friends or family

Provide, encourage, and help with prayer or meditation; use uplifting stories or music in accordance with patient's preference.

Refer and collaborate with spiritual counselor to help affirm the individual and resolve feelings of anger, isolation, guilt and past life hurts.

Help individual to realize that there is a forgiving and all-loving God. *Many persons with AIDS feel a sense of alienation with their formal source of faith or religion and have a picture of God as punishing and unforgiving. Faith system can be a primary source of being connected with a power beyond oneself and feeling a sense of love and oneness with others.*

REFERENCES

Bufford RK, Paloutzian RF, Ellison CW: Norms for the spiritual well-being scale, *J Psychology Theology* 19(1):56-70, 1991.

Carson V, Soeken KL, Shanty J, Terry L: Hope and spiritual well-being: essentials for living with AIDS, *Perspec Psychiatr Care* 26(2):2834, 1990.

Fryback PB: Health for people with a terminal diagnosis, *Nurs Sci Q* 6(3):147-159, 1993.

Heliker D: Reevaluation of a nursing diagnosis; spiritual distress. *Nurs Forum* 27(4):15-20, 1992.

Landau-Stanton J, Clements CD, Tartaglia AE: Spiritual, cultural and community systems. In Landau-Stanton JB, Clements C: *AIDS health and mental health,* New York, 1993, Brunner/Mazel.

Peri TAC: Promoting spirituality in persons with acquired immunodeficiency syndrome: a nursing intervention. *Holistic Nurs Pract* 10(1):68-76, 1995.

Reed PG: An emerging paradigm for the investigation of spirituality in nursing, *Res Nurs Health* 15:349-357, 1992.

Smucker C: A phenomenological description of the experience of spiritual distress. In Rantz MJ, Lemone P: *Classification of nursing diagnoses: proceedings of the eleventh conference,* Glendale, Calif, 1995, CINAHL Information Systems.

Wesorick B: Consensual validation of interventions categorized by nursing diagnosis. In Rantz MJ, Lemone P: *Classification of nursing diagnoses: proceedings of the eleventh conference,* Glendale, Calif, 1995, CINAHL Information Systems.

Spiritual distress (distress of the human spirit)—cont'd

Spiritual well-being, potential for enhanced

CLINICAL CONDITION/ MEDICAL DIAGNOSIS	RELATED FACTORS
A 47 year-old business executive receiving daily radiation after mastectomy	Expresses renewed appreciation of life; wishes to reestablish relationships with estranged family members

Patient goals
Expected outcomes
    Associated nursing/collaborative interventions *and scientific rationale*

Find greater self-awareness and acceptance as evidenced by the following:

Discusses the meaning of health in her life
Formulates new goals
Expresses hope for the future

Use "kything" to bring about a spiritual connection. The process of kything includes: choosing to be a healing force in an individual's life; becoming quiet and centered; holding individual in awareness; and joining self with other in spirit.

Ask individual to tell her story and describe what is most meaningful in her life. *Meanings change as life unfolds.*

Seek to understand the situation as it is being experienced by the individual; remain focused on what individual is relating.

Assess the individual's inner strengths and ability to seek meaning and fulfillment in life (e.g., use Assessing the Spiriting Process too).

Help individual uncover the meaning of health in her life through the reassessment of priorities. *Priorities change when individuals face their own mortality.*

Help individual find things to hope for. *Hope enables individuals to continue to enjoy their lives.*

Renew relationships with family members as evidenced by the following:

Writes a personal letter to each family member expressing desire to spend time with them and recalls enjoyment of past experiences
Follows letter with personal telephone contact to arrange a family meeting at their convenience
Modifies daily activities to provide more time to build family relationships

Help individual to use inner strength to make first move toward reconnecting with family. *Facing own mortality increases significance of family, friendships, and love.*

Identify caring behaviors in nurse-patient relationship and use as basis for teaching new caring behaviors. *Caring and being cared for promotes an individual's survival.*

Seek opportunity to help family members recognize individual's need for renewed relationships.
Connectedness is a central theme and critical attribute of spiritual perspective. Connectedness is a significant, shared and meaningful personal relationship with another.

REFERENCES

Bauer T, Barron CR: Nursing interventions for spiritual care: preferences of the community-based elderly, *J Holistic Nurs* 13(3):268-279, 1995.

Burkhardt MA, Nagai-Jacobson MG: Reawakening spirit in clinical practice, *J Holistic Nurs* 12(1):9-21, 1994.

Dossey B, Frisch NC, Guzzetta CE, Burkhardt MA: American Holistic Nurses Association. In Carroll-Johnson RM, Paquette M: *Classification of nursing diagnoses: proceedings of the tenth conference,* Philadelphia, 1994, JB Lippincott.

Fryback PB: Health for people with a terminal diagnosis: *Nurs Sci Q* 6(3):147-159, 1993.

Haase JC and others: Simultaneous concept analysis of spiritual perspective, hope, acceptance and self-transcendence, *Image: J Nurs Scholar* 24(2):141-147, 1992.

Kaye J, Robinson KM: Spirituality among caregivers, *Image: J Nurs Scholar* 26(3):218-221, 1994.

Mansen TJ: The spiritual dimension of individuals: conceptual development, *Nurs Diagn* 4(4):140-147, 1993.

Newman MA: Theory for nursing practice, *Nurs Sci Q* 7(4):153-157, 1994.

Ray V: *Green spirituality: reflections on belonging to a world beyond myself,* New York, 1992, HarperCollins.

Reed PG: An emerging paradigm for the investigation of spirituality in nursing, *Res Nurs Health* 15(5):349-357, 1992.

Spiritual well-being, potential for enhanced—cont'd

427

Suffocation, risk for

CLINICAL CONDITION/ MEDICAL DIAGNOSIS	RISK FACTORS
Alcohol abuse	Smokes in bed; frequent emesis

Patient goals
Expected outcomes
> Associated nursing/collaborative interventions *and scientific rationale*

Recognize increased risk of suffocation as evidenced by the following:

Permanently removes all smoking materials from bedside
Establishes a separate area in home for smoking; outside when weather is mild
> Teach patient/spouse dangers of smoking in bed.
> Teach patient/spouse dangers of secondhand smoke.
> Refer patient to smoking cessation clinic.

Verbalizes understanding of risks associated with drinking behaviors
Spouse demonstrates side-lying position and use of supports to keep patient on side following bouts of drinking.
> Use anatomic drawings to teach patient/spouse danger in inhaling expelled gastric contents.
> Teach spouse to position patient on side to avoid inhaling own vomit. *Knowledge of safety measures will help spouse to reduce risk of suffocation.*

Participate in alcohol rehabilitation program as evidenced by the following:

Acknowledges problem with alcohol abuse
Verbalizes knowledge of adverse effects of excessive drinking
> Offer patient and spouse opportunity to discuss their perceptions of patient's drinking behavior.
> Assist patient in examining consequences of drinking behavior. *A sustained state of alcoholic denial*

of the consequences of drinking prevents voluntary seeking of treatment.

Joins Al-Anon (spouse)

Enters alcohol treatment program (patient)

Provide patient and spouse with list of alcohol treatment programs in the community.

Negotiate weekly telephone follow-up with patient/spouse.

REFERENCES

Hall JM: How lesbians recognize and respond to alcohol problems: a theoretical model of problematization, *Adv Nurs Sci* 16(3):46-63, 1994.

Hawks JH, Lindeman J, Bartek JK: A validation study, altered family processes: alcoholism. Abstract. In Carroll-Johnson RM, Paquette M, eds: *Classification of nursing diagnoses: proceedings of the tenth conference,* Philadelphia, 1994, JB Lippincott.

Hughes TL: Research on alcohol and drug use among women: A review and update. In McElmurry BJ, Parker RS, eds: *Ann Rev Women's Health,* New York, 1993, National League for Nursing Press.

O'Connell KA: Smoking cessation. In Bulechek GM, McCloskey JC, eds: *Nursing interventions: essential nursing treatments,* Philadelphia, 1992, WB Saunders.

O'Connell KA: Smoking cessation: research on relapse crises, *Annu Rev Nurs Res* 8:83-100, 1990.

Sullivan EJ and Handley SM: Alcohol and drug abuse in nurses. *Annu Rev Nurs Res* 10:113-125, 1992.

Sullivan EJ and Handley SM: Alcohol and drug abuse, *Annu Rev Nurs Res* 1993, 11:281-297, 1993.

Wing DM: Transcending alcoholic denial, *Image: J Nurs Scholar* 27(2):121-126, 1995.

Swallowing, impaired

CLINICAL CONDITION/ MEDICAL DIAGNOSIS	RELATED FACTORS
Right cerebrovascular accident (CVA) with paralysis of left side of face and mouth.	Decreased gag reflex and oral sensations; delayed swallow mechanism.

Patient goals
Expected outcomes
    Associated nursing/collaborative interventions *and scientific rationale*

Swallow food and liquids safely as evidenced by the following:

Swallows without aspirating

Feed patient only when alert. *Lethargy hinders safe swallowing.*

Supervise during feeding *to promote safe swallowing.*

Check affected side of mouth for pocketing during and after meals. *Pocketing of food may occur on the affected side of mouth because of paralysis or weakness leading to high risk for aspiration.*

Place emergency equipment at patient's bedside and meal site *in case of choking.*

Minimize distractions in the environment *to keep patient focused on safe swallowing technique.*

Allow enough time to eat. *Rushing decreases compliance with swallowing precautions.*

Feed patient one small bolus of food at a time, starting with ¼ to ½ teaspoon and never exceeding 1 teaspoonful. *Small boluses are easier to swallow and manipulate for patients with impaired oral control.*

Avoid mixing food textures, such as beef barley soup. *Varied food textures are more difficult for dysphagic patients to manage and may increase risk for aspiration.*

Place foods on unaffected side of mouth *to promote optimal oral control and allow patient to sense where food is in mouth.*

Use verbal cueing, naming each bite of food, where placed, and when to swallow. *Cueing assists patient with sequencing.*

Reinforce swallowing techniques with patient at every meal. *Frequent reinforcement of correct technique improves carryover.*

Follow recommendations of speech therapist for compensatory strategies *to reduce risk of aspiration and improve swallowing efficiency.*

Position patient upright with head flexed slightly forward in chin tuck position at mealtimes. *Chin tuck position reduces the likelihood of aspiration during swallowing by maximizing airway closure and esophageal opening and decreasing the speed of bolus transit.*

Keep patient in upright position for at least ½ hour after meals. *This position reduces the risk of aspiration.*

Encourage patient to rotate head toward the affected side. *This position causes bolus to lateralize away from direction of rotation when swallowing, thus directing bolus to functional side.*

Encourage double swallow technique. *It decreases likelihood of aspiration.*

Provide rest periods before and during feeding *to ensure optimal participation in eating.*

Praise small gains in ability to swallow. *Positive reinforcement enhances confidence in swallowing ability.*

Monitor for signs of aspiration (fever, coughing, choking on small amounts of food, upper airway congestion, wet voice quality). *Aspiration is a common complication for dysphagic patients, requiring continual monitoring.*

Collaborate with dietician and speech therapist to develop a plan for introduction and progression of fluids. Introduce thick liquids first. Progressively add thin liquids, beginning with juices with the most taste (citrus) and most sensation (carbonated beverages). Use thickening agents as needed. Add thin liquids without much lasting taste (water and tea). *Thick liquids provide more sensation in the dysphagic patient's mouth and throat and are therefore easier to control and swallow.*

Collaborate with dietician and speech therapist to develop a plan for introduction and progression of foods. Introduce foods with pureed consistency first. Progressively add soft (ground) foods, then solid foods beginning with those that require the least chewing. *Foods that are cohesive and soft are easiest to control in the mouth and swallow safely.*

Maintain adequate nutrition and hydration as evidenced by the following:

Maintains stable weight

Encourage intake of 2000 calories every 24 hours. *Adequate intake prevents weight loss and decreases risk of muscular wasting.*

Provide mouth care before and after meals. *Mouth care stimulates salivation.*

Consider supplemental tube feedings if oral intake less than body requirements. *Early attention to maintaining adequate nutrition decreases length of stay and complications in post CVA patients.*

Schedule tube feedings in such a manner as *to avoid interference with oral feeding and to facilitate stimulation of appetite.*

Determine patient's food preferences from patient and family members *to increase the probability of sufficient nutritional intake.*

Provide high-calorie nutritional supplement 2 hours after meals and at bedtime. *Providing nutritional supplements enhances the likelihood of attaining and maintaining desired nutritional status.*

Provide small frequent meals. *Small meals enhance the likelihood of maximal caloric intake.*

Weigh patient at least twice a week.

Monitor caloric intake, serum albumin and protein. *Monitoring promotes early recognition of inadequate nutrition/hydration.*

Maintains minimum fluid intake of 1500 ml every 24 hours

Monitor intake and output. *Monitoring decreases the risk of dehydration.*

Determine patient's liquid preferences from patient and family members *to increase the likelihood of required fluid intake.*

Evaluate need for supplemental tube feeding *to maintain adequate nutrition and hydration.*

Learn safe swallowing techniques and participate in care management as evidenced by the following:

Family members assist patient with feeding with less supervision over time

Reassure family members about actual or potential improvements in swallowing. *Progress may be slow, so indications reflecting improvement need to be highlighted for family.*

Reinforce with patient and family that swallowing problems may be temporary. *Accurate, hopeful information may help the patient and family cope with the present impairment.*

Collaborate with speech therapist to teach and reinforce knowledge and understanding of compensatory swallowing techniques.

Provide written resources for future reference.

Family members describe and demonstrate pertinent safety techniques

Family members provide encouragement and support during meals

Instruct family about diet modification for home use in collaboration with dietician. *Assistance may be required to translate hospital techniques to home environment.*

Teach Heimlich maneuver to family members *to prepare for possible emergency.*

Collaborate with speech therapist and family to ensure that family members participate in patient's swallowing therapy sessions. *Observation and practice with patient's swallowing therapy will decrease anxiety.*

Swallowing, impaired—cont'd

REFERENCES

Bronstein K, Popovich J, Stewart-Amidel C: *Promoting stroke recovery,* St Louis, 1991, Mosby.

Cochran I and others: Stroke care: piecing together the long-term picture, *Nursing 94* June: 34-41, 1994.

Cole-Arvin C, Notich L, Underhill A: Identifying and managing dysphagia, *Nursing 94* January:48-49, 1994.

DePippo K, Holas M, Reding M, Mandel F, Lesser M: Dysphagia therapy following stroke: a controlled trial, *Neurology* 44:1655-1660, 1994.

Lugger K: Dysphagia in the elderly stroke patient, *J Neurosci Nurs* April, 1994 26(2):78-84, 1994.

Moore K: Stroke: the long road back, *RN* 50-54, 1994.

Saltzman LS, Rosenberg CH, Wolf RH: Brainstem infarct with pharyngeal dysmotility and paralyzed vocal cord—management with a multidisciplinary approach, *Arch Phys Med Rehabil* 74(2):214, 1993.

Welch MV and others: Changes in pharyngeal dimensions effected by chin tuck, *Arch Phys Med Rehabil* 74(2):178, 1993.

Swallowing, impaired—cont'd

Thermoregulation, ineffective

CLINICAL CONDITION/
MEDICAL DIAGNOSIS   RELATED FACTORS

Premature infant   Immature thermoregulatory system

Patient goals
Expected outcomes
   Associated nursing/collaborative interventions *and*
      scientific rationale

Establish normothermia as evidenced by the following:

Maintains temperature within normal range

Adjust environmental temperature to infant's needs by using an incubator or radiant warmer; avoiding drafts and cold environmental temperatures; keeping infant clothed in undershirt, diaper, and gown in order to increase resistance to nonevaporative heat loss; keeping head covered *because up to 60% of heat loss occurs this way.*

Initiate kangaroo care.

Provide warm humidified oxygen 32° to 36° C.

Administer intravenous (IV) fluids at room temperature.

Monitor for and report the following signs and symptoms of hypothermia: poor feeding, increased or decreased spontaneous activity, weak cry, decreased muscle tone, difficult arousal, irritability, lethargy, cyanosis, pallor, respiratory distress, bradycardia.

Monitor the following laboratory values that may be affected by thermal instability: decreased serum pH level, which indicates presence of acidosis, *because acidosis may result from increased oxygen demands to generate heat;* decreased blood glucose *because hyperglycemia may result from increased use of carbohydrate stores in an effort to generate heat.*

Thermoregulation, ineffective

435

REFERENCES

Lawson L: Hypothermia and trauma injury; temperature monitoring and rewarming strategies, *Crit Care Nurse Q* 15(1):21, 1992.

Ludington-Hoe SM, et al: Kangaroo care: research results, and practice implications and guidelines, *Neonatal Netw* 13(1):19-27, 1994.

Merenstein GB, Gardner SL: *Handbook of neonatal intensive care,* ed 3, St Louis, 1993, Mosby.

Roncoli M, Medoff-Cooper B: Thermoregulation in low birth-weight infants, *NAACOG'S Clin Iss* 3(1):25, 1992.

Stevens T: Managing postoperative hypothermia, rewarming and its complications, *Crit Care Nurse Q* 16(1):60, 1993.

Thomas K: Thermoregulation in neonates, *Neonatal Netw* 13(2):15, 1994.

Thermoregulation, ineffective—cont'd

Thought processes, altered

CLINICAL CONDITION/ MEDICAL DIAGNOSIS	RELATED FACTORS
Borderline Personality Disorder	Coping with feelings of distress
	Negative self-evaluation

**Patient goals
Expected outcomes**
   Associated nursing/collaborative interventions *and
      scientific rationale*

Maintains contact with mental health and medical systems instead of constant antagonism and discontinuing treatment as evidenced by the following:

Seeks assistance for specific problems or situations

   Assist in clarifying situation by asking who, what, when, where, why, and how. *Remaining focused on problems of daily living assists patient in perceiving situations in several contexts not just good or bad in relation to the self; it promotes seeing world as less dangerous.*

   Provide weekly contact to focus on events and teach tolerance of one's emotional state. *Becoming aware of one's own anger, disappointment, etc. enables patient to express emotions and learn new ways to manage the range of emotions patient will begin to perceive self as less powerless to cope.*

Demonstrates cognitive ability to track the consequences of certain stressful events on emotions and thought about self

   Teach to monitor self in relation to causes of stress or problems and behaviors occurring as result of inaccurate facts, and to note the changes needed modify stressor, change behavioral response to stressor, or change automatic thoughts. *All these techniques contribute to increasing a sense of self and one's ability to act in a responsible manner.*

   Assist to determine what is helpful, less helpful, and even harmful.

Thought processes, altered

Demonstrates the use of one or two coping strategies to handle feelings of distress, particularly stopping suicidal behaviors

Teach ways to provide self with structure. Make list and post on wall, draw a circle and place self inside, use a room or chair to make boundaries more concrete. *"Concretizing" the structure assists a person in achieving a sense of self, a feeling of control of self especially when feelings of anxiety are increasing.*

Teach coping strategies to focus on behavior (e.g., recording automatic thoughts, asking another about personal interpretations of situation, relaxation techniques, role playing) and to use cognitive process (e.g., catching and stopping automatic thought, active problem solving).

Teach how to reward self in concrete ways (e.g., going to a special movie), as well as use of cognitive methods (e.g., "That was a good idea").

REFERENCES

Beck AT: *Cognitive therapy of personality disorders,* New York, 1990, Guilford Press.

Gunderson JG, Links P: Borderline personality disorder. In Gabbard GO, ed: *Treatments of psychiatric disorders,* Vol II, ed 2, Washington DC, 1995, American Psychiatric Press.

Greene H, Ugarriza DN: The 'stable unstable' borderline personality disorder: history, theory and nursing intervention, *J Psychosoc Nurs Ment Health Serv* 33(12):26-30, 1996.

Lineham MM: *Cognitive-behavioral treatment of borderline personality disorder,* New York, 1993, Guilford Press.

Miller SG: Borderline personality disorder from the patient's perspective, *Hosp Commun Psychiatry* 45(12):1215-1219, 1994.

Paris J: *Borderline personality disorder,* Washington DC, 1994, American Psychiatric Press.

Stein KF: Affect instability in adults with a borderline personality disorder, *Arch Psychiatr Nurs* 10(1):32-40, 1996.

Thought processes, altered—cont'd

Tissue integrity, impaired

CLINICAL CONDITION/ MEDICAL DIAGNOSIS	RELATED FACTORS
Venostasis ulcers	Venous pooling

Patient goals
Expected outcomes
   Associated nursing/collaborative interventions *and*
      scientific rationale

Attain tissue healing as evidenced by the following:

Reduced edema surrounding lesion
Intact skin of lower extremity
   Assess lesion for depth (partial or full thickness)
      and healing phase (e.g., granulation, epithe-
      lization).
   Remove constrictive clothing.
   Provide physiologic and aseptic environment for
      lesion.
   Avoid cytotoxic solutions.
   Consult physician concerning moisture-retentive
      dressings.
   Consult physician concerning medications (e.g.,
      diuretic therapy).
Wound free of purulent and necrotic material
   Clean lesion with nonirritating solutions (e.g., nor-
      mal saline)
   Remove purulent drainage and necrotic tissue.
   Consult physician concerning debridement strate-
      gies (e.g., sharp, mechanical, enzymatic and/or
      autolytic)
Wound care performed by patient or significant other
   Teach patient or significant other to perform
      wound care and to detect symptoms and signs
      of infection or increased inflammation.
   Teach patient to avoid constrictive clothing (e.g.,
      shoes, stockings, tight-waisted undergarments).
Circulatory exercises and postural maneuvers per-
formed by patient
   Demonstrate and assist patient in performing

Tissue integrity, impaired

439

lower extremity exercises and deep breathing exercises sequentially, to activate skeletal muscle pump and respiratory pump in lying or standing position.

Elevate extremity when patient is in sitting position.

Teach patient to avoid crossing legs. *Gravity affects venous flow and lymph in the lower extremities. Crossing legs impedes venous return and promotes venostatis that leads to edema formation and impaired tissue perfusion.*

Develop an exercise schedule with patient that includes a comfortable combination of walking and rest periods and that avoids standing still for prolonged periods.

Consult physician about compressive stockings or pneumatic leggings. *If venous insufficiency is severe, long-term ambulatory elastic compression stocking therapy may be used to facilitate venous return and promote healing or prevent recurrence of ulceration.*

REFERENCES

Bishop JB and others: A prospective randomized evaluator-blinded trial of two potential wound healing agents for the treatment of venous stasis ulcers, *J Vasc Surg,* 16(2):251-257, 1992.

Harris AH and others: Managing vascular leg ulcers Part 1: assessment, *Am J Nurs* 96(1):38-43, 1996.

Harris AH and others: Managing vascular leg ulcers part 2: treatment, *Am J Nurs* 96(2):40-46, 1996.

Kikta MJ and others: A prospective, randomized trial of Unna's boots versus hydroactive dressing in the treatment of venous stasis ulcers, *J Vasc Surg* 7(3):478-483, 1988.

Korstanje MJ: Venous stasis ulcers. Diagnostic and surgical considerations, *Dermatol Surg* 21(7):635-640, 1995.

Mayberry JC and others: Fifteen-year results of ambulatory compression therapy for chronic venous ulcers, *Surgery* 109(5):575-581, 1991.

McCulloch JM and others: Intermittent pneumatic compression improves venous ulcer healing, *Adv Wound Care* 7(4):22-25, 1994.

Mofffatt CJ, O'Hare L: Venous leg ulceration: Treatment by high compression bandaging, *Ostomy/Wound Manag* 41(4):16-25, 1995.

US Department of Health and Human Services: Clinical practice guideline No. 3, pressure ulcers in adults: prediction and prevention, AHCPR Publication No. 92-0047, 1992.

US Department of Health and Human Services: Clinical practice guideline No. 15, pressure ulcer treatment, AHCPR Publication No. 95-0653, 1994.

Tissue perfusion, altered (peripheral)

CLINICAL CONDITION/ MEDICAL DIAGNOSIS	RELATED FACTORS
Arterial occlusive disease	Interruption of arterial flow

> **Patient goals**
> **Expected outcomes**
> Associated nursing/collaborative interventions *and scientific rationale*

Manifest decreasing signs and symptoms of tissue damage as evidenced by the following:

Decreased claudication, with warmth and good color of extremities, no ulcers

Encourage ambulation, if possible.

Instruct on exercise program of active or passive ROM to extremities every 2 hours as appropriate. *Exercise promotes adequate circulation and formation of collateral blood vessels.*

Keep legs level with or slightly lower than heart. *Gravity promotes arterial circulation and reduces pain.*

Avoid prolonged exposure to cold environmental temperature; room temperature should be 72° to 74° F. *Cold temperatures cause vasoconstriction.*

Avoid pressure on extremities by use of water mattress, foot cradle, keeping heels off bed.

Administer and teach patient about pain medication and agents that decrease blood viscosity.

Modify lifestyle to decrease signs and symptoms of peripheral vascular disorder as evidenced by the following:

Verbalizes knowledge of therapeutic measures

Assist patient in controlling risk factors. Instruct patient to:

- Stop smoking *because smoking constricts blood vessels, inhibits ability of blood to carry oxygen by increasing carbon monoxide levels, and results in*

Tissue perfusion, altered (peripheral)

increased platelet adhesiveness and thrombus formation

- Eat low fat–low cholesterol diet *because lipids attach to the arterial wall, causing atherosclerotic lesions*
- Exercise *because sedentary lifestyle decreases arterial patency and prevents collateral circulation from developing*
- Control blood pressure *because hypertension causes a high-pressure arterial system, which damages the intimal endothelium and makes it more permeable to lipid penetration and plaque formation*
- Use proper foot care, wear protective shoes, and inspect feet daily

Instruct patient about signs and symptoms to report to physician, such as cuts, rashes, ulcers, reddened areas, increased pain.

Give patient list of community resources.

Discuss the patient's and significant others' responses to the disease, such as anxiety, powerlessness, depression and fears such as of increased pain, inability to walk, and amputation.

REFERENCES

Beaver B: Health education and the patient with peripheral vascular disease, *Nurs Clin North Am* 21(2):265, June 1986.

Burch KO: PVD: nurse-patient interventions, *J Vascular Nurs* 9(4):13, 1991.

Crosby F, et al: Well-being and concerns of patients with peripheral arterial occlusive disease, *J Vascular Nurs* 11(1):5, 1993.

Herman JA: Nursing assessment and nursing diagnosis in patients with peripheral vascular disease, *Nurs Clin North Am* 21(2):219, June 1986.

Hiatt W, Regensteiner J: Nonsurgical management of peripheral arterial disease, *Hosp Pract* 28(2):59, 1993.

Turner J: Nursing intervention in patients with peripheral vascular disease, *Nurs Clin North Am* 21(2):233, June 1986.

Warbinek E, Wyness MA: Designing nursing care for patients with peripheral vascular occlusive disease—Part II: nursing assessment and standard care plans, *Cardiovasc Nurs* 22(2):6, 1986.

Tissue perfusion, altered (peripheral)—cont'd

Trauma, risk for (falling)

CLINICAL CONDITION/ MEDICAL DIAGNOSIS	RISK FACTORS
Degenerative joint disease	Sedentary lifestyle; household clutter; narrow, poorly lighted hallways

Patient goals
Expected outcomes
  Associated nursing/collaborative interventions *and scientific rationale*

Increase activity level as evidenced by the following:

Obtains and uses a walker
Increases walking distance 10 feet per week
Walks outdoors when visitors or family members are willing to provide assistance

Refer patient for free loan of walker from community resource such as church.

Develop with patient a plan to increase walking distance to tolerance level. *Increased activity will strengthen muscles and decrease risk of falling.*

Increase safety while maintaining an independent lifestyle as evidenced by the following:

Obtains information about "life-line" to summon help when needed
Negotiates with neighbors to check on him periodically

Discuss with patient advantages of "life-line" over portable telephone to summon help. *Life-line enables the patient to summon help from any room and outdoors.*

Provide information about home health services to assist with activities of daily living as needed.

Adapt to home environment to reduce risk of falling as evidenced by the following:

Obtains assistance from family members to sort and store items that are creating a hazard in hallways

Trauma, risk for (falling)

443

Keep an updated list of where items are stored
Hallways are clear and well-lighted
Collaborates with family to complete risk assessment profile

Assist patient with examination of hazards in environment.

Teach patient to keep flashlight at bedside in case of power failure during the night. *Most falls occur between the patient's bed and the bathroom.*

Educate patient and family members about risk factors that contribute to falls.

Use a "risk assessment for falls scale" to alert patient and family to internal and external risk factors.

REFERENCES

Fitzmaurice JB and others: Use of an innovation diffusion model to disseminate guidelines on risk for injury due to slips and falls. In Rantz MJ, Lemone P, editors: *Classification of nursing diagnoses: proceedings of the eleventh conference,* Glendale, Calif, 1995, CINAHL Information Systems.

Hogue CC, Studenski S, Duncan P: Assessing mobility: the first step in preventing falls. In Gunk SG and others, eds: *Key aspects of recovery: improving nutrition, rest and mobility,* New York, 1990, Springer.

Janken JI, Reynolds BA: Identifying patients with the potential for falling. In McLane AM, ed: *Classification of nursing diagnosis: proceeding of the seventh conference,* St Louis, 1987, Mosby.

McCloskey JC, Bulechek GM: Fall prevention. In *Nursing interventions classification (NIC),* ed 2, St Louis, 1996, Mosby.

Morse JM: Nursing research on patient falls in health care institutions, *Annu Rev Nurs Res* 11:299-316, 1993.

Ross JER, Watson CA, Glydenvand TA, Reinboth JAL: Potential for trauma. In Mass M, Buckwalter KC, Hardy M: *Nursing diagnoses and interventions for the elderly,* Redwood City, Calif, 1991, Addison-Wesley.

Spellbring AM: Assessing elderly patients at high risk for falls: a reliability study, *J Nurs Qual Assur* 6(3):30-35, 1992.

Whedon MB, Shedd P: Prediction and prevention of patient falls, *Image J Nurs Schol* 21:108-114, 1989.

Trauma, risk for (falling)—cont'd

Unilateral neglect

CLINICAL CONDITION/ MEDICAL DIAGNOSIS	RELATED FACTORS
Right-sided cerebrovascular accident (CVA) with hemianopia	Disturbed perceptual ability

Patient goals
Expected outcomes
    Associated nursing/collaborative interventions *and*
      scientific rationale

Have realistic awareness of perceptual deficit as evidenced by the following:

Verbalizes realistic estimation of degree of deficit, e.g., does not ignore or underestimate deficit

Explain to patient that one side is being neglected.
Encourage patient to share own perception and provide realistic feedback *to assist the patient to understand and acknowledge the condition.*

Be protected from injury as evidenced by the following:

Experiences no accidents

Provide a safe environment by regularly orienting patient to environment; removing excess furniture and equipment; providing good lighting; placing call bell and frequently used objects on unaffected side within easy reach; keeping side rail up on affected side. *Structuring the environment to decrease hazards is essential to safety.*

Absence of injury resulting from deficit

Supervise or assist in transferring and ambulating.
Protect neglected side during activities and teach patient to assume this responsibility; teach patient to check position of limbs on affected side *to prevent unfelt trauma.*

Note perceptual deficit on patient record and in patient's room to inform caregivers. *Continuity*

Unilateral neglect

of safe care is enhanced when all caregivers are aware of the patient's perceptual deficits.

Acquire knowledge and skill to decrease or cope with deficit as evidenced by the following:

Responds to verbal, visual, and tactile cues to decrease neglect of affected side; scans and protects affected side

Teach patient to scan affected side; place clock or some frequently used item on side of deficit *to help establish a pattern of scanning.*

Use "cueing" to affected side (e.g., place red line in margin of books on affected side, small bells on limbs of affected side) and monocular patching of eye on affected side.

Spend time with patient, manipulating affected side and encouraging patient to use it. (1) Have patient handle ignored limbs on unaffected side. (2) Increase stimulation to affected side by touching or massaging with scented lotion. *Verbal, visual, and tactile cues to decrease neglect of the affected side reinforce each other in enhancing perceptual functioning.*

Compensates for perceptual loss

Assist compensation for perceptual deficit by arranging environment within patient's perceptual field.

Use visual and verbal communication regarding limb placement on affected side.

Demonstrates increased participation and independence in activities of daily living (ADLs)

Promote conscious attention, after initial stress, to neglected side by placing frequently used items on that side; position patient so that affected side is in view; talk to patient from that side. *Activities that direct attention to the neglected side can increase awareness and use of that side.*

Place food tray toward unaffected side; teach patient to rotate place periodically.

Encourage patient to perform ADLs such as toothbrushing in front of a mirror; supervise and give feedback.

Verbalizes feelings of progress in regard to perceptual deficit

Assess regularly for degree of deficit and adaptation to deficit; assess contributing factors.

Decrease confusing stimuli; avoid relocation; maintain consistency of caregivers and consistency of routine for self-care; explain procedures and treatment well in advance. *An established plan of care by consistent caregivers can decrease distortions in perception and subsequent disorientation.*

Include family in rehabilitation process *so that they understand it, support it, and can continue it in home environment.*

REFERENCES

Kalbach LR: Unilateral neglect: mechanisms and nursing care, *J Neurosci Nurs* 23:125, 1991.

Rubio KB, Van Deusen J: Relation of perceptual and body image dysfunction to activities of daily living of persons after stroke, *Am J Occup Ther* 49(6):551, 1995.

Warren M: A hierarchical model for evaluation and treatment of visual perceptual dysfunction in adult acquired brain injury, Part 1 and 2, *Am J Occup Ther* 47(1):42, 1993.

Webster JS and others: Rightward orienting bias, wheelchair maneuvering, and fall risk, *Arch Phys Med Rehabil* 76(10):924, 1995.

Unilateral neglect—cont'd

Urinary elimination, altered

CLINICAL CONDITION/ MEDICAL DIAGNOSIS	RELATED FACTORS
Long-term use of a Foley catheter	Diminished urinary sphincter control; social isolation

Patient goals
Expected outcomes
   Associated nursing/collaborative interventions *and scientific rationale*

Establish a normal pattern of urinary elimination as evidenced by the following;

Adheres to established voiding schedule
Decrease in number of episodes of involuntary loss of urine

   Establish a regular voiding schedule with patient; start with every 2 hours.

   Teach and monitor use or voiding record *to identify changes in pattern of urination and decrease in involuntary loss of urine.*

   Teach and monitor use of pelvic floor exercises (PFEs).

Provide written instructions:
   - Sit or stand without tensing muscles of legs, buttocks, or abdomen
   - Contract and relax circumvaginal muscles and urinary and anal sphincters for 3-4 seconds and repeat in a staccato fashion.
   - Do PFEs 25 to 30 times, three times a day. *PFEs strengthen the circumvaginal muscles, urinary sphincter, and external anal sphincter.*

Drinks six to eight glasses of water per day

   Collaborate with patient to establish a pattern of fluid intake *to maintain hydration* (e.g., 200 mL every 2 hours during day).

   Suggest patient drink 120 mL cranberry juice per day.

Skin in perineal area is clean and dry
No redness or discomfort in perineal area

Teach patient protective skin care (e.g., use Desitin ointment on skin in vulnerable areas).

Provide information about continence aids. *Use of continence aids helps to alleviate patient's anxiety and contributes to continence.*

Experience decrease in social isolation as evidenced by the following:

Makes short trips to family member's home
Reports increase in self-confidence
Contacts employer to plan for return to work

Encourage short trips to friends and relatives.

Suggest regular use of panty liners *to increase confidence.*

Assist patient with design of a plan for eventual return to work; help patient make initial contact with employer.

REFERENCES

Dowd TT: Discovering older women's experience of urinary incontinence, *Res Nurs Health* 14(3):179-186, 1991.

McCloskey JC, Bulechek GM, editors: Urinary bladder training. *Nursing interventions classification (NIC),* ed 2, St Louis, 1996, Mosby.

McCloskey JC, Bulechek GM, editors: Urinary habit training. In *Nursing interventions classification (NIC),* ed 2, St Louis, 1996, Mosby.

McCormick KA, Palmer MH: Urinary incontinence in older adults. *Annu Rev Nurs Res* 10:25-53, 1992.

Mitteness LS: Urinary incontinence: a perspective on symptom management. In Larson PJ, ed: *Symptom management proceedings,* San Francisco, 1992, University of California.

Palmer MH, Bone LR, Fahey M, Mamom J, Steinwachs D: Detecting urinary incontinence in older adults during hospitalization, *Appl Nurs Res* 5(4):174-180, 1992.

Sampselle CM, DeLancey JO: The urine stream interruption test and pelvic muscle function, *Nurs Res* 41(2):73-77, 1992.

Specht J and others: Urinary incontinence. In Maas M, Buckwalter KC, Hardy M: *Nursing diagnosis and interventions for the elderly,* Redwood City, Calif, 1991, Addison-Wesley.

Talbot LA: Coping with urinary incontinence: development and testing of a scale, *Nurs Diagn* 5(3):127-132, 1994.

Urinary elimination, altered—cont'd

Urinary retention

CLINICAL CONDITION/
MEDICAL DIAGNOSIS

RELATED FACTORS

Bowel resection;
moderate prostatic
hypertrophy

Disruption of usual voiding pattern;
limited activity

Patient goals
Expected outcomes
    Associated nursing/collaborative interventions *and*
      scientific rationale

Reestablish usual voiding pattern as evidenced by the following:

Voids every 3 to 4 hours
Uses Credé's maneuver to facilitate complete emptying of bladder (with physician's approval)
Verbalizes understanding of prostatic hypertrophy in development of urinary retention

> Use 100% silicone catheter for indwelling catheter in immediate postoperative period.
>
> Select appropriate catheter size. *Catheter that is too large obstructs seminal ducts and may lead to epididymitis or prostatitis; usual size is 16-18 French in male. French catheter scale: each graduation is ⅓ mm. Catheter that is too narrow is difficult to insert and permits retrograde extension of bacteria.*
>
> Teach patient methods to stimulate voiding; stroke lower abdomen or inner thighs; pour warm water over perineum; run water in sink; tap over symphysis pubis. *Stimulation of primitive reflexes facilitates voiding after removal of catheter.*
>
> Teach patient and family the pathophysiology of prostatic hypertrophy in relation to urinary retention.

Adhere to health practices to prevent urinary infection as evidenced by the following:

Maintains adequate oral intake by taking 8 oz of fluid with meals, between meals, and in early evening

Urinary retention

Takes superphysiologic amounts of vitamin C, at least 1000 mg daily

Provide patient with oral and or intravenous intake of 2000-2500 ml unless contraindicated.

Teach patient and family to maintain acid urine with use of vitamin C or large quantities of cranberry juice. *Keeping urine acidic helps to prevent bladder infections.*

No signs or symptoms of infection after removal of catheter as evidenced by the following:

Reports absence of burning, frequency, and urgency
Urinalysis confirms the absence of bacteria in urine

Monitor patient for signs and symptoms of urinary tract infection.

Obtain daily urinalysis if catheter remains in for more than 48 hours.

Obtain midstream voided specimen 24 hours after removal of catheter and with any signs or symptoms of urinary tract infection, such as burning, frequency, urge incontinence.

Instruct patient and family to call physician if signs or symptoms of infection develop after discharge from hospital.

Increase level of activity as evidenced by the following:

Walks with assistance 4 to 5 times a day
Requests pain medication ½ hour before walking in early postoperative period
Stands to void or walks to bathroom after removal of catheter

Collaborate with patient to establish increasing activity schedule.

Provide pain medication ½ hour before walking and initial voiding attempts after removal of catheter.

Have patient stand to void or walk to bathroom after removal of catheter.

REFERENCES

Kinney AB, Blount M: Effect of cranberry juice on urinary pH, *Nurs Res* 28:287, 1979.

Kinney AB, Blount M, Dowell M: Urethral catheterization: pros and cons of an invasive but sometimes essential procedure, *Geriatr Nurs*, 1:258, 1980.

McCloskey JC, Bulechek GM, editors: Urinary retention care. In *Nursing interventions classification (NIC)*, ed 2, St Louis, 1996, Mosby.

McCloskey JC, Bulechek GM, editors: Urinary catheterization. In *Nursing interventions classification (NIC)*, ed 2, St Louis, 1996, Mosby.

McCloskey JC, Bulechek GM, editors: Urinary catheterization: intermittent. In *Nursing interventions classification (NIC)*, ed 2, St Louis, 1996, Mosby.

McCloskey JC, Bulechek GM, editors: Urinary elimination management. In *Nursing interventions classification (NIC)*, ed 2, St Louis, 1996, Mosby.

Voith AM, Smith DA: Validation of the nursing diagnosis of urinary retention, *Nurs Clin North Am* 20:723, 1985.

Urinary retention—cont'd

Ventilation, inability to sustain spontaneous

CLINICAL CONDITION/ MEDICAL DIAGNOSIS	RELATED FACTORS
Chronic respiratory failure; respiratory muscle dysfunction/ weakness	Imbalance between ventilatory capacity and ventilatory demand because of decreased capacity and/or increased ventilatory demand

Patient goals
Expected outcomes
> Associated nursing/collaborative interventions *and scientific rationale*

Demonstrate decreased ventilatory demand as evidenced by the following:

Effective breathing pattern
Respiratory rate within normal limits
No accessory muscle use
Ti/Ttot* and Vd/Vt* within normal limits
Normal lung compliance
Arterial CO_2 and O_2 concentrations within normal limits
Body temperature within normal limits
Work of breathing (measured) within normal limits
No air trapping at end of expiration (Auto-PEEP)*
Normal, clear breath sounds
> Set ventilator to maximize expiratory time (increase inspiratory flow rate or decrease delivered tidal volume). *This setting will decrease occurrence of air trapping or intrinsic PEEP, thus decreasing WOB.* *
>
> Avoid excessive carbohydrate caloric intake.
> Monitor body temperature and treat fever.
> Maintain infection control procedures.
> *Decreased metabolic demands will decrease the ventilatory workload.*

---

* Abbreviations: *PEEP,* positive-end expiratory pressure; *WOB,* work of breathing; *ROM,* range of motion; *Ti,* inspiratory time; *Ttot,* total respiratory time; *Vd,* dead space; *Vt,* tidal volume.

Ventilation, inability to sustain spontaneous

Provide calm, quiet, and comfortable environment.

Administer analgesic and anxiolytic medication as needed

Teach relaxation and stress reduction techniques.

Monitor acid/base status of body fluids and treat alterations.

Anxiety, pain, stress, hypoxemia, and acidosis increase respiratory drive, thus increasing ventilatory demand and WOB.* Avoiding these conditions decreases demand and WOB.

Maintain airway patency and clearance by checking size of endotracheal tube and suctioning airway as needed. *Decreased air flow resistance minimizes WOB.*

Schedule physical activities and exercise routines, as tolerated: up to chair, ambulate, assist with hygiene, and active and passive ROM* and bed exercise. *Prevent muscle deconditioning and provide patient with diversionary activities. Muscle deconditioning will contribute to increased ventilatory demand. Diversion helps decrease anxiety.*

Achieve optimal ventilatory capability as evidenced by the following:

Maximal inspiratory and expiratory pressures within normal limits

Tidal volume and vital capacity within normal limits

Respiratory rate within normal limits

Assess nutritional status. Correct nutritional deficits. *Optimal muscle performance depends on adequate supply of nutrients for energy production and protein for muscle tissue repair. In addition, malnutrition blunts respiratory drive.*

Position to allow maximal thoracic excursion *to allow diaphragm to contract from optimum length for maximum contractibility.*

Monitor acid/base of body fluids and correct alterations. *Alkalosis blunts respiratory drive.*

* Abbreviations: *PEEP,* positive-end expiratory pressure; *WOB,* work of breathing; *ROM,* range of motion; *Ti,* inspiratory time; *Ttot,* total respiratory time; *Vd,* dead space; *Vt,* tidal volume.

Ventilation, inability to sustain spontaneous—cont'd

Monitor effects of sedative agents. *Sedatives can blunt respiratory drive.*

Promote normal rest/sleep patterns. Pace activities to allow rest periods. *Rest allows energy reserves to be replenished. Sleep deprivation blunts respiratory drive.*

Provide mechanical ventilatory support at a level that provides rest of respiratory muscles. Use appropriate settings. Apply appropriate mode of ventilation. *Rest is only specific treatment for muscle fatigue. Maximal rest allows complete recovery from fatigue. Improper ventilator settings, type, and cycling, as well as high resistance valves and circuitry add to workload and prevent complete rest and recovery of muscle function.*

Provide inspiratory muscle training, if appropriate. *This increases strength and endurance, and prevents further deconditioning of respiratory muscles.*

Maintain relative balance between ventilatory capacity and demand as evidenced by the following:

Stable or increasing amount of ventilator free time (number of hours off ventilator in 24 hours)

Appears comfortable while on ventilator

Actively participates in care

Expresses satisfaction with care

Provide environment conducive to collaborative patient care management and that uses resources and staff mix appropriate to the care needs of the patient. *Patient outcomes are more likely to be achieved through collaborative care planning and management using adequate numbers of appropriately prepared providers.*

Involve patient and significant others in care planning and management *to increase patient motivation and the likelihood of attainment of expected outcomes.*

REFERENCES

Baldwin-Myers A and others: *Standards of care for the ventilator-assisted individual: a comprehensive management plan from hospital to home,* Loma Linda, Calif, undated, Loma Linda University Medical Center.

Ventilation, inability to sustain spontaneous—cont'd

Benotti PN, Bistrian B: Metabolic and nutritional aspects of weaning from mechanical ventilation, *Crit Care Med* 17:181-185, 1989.

Burns SM, Clochesy J, Goodnough-Hanneman S, Ingersoll G, Knebel AR, Shekleton ME: Weaning from long-term mechanical ventilation, *Am J Crit Care* 4(1):4-22, 1995.

Daly BJ and others: Development of a special care unit for chronically critically ill patients, *Heart Lung* 20:45-52, 1991.

Geisman LK, Ahrens T: Auto-PEEP: An impediment to weaning in the chronically ventilated patient, *AACN Clin Iss Crit Care Nurs* 2(3):391-397, 1991.

Gracey DR and others: Outcomes of patients admitted to a chronic ventilator-dependent unit in an acute care hospital, *Mayo Clinic Proceedings* 67:131-136, 1992.

Kastens VM: Nursing management of "Auto-PEEP," *Focus Crit Care* 18(5):419-421, 1991.

Knebel AR: When weaning from mechanical ventilation fails, *Am J Crit Care* 1(3):19-29, 1992.

Lundberg JA, Noll ML: The long term acute care hospital: A new option for ventilator dependent individuals, *AACN Clin Iss Crit Care Nurs* 1(2):280-288, 1990.

Marini JJ: The physiologic determinants of ventilator dependency, *Resp Care* 31:271-282, 1986.

Marini JJ: Weaning from mechanical ventilation, *New Engl J Med* 324(21):1496-1498, 1991.

Shekleton ME: Respiratory muscle conditioning and the work of breathing: A critical balance in the weaning patient, *AACN Clin Iss Crit Care Nurs* 2(3):405-414, 1991.

Stewart KH and others: Quality of care in weaning from mechanical ventilation, *J Nurs Qual Care* 6(4):44-50, 1992.

Thompson KS and others: Building a critical path for ventilator dependency, *Am J Nurs* 28-31, 1991.

Thorens JB and others: Influence of the quality of nursing on the duration of weaning from mechanical ventilation in patients with chronic obstructive pulmonary disease, *Crit Care Med* 23(11):1807-1815, 1995.

Ventilation, inability to sustain spontaneous—cont'd

Ventilatory weaning response, dysfunctional (DVWR)

CLINICAL CONDITION/ MEDICAL DIAGNOSIS	RELATED FACTORS
Acute respiratory failure	Physiologic and psychologic readiness to wean from mechanical ventilation

Patient goals
Expected outcomes
  Associated nursing/collaborative interventions *and scientific rationale*

Achieve stable, optimal physiologic status as evidenced by the following:

Alert and rested appearance

Heart rate and rhythm, blood pressure, respiratory rate, tidal volume, electrolytes (especially K^+, Mg^{++}, PO_4), Hgb, Hct, arterial blood gases, weaning parameters, serum albumin, and albumin/globulin ratio within normal limits

Balanced intake and output

Weight stable and within target ideal body weight range

No complaints of dyspnea

Effective airway clearance; normal, clear breath sounds; minimal secretions

Effective breathing pattern; complete, equal, bilateral chest excursion and no paradoxical breathing

No complaints of pain

  Assess and monitor respiratory, hemodynamic, metabolic, hydration, and central nervous system parameters. *Ventilatory and hemodynamic stability and decreased metabolic demand help to minimize work of breathing.*

  Maintain proper ventilator settings. *Inappropriate settings can increase ventilatory workload and predispose respiratory muscles to fatigue. Appropriate settings promote rest of respiratory muscles.*

  Encourage adequate intake of food and fluids. Provide nutritional supplementation as needed.

Ventilatory weaning response, dysfunctional (DVWR)

457

Obtain nutritional consultation.

Normal muscle performance and adequate energy supply depend on matching nutritional requirements to metabolic needs.

Promote normal rest/sleep patterns. Schedule weaning trial in AM or when patient feels rested. Allow 1- to 2-hour rest periods before weaning trial after other activities. *Rest is necessary to replenish depleted energy reserves and promote optimal muscle and organ system function.*

Maintain airway patency and clearance:
- Check size of endotracheal tube.
- Check placement of endotracheal tube.
- Suction airway as needed before weaning trial.

Decreased air flow resistance minimizes the work of breathing.

Position with head elevated, back straight from waist (in chair, on side of bed, in high Fowler's position). *Maximal thoracic excursion allows increased lung volumes, thus increasing ventilation to participate in gas exchange.*

Promote comfort and relieve pain:
- Teach relaxation techniques.
- Provide diversionary activities.
- Administer analgesic medication.

Discomfort and pain increase anxiety and cause ineffective breathing patterns such as "splinted" respiration or rapid, shallow breathing that increases dead space.

Demonstrate feelings of control and independence and minimal anxiety as evidenced by the following:

Calm, relaxed appearance
Verbalizes understanding of weaning plans
States satisfaction with answers to questions
Expresses minimal feelings of anxiety and powerlessness

Discuss weaning plan with patient and significant others.

Explain procedures to be followed.

Solicit and answer questions.

Reassure that continuous monitoring will occur during weaning trial.

Reassure that multiple weaning trials are normal and expected.

Explain alarm systems and all safety measures being implemented.

Increased understanding will promote cooperation with plan and increase belief in ability and motivation to succeed, as well as decrease anxiety about weaning trial.

During weaning trial: tolerate decreased ventilatory rate or level of pressure support or total discontinuation of mechanical ventilatory support as evidenced by the following:

Stable breathing pattern with minimal initial increase in respiratory rate and decrease in tidal volume

Stable blood pressure, heart rate, and rhythm

Stable arterial blood gas levels

Breath sounds clear

Quiet, comfortable breathing without complaints of dyspnea, fatigue, or excessive warmth or discomfort

Skin of face and peripheral extremities remains warm and dry and pink in color

Communicate confidence in patient's readiness and ability to wean.

Provide comfortable and calm lighting, temperature, and support persons.

These actions increase patient's level of confidence in self and decrease anxiety level.

Implement collaboratively developed individualized weaning plan that includes goals, methods, and time frames. *Use of a plan that incorporates weaning protocols agreed on by all health-care team members promotes consistency of approach and increases weaning success rate.*

Remain with patient and monitor status continuously during weaning trial. *Promote safety, because change can occur rapidly and may require immediate intervention.*

Ventilatory weaning response, dysfunctional (DVWR)—cont'd

Suction airway as needed during weaning trial *to maintain airway patency and decrease resistance to air flow, thus minimizing work of breathing.*

Provide fan at bedside. *Sensation of coolness and blowing air lessens feelings of shortness of breath.*

Communicate progress in achieving weaning goals to patient and significant others as weaning process continues. *Positive feedback increases motivation.*

REFERENCES

Anderson J, O'Brien M: Challenges for the future: the nurse's role in weaning patients from mechanical ventilation, *Inten Crit Care Nurs* 11(1):2-5, 1995.

Birdsall C: Searching for the best weaning method, *Crit Care Specialist* 1:6-7, 1993.

Bridges EJ: Transition from ventilatory support: knowing when the patient is ready to wean, *Crit Care Nurs Q* 15(1):14-20, 1992.

Burns SM, Burns JE, Truwit JD: Comparison of five clinical weaning indices, *Am J Crit Care* 3(5):342-352, 1994.

Calhoun CJ, Specht NL: Standardizing the weaning process, *AACN Clin Iss Crit Care Nurs* 2(3):398-404, 1991.

Carroll KC, Magruder CC: The role of analgesics and sedatives in the management of pain and agitation during weaning from mechanical ventilation, *Crit Care Nurs Q* 15(4):68-77, 1993.

Goodnough-Hanneman S: Multidimensional predictors of success or failure with early weaning from mechanical ventilation after cardiac surgery, *Nurs Res* 43(1):4-10, 1994.

Goodnough-Hanneman S and others: Weaning from short-term mechanical ventilation, *Am J Crit Care* 3(6):421-443, 1994.

Henneman EA: The art and science of weaning from mechanical ventilation, *Focus Crit Care* 18(6):490-501, 1991.

Jenny J, Logan J: Promoting ventilator independence: a grounded theory perspective, *Dimens Crit Care Nurs* 13(1):29-37, 1994.

Knebel AR: Weaning from mechanical ventilation: Current controversies, *Heart Lung* 20(4):321-331, 1991.

Knebel AR, Janson-Bjerklie SL, Malley JD, Wilson AG, Marini JJ: Comparison of breathing comfort during weaning with two ventilatory modes, *Am J Respir Crit Care Med*, 149(1):14-18, 1994.

Logan J, Jenny J: Deriving a new nursing diagnosis through qualitative research: Dysfunctional ventilatory weaning response, *Nurs Diagn* 1(1):37-43, 1990.

Sabau D and others: Therapist driven weaning protocol evaluation in the cardiovascular recovery room, *Crit Care Med* 22(1):A226, 1994.

Weilitz PB: Weaning a patient from mechanical ventilation, *Crit Care Nurs* 13(4):33-40, 1993.

Ventilatory weaning response, dysfunctional (DVWR)—cont'd

Violence, risk for: directed at others*

CLINICAL CONDITION/ MEDICAL DIAGNOSIS	RISK FACTORS
Antisocial personality disorder	Antisocial character

Patient goals
Expected outcomes
　　Associated nursing/collaborative interventions *and*
　　　　scientific rationale

Experience a reduced probability for violence as evidenced by the following:

Verbalizes less aggression, decreases use of coercive or intimidating interaction style, verbalizes anger appropriately, refrains from harming others, and controls own behavior

Monitor patient for the following: verbal aggression (e.g., anger/shouting), coercive or intimidating interaction style, and physical aggression against others. *Early interventions in the preceding factors can prevent a serious violent episode.*

Medicate as needed *to assist patient in controlling aggressive/violent behavior.*

Observe for side effects of drugs/medications *because violence can be precipitated by them.*

Assess for evidence of past physical aggression against other/objects, life stressors, and family violence. *A past history or any of the preceding additional risk factors predisposes an individual to coping with life or obtaining a desired end through violence.*

Determine parental discipline patterns the patient experienced. *The more abusive, the greater potential for violence.*

Avoid a tone of voice that suggests nagging, pessimism, indifference, or hostility. Also avoid direct confrontation and response to abusive language with abusive language. *Patients respond*

Violence, risk for: directed at others

461

to these staff behaviors defensively (sometimes violently) because they are perceived as a threat to the self.

Avoid extensive eye-to-eye contact, especially when anger is intensifying. *Eye contact can be perceived as an assertion of dominance over the individual and can lead to defensive violence.*

Respond to questions asked by patient. *This increases the patient's feeling of worth and decreases the need for violence to obtain what is desired.*

Demonstrates positive regard for others, and demonstrates constructive coping skills in dealing with stress and frustration.

Monitor patient for the following: strong interest in and/or availability of weapons and ideas of persecution. *These are predisposing factors that can lead to violence.*

Monitor patient for a value system in which violence is viewed as an acceptable response, for perceptions of self and environment, and for variations in interpersonal perceptions. *If the perceptual variation is disturbing to the individual, violence may be used to force greater congruence of perceptions.*

Determine patient's perception regarding the need for violence *as this relates to the patient's belief about using violence.*

Identifies therapeutic resources available to help change behavior and verbalizes need to decrease the use of violence

Provide one-to-one supportive counseling *to identify coping mechanisms and to recognize consequences of violent behavior.*

Provide nurse-group psychotherapy *to eliminate interpersonal dysfunctions, develop better communication skills, and foster socialization.*

Provide positive reinforcement of behaviors that help to decrease/control violent behavior *because this rewards the patient's attempts to use socially acceptable behaviors.*

Violence, risk for: directed at others—cont'd

462

Recommend or provide family therapy *to resolve family issues/conflicts and to empower the family in coping with and establishing sanctions for the violent family member.*

Provide health teaching in the following areas:

- Accepting accountability for own behavior (e.g., if patient injures others or breaks something, he/she must provide restitution within the limits of program)
- Recognizing impending violence and taking action for aborting the violent behavior
- Learning alternate coping mechanisms, such as negotiating skills, socially acceptable ways of expressing feelings of anger and hostility, and/or stress-reducing and relaxation skills. *Alternative coping mechanisms for stress or perceived threats decrease the need to use violence for coping.*

Responds to ward milieu nonviolently

Create a unit environment that is light, open, and uncrowded with a low noise level and adequate staffing *so that the patient can feel safe and know that the staff can control any violence that occurs. The low noise level decreases arousal/agitation as increases in these can lead to violence.*

Establish hospital unit norm against physical harm to others with set sanctions for infractions. *The expectation that violence will not be tolerated decreases violence.*

- Provide staff education on managing assaultive-aggressive behavior *to decrease probability of patient/staff injuries.*
- Provide staff training on what will be perceived as aggression/assaultiveness *to prevent the splitting of the staff by patient manipulation.*
- Restrain/seclude as needed *to prevent injuries and to assist the patient to regain control of his/her behavior.*

Provide opportunities for aerobic exercises three to seven times per week. *This uses a socially acceptable way of expressing angry feelings, decreasing agitation, and maintaining health.*

Violence, risk for: directed at others—cont'd

REFERENCES

AAN Working Paper: Violence as a nursing priority: policy implications, *Nurs Outlook* 41(2):83, 1993.

Estoff SE, Zimmer C, Lachicotte WS, Benoit J: The influence of social networks and social support on violence by persons with serious mental illness, *Hosp Community Psychiatry* 45:669-679, 1994.

Garza-Trevina ES: Neurobiological factors in aggressive behavior, *Hosp Community Psychiatry* 45:690-699, 1994.

Junginger J: Command hallucinations and the prediction of dangerousness, *Psychiatr Serv* 46:911-914, 1995.

Morrison EF: A comparison of perceptions of aggression and violence by psychiatric nurses, *J Nurs Stud* 30(3):261, 1993.

Morrison EF: The measurement of aggression and violence in hospitalized psychiatric patients, *J Nurs Stud* 30(1):51, 1993.

Larson L: High risk for violence: self-directed or directed at others. In McFarland GK, McFarland EA, eds: *Nursing diagnosis and intervention: planning for patient care,* ed 3, St Louis, 1997, Mosby.

Madela EN, Poggenpoel M: The experience of a community characterized by violence: implications for nursing, *J Adv Nurs* 18(5):691, 1993.

Violence, risk for: directed at others—cont'd

*In 1996 NANDA split the diagnosis "Violence, risk for: self-directed or directed at others" into two diagnoses, "Violence, risk for: self-directed" and "Violence, fisk for: directed at others." This care plan represents the diagnosis "Violence, risk for: directed at others."

NURSING DIAGNOSES

With Associated NIC Nursing Interventions

Since the early 1970s, nurse leaders have been involved in the identification, development, and classification of nursing diagnoses. Current ongoing developmental work is coordinated by the North American Nursing Diagnosis Association (NANDA) resulting in a current list of 137 nursing diagnoses (NANDA, 1996).* More recently, the development and classification of nursing interventions has been coordinated by faculty at the University of Iowa resulting in the Nursing Interventions Classification (NIC), which currently lists 433 interventions (McCloskey and Bulechek, 1996). Members of the Iowa Intervention Project proceeded to matchup the nursing interventions with nursing diagnoses (Daly, 1996). Section Three of the Pocket Guide is drawn from the result of this work. NANDA nursing diagnoses are listed in alphabetical order. Linked to each nursing diagnosis are one or more of the general NIC nursing interventions with definitions that are further delineated by specific activities in NIC (see McCloskey and Bulechek, 1996, for a comprehensive list of all NIC interventions with definitions and activities). When developing a nursing care plan, the prototype nursing care plans found in Section Two can be augmented by referring to the nursing diagnosis under consideration in Section Three and reviewing the suggested nursing interventions.

REFERENCES

Daly JM, and others: A care planning tool that proves what we do, *RN* 26-29, 1996.

McCloskey JC, Bulechek GM, eds: *Nursing interventions classification (NIC)*, ed 2, St Louis, Mosby, 1996.

North American Nursing Diagnosis Association: *NANDA nursing diagnosis: definitions and classification 1997-1998*, Philadelphia, 1996, The Association.

*The NANDA diagnoses Self-Care Deficit and Sensory/Perceptual Alteration are counted individually by specified type.

Activity intolerance

ACTIVITY THERAPY   Prescription of and assistance with specific physical, cognitive, social, and spiritual activities to increase the range, frequency, or duration of an individual's (or group's) activity

ENERGY MANAGEMENT   Regulating energy use to treat or prevent fatigue and optimize function

Activity intolerance, risk for

EMOTIONAL SUPPORT   Provision of reassurance, acceptance, and encouragement during times of stress

ENERGY MANAGEMENT   Regulating energy use to treat or prevent fatigue and optimize function

Adaptive capacity, decreased: intracranial

CEREBRAL EDEMA MANAGEMENT   Limitation of secondary cerebral injury resulting from swelling of the brain tissue

CEREBRAL PERFUSION PROMOTION   Promotion of adequate perfusion and limitation of complications for a patient experiencing or at risk for inadequate cerebral perfusion

INTRACRANIAL PRESSURE (ICP) MONITORING   Measurement and interpretation of patient data to regulate intracranial pressure

NEUROLOGIC MONITORING   Collection and analysis of patient data to prevent or minimize neurologic complications

Adjustment, impaired

COPING ENHANCEMENT   Assisting a patient to adapt to perceived stressors, changes, or threats that interfere with meeting life demands and roles

Airway clearance, ineffective

AIRWAY MANAGEMENT   Facilitation of patency of air passages

AIRWAY SUCTIONING   Removal of airway secretions by inserting a suction catheter into the patient's oral airway and/or trachea

Anxiety

ANXIETY REDUCTION   Minimizing apprehension, dread, foreboding, or uneasiness related to an unidentified source of anticipated danger

Aspiration, risk for

ASPIRATION PRECAUTIONS   Prevention or minimization of risk factors in the patient at risk for aspiration

Body image disturbance

BODY IMAGE ENHANCEMENT   Improving a patient's conscious and unconscious perceptions and attitudes toward his or her body

Body temperature, altered, risk for

TEMPERATURE REGULATION   Attaining and/or maintaining body temperature within a normal range
TEMPERATURE REGULATION: INTRAOPERATIVE   Attaining and/or maintaining desired intraoperative body temperature
VITAL SIGNS MONITORING   Collection and analysis of cardiovascular, respiratory, and body temperature data to determine and prevent complications

Bowel incontinence

BOWEL INCONTINENCE CARE   Promotion of bowel continence and maintenance of perinatal skin integrity
BOWEL INCONTINENCE CARE: ENCOPRESIS   Promotion of bowel continence in children
BOWEL TRAINING   Assisting the patient to train the bowel to evacuate at specific intervals

Breastfeeding, effective

BREASTFEEDING ASSISTANCE   Preparing a new mother to breastfeed her infant

Breastfeeding, ineffective

LACTATION COUNSELING   Use of an interactive helping process to assist in maintenance of successful breastfeeding

Breastfeeding, interrupted

BOTTLE FEEDING   Preparation and administration of fluids to an infant through a bottle

EMOTIONAL SUPPORT   Provision of reassurance, acceptance, and encouragement during times of stress

LACTATION COUNSELING   Use of an interactive helping process to assist in maintenance of successful breastfeeding

Breathing pattern, ineffective

AIRWAY MANAGEMENT   Facilitation of patency of air passages

RESPIRATORY MONITORING   Collection and analysis of patient data to ensure airway patency and adequate gas exchange

Cardiac output, decreased

CARDIAC CARE   Limitation of complications resulting from an imbalance between myocardial oxygen supply and demand for a patient with symptoms of impaired cardiac function

CARDIAC CARE: ACUTE   Limitation of complications for a patient recently experiencing an episode of an imbalance between myocardia oxygen supply and demand resulting in impaired cardiac function

CIRCULATORY CARE: MECHANICAL ASSIST DEVICE   Temporary support of the circulation through the use of mechanical devices or pumps

HEMODYNAMIC REGULATION   Optimization of heart rate, preload, afterload, and contractility

SHOCK MANAGEMENT: CARDIAC   Promotion of adequate tissue perfusion for a patient with severely compromised pumping function of the heart

Caregiver role strain

CAREGIVER SUPPORT   Provision of the necessary information, advocacy, and support to facilitate primary patient care by someone other than a health care professional

Caregiver role strain, risk for

CAREGIVER SUPPORT   Provision of the necessary information, advocacy, and support to facilitate primary patient care by someone other than a health care professional

Communication, impaired verbal

ACTIVE LISTENING   Attending closely to and attaching significance to a patient's verbal and nonverbal messages

COMMUNICATION ENHANCEMENT: HEARING DEFICIT   Assistance in accepting and learning alternate methods for living with diminished hearing

COMMUNICATION ENHANCEMENT: SPEECH DEFICIT   Assistance in accepting and learning alternate methods for living with impaired speech

Community coping, potential for enhanced

ENVIRONMENTAL MANAGEMENT: COMMUNITY   Monitoring and influencing of the physical, social, cultural, economic, and political conditions that affect the health of groups and communities

HEALTH EDUCATION   Developing and providing instruction and learning experiences to facilitate voluntary adaptation of behavior conducive to health in individuals, families, groups, or communities

HEALTH POLICY MONITORING   Surveillance and influence of government and organization regulations, rules, and standards that affect nursing systems and practices to ensure quality care of patients

Community coping, ineffective

ENVIRONMENTAL MANAGEMENT: COMMUNITY   Monitoring and influencing of the physical, social, cultural, economic, and political conditions that affect the health of groups and communities

HEALTH EDUCATION   Developing and providing instruction and learning experiences to facilitate voluntary adaptation of behavior conducive to health in individuals, families, groups, or communities

HEALTH POLICY MONITORING   Surveillance and influence of government and organization regulations, rules, and standards that affect nursing systems and practices to ensure quality care of patients

Confusion, acute

DELIRIUM MANAGEMENT   Provision of a safe and therapeutic environment for the patient who is experiencing an acute confusional state

DELUSION MANAGEMENT   Promoting the comfort, safety, and reality orientation of a patient experiencing false, fixed beliefs that have little or no basis in reality

Confusion, chronic

DEMENTIA MANAGEMENT   Provision of a modified environment for the patient who is experiencing a chronic confusional state

MOOD MANAGEMENT   Providing for the safety and stabilization of a patient who is experiencing dysfunctional mood

Constipation

CONSTIPATION/IMPACTION MANAGEMENT   Prevention and alleviation of constipation/impaction

Constipation, colonic

CONSTIPATION/IMPACTION MANAGEMENT   Prevention and alleviation of constipation/impaction

Constipation, perceived

BOWEL MANAGEMENT   Establishment and maintenance of a regular pattern of bowel elimination

Coping, defensive

SELF-AWARENESS ENHANCEMENT   Assisting a patient to explore and understand his or her thoughts, feelings, motivations, and behaviors

Coping, family: potential for growth

DEVELOPMENTAL ENHANCEMENT   Facilitating or teaching parents/caregivers to facilitate the optimal gross motor, fine motor, cognitive, social, and emotional growth of preschool and school-age children

FAMILY SUPPORT   Promotion of family values, interests, and goals

NORMALIZATION PROMOTION   Assisting parents and other family members of children with chronic illnesses or disabilities in providing normal life experiences for their children and families

PASS FACILITATION   Arranging a leave for a patient from a health care facility

Coping, ineffective family: compromised

FAMILY INVOLVEMENT   Facilitating family participation in the emotional and physical care of the patient

FAMILY MOBILIZATION   Use of family strengths to influence patient's health in a positive direction

FAMILY SUPPORT   Promotion of family values, interests, and goals

Coping, ineffective family: disabling

FAMILY SUPPORT   Promotion of family values, interests, and goals

FAMILY THERAPY   Assisting family members to move their family toward a more productive way of living

Coping, ineffective individual

COPING ENHANCEMENT   Assisting a patient to adapt to perceived stressors, changes, or threats that interfere with meeting life demands and roles

DECISION-MAKING SUPPORT   Providing information and support for a patient who is making a decision regarding health care

Decisional conflict (specify)

DECISION-MAKING SUPPORT   Providing information and support for a patient who is making a decision regarding health care

Denial, ineffective

ANXIETY REDUCTION   Minimizing apprehension
dread, foreboding, or uneasiness related to an
unidentified source of anticipated danger

COUNSELING   Use of an interactive helping process
focusing on the needs, problems, or feelings of the
patient and significant others to enhance or support coping, problem-solving, and interpersonal
relationships

Diarrhea

DIARRHEA MANAGEMENT   Prevention and alleviation
of diarrhea

Disuse syndrome, risk for

ENERGY MANAGEMENT   Regulating energy use to
treat or prevent fatigue and optimize function

Diversional activity deficit

RECREATION THERAPY   Purposeful use of recreation to
promote relaxation and enhancement of social
skills

SELF-RESPONSIBILITY FACILITATION   Encouraging a
patient to assume more responsibility for own
behavior

Dysreflexia

DYSREFLEXIA MANAGEMENT   Prevention and elimination of stimuli that cause hyperactive reflexes and
inappropriate autonomic responses in a patient
with a cervical or high thoracic cord lesion

Energy field disturbance

THERAPEUTIC TOUCH   Directing one's own interpersonal energy to flow through the hands to help or
heal another

Environmental interpretation syndrome, impaired

DEMENTIA MANAGEMENT   Provision of a modified
environment for the patient who is experiencing a
chronic confusional state

ENVIROMENTAL MANAGEMENT   Manipulation of the
   patient's surroundings for therapeutic benefit

Family processes, altered: alcoholism

FAMILY PROCESS MAINTENANCE   Minimization of
   family process disruption effects
SUBSTANCE ABUSE TREATMENT   Supportive care of
   patient/family members with physical and psychosocial problems associated with the use of
   alcohol or drugs

Family processes, altered

FAMILY INTEGRITY PROMOTION   Promotion of family
   cohesion and unity
FAMILY PROCESS MAINTENANCE   Minimization of
   family process disruption effects
NORMALIZATION PROMOTION   Assisting parents and
   other family members of children with chronic
   illnesses or disabilities in providing normal experiences for their children and families

Fatigue

ENERGY MANAGEMENT   Regulating energy use to
   treat or prevent fatigue and optimize function

Fear

ANXIETY REDUCTION   Mimimizing apprehension,
   dread, foreboding, or uneasiness related to an
   unidentified source of anticipated danger
COPING ENHANCEMENT   Assisting a patient to adapt
   to perceived stressors, changes, or threats that
   interfere with meeting life demands and roles
SECURITY ENHANCEMENT   Intensifying a patient's
   sense of physical and psychologic safety

Fluid volume deficit

ELECTROLYTE MANAGEMENT   Promotion of electrolyte balance and prevention of complications
   resulting from abnormal or undesired serum electrolyte levels

FLUID MANAGEMENT   Promotion of fluid balance and prevention of complications resulting from abnormal or undesired fluid levels

FLUID MONITORING   Collection and analysis of patient data to regulate fluid balance

HYPOVOLEMIA MANAGEMENT   Expansion of intravascular fluid volume in a patient who is volume depleted

INTRAVENOUS (IV) THERAPY   Administration and monitoring of IV fluids and medications

SHOCK MANAGEMENT: VOLUME   Promotion of adequate tissue perfusion for a patient with severely compromised intravascular volume

Fluid volume deficit, risk for

AUTOTRANSFUSION   Collecting and reinfusing blood that has been lost intraoperatively or postoperatively from clean wounds

ELECTROLYTE MANAGEMENT   Promotion of electrolyte balance and prevention of complications resulting from abnormal or undesired serum electrolyte levels

FLUID MANAGEMENT   Promotion of fluid balance and prevention of complications resulting from abnormal or undesired fluid levels

FLUID MONITORING   Collection and analysis of patient data to regulate fluid balance

HYPOVOLEMIA MANAGEMENT   Expansion of intravascular fluid volume in a patient who is volume depleted

INTRAVENOUS (IV) THERAPY   Administration and monitoring of IV fluids and medications

SHOCK MANAGEMENT: VOLUME   Promotion of adequate tissue perfusion for a patient with severely compromised intravascular volume

Fluid volume excess

FLUID MANAGEMENT   Promotion of fluid balance and prevention of complications resulting from abnormal or undesired fluid levels

FLUID MONITORING   Collection and analysis of patient data to regulate fluid balance

Gas exchange, impaired

ACID-BASE MANAGEMENT Promotion of acid-base balance and prevention of complications resulting from acid-base balance

AIRWAY MANAGEMENT Facilitation of patency of air passages

Grieving, anticipatory

GRIEF WORK FACILITATION Assistance with the resolution of a significant loss

GRIEF WORK FACILITATION: PERINATAL DEATH Assistance with the resolution of a perinatal loss

Grieving, dysfunctional

GRIEF WORK FACILITATION Assistance with the resolution of a significant loss

GRIEF WORK FACILITATION: PERINATAL DEATH Assistance with the resolution of a perinatal loss

Growth and development, altered

DEVELOPMENTAL ENHANCEMENT Facilitating or teaching parents/caregivers to facilitate the optimal gross motor, fine motor, language, cognitive, social and emotional growth of preschool and school-aged children

NUTRITIONAL MONITORING Collection and analysis of patient data to prevent or minimize malnourishment

NUTRITION THERAPY Administration of food and fluids to support metabolic processes of a patient who is malnourished or at high risk for becoming malnourished

SELF-RESPONSIBILITY FACILITATION Encouraging a patient to assume more responsibility for own behavior

Health maintenance, altered

HEALTH SYSTEM GUIDANCE Facilitating a patient's location and use of appropriate health services

SUPPORT SYSTEM ENHANCEMENT Facilitation of support to patient by family, friends, and community

Health-seeking behaviors (specify)

HEALTH EDUCATION   Developing and providing instruction and learning experiences to facilitate voluntary adaptation of behavior conducive to health in individuals, families, groups, or communities

SELF-MODIFICATION ASSISTANCE   Reinforcement of self-directed change initiated by the patient to achieve personally important goals

Home maintenance management, impaired

HOME MAINTENANCE ASSISTANCE   Helping the patient/family to maintain the home as a clean, safe, and pleasant place to live

Hopelessness

HOPE INSTILLATION   Facilitation of the development of a positive outlook in a given situation

Hyperthermia

FEVER TREATMENT   Management of a patient with hyperpyrexia caused by nonenvironmental factors

MALIGNANT HYPERTHERMIA PRECAUTIONS   Prevention or reduction of hypermetabolic response to pharmacological agents used during surgery

TEMPERATURE REGULATIONS   Attaining and/or maintaining body temperature within a normal range

TEMPERATURE REGULATION: INTRAOPERATIVE   Attaining and/or maintaining desired intraoperative body temperature

VITAL SIGNS MONITORING   Collection and analysis of cardiovascular, respiratory, and body temperature data to determine and prevent complications

Hypothermia

HYPOTHERMIA TREATMENT   Rewarming and surveillance of a patient whose core body temperature is below 35° C

TEMPERATURE REGULATION   Attaining and/or maintaining body temperature within a normal range

TEMPERATURE REGULATION: INTRAOPERATIVE   Attaining and/or maintaining desired intraoperative body temperature

VITAL SIGNS MONITORING   Collection and analysis of cardiovascular, respiratory, and body temperature data to determine and prevent complications

Incontinence, functional

URINARY HABIT TRAINING   Establishing a predictable pattern of bladder emptying to prevent incontinence for persons with limited cognitive ability who have urge, stress, or functional incontinence

URINARY INCONTINENCE CARE   Assistance in promoting continence and maintaining perineal skin integrity

Incontinence, reflex

URINARY BLADDER TRAINING   Improving bladder function for those with urge incontinence by increasing the bladder's ability to hold urine and the patient's ability to suppress urination

URINARY CATHETERIZATION: INTERMITTENT   Regular periodic use of a catheter to empty the bladder

Incontinence, stress

PELVIC FLOOR EXERCISE   Strengthening the pubococcygeal muscles through voluntary, repetitive contraction to decrease stress or urge incontinence

URINARY INCONTINENCE CARE   Assistance in promoting continence and maintaining perineal skin integrity

Incontinence, total

URINARY INCONTINENCE CARE   Assistance in promoting continence and maintaining perineal skin integrity

Incontinence, urge

URINARY HABIT TRAINING   Establishing a predictable pattern of bladder emptying to prevent incontinence for persons with limited cognitive ability who have urge, stress, or functional incontinence

URINARY INCONTINENCE CARE   Assistance in promoting continence and maintaining perineal skin integrity

Infant behavior, disorganized

ENVIRONMENTAL MANAGEMENT   Manipulation of
the patient's surroundings for therapeutic benefit

Infant behavior, disorganized: risk for

ENVIRONMENTAL MANAGEMENT   Manipulation of
the patient's surroundings for therapeutic benefit

NEWBORN MONITORING   Measurement and interpretation of physiologic status of the neonate the
first 24 hours after delivery

POSITIONING   Moving the patient or a body part to
provide comfort, reduce the risk of skin breakdown, promote skin integrity, and/or promote
healing

SURVEILLANCE   Purposeful and ongoing acquisition,
interpretation, and synthesis of patient data for
clinical decision-making

Infant behavior, organized: potential for enhanced

ENVIRONMENTAL MANAGEMENT: ATTACHMENT
PROCESS   Manipulation of the patient's surroundings to facilitate the development of the parent-
infant relationship

SLEEP ENHANCEMENT   Facilitation of regular sleep/
wake cycles

Infant feeding pattern, ineffective

ENTERAL TUBE FEEDING   Delivering nutrients and
water through a gastrointestinal tube

LACTATION COUNSELING   Use of an interactive helping process to assist in maintenance of successful
breastfeeding

NONNUTRITIVE SUCKING   Provision of sucking opportunities for infant who is gavage fed or who can
receive nothing by mouth

TUBE CARE: UMBILICAL LINE   Management of a newborn with an umbilical catheter

Infection, risk for

IMMUNIZATION/VACCINATION ADMINISTRATION
Provision of immunizations for prevention of
communicable disease

INFECTION CONTROL   Minimizing the acquisition
and transmission of infectious agents
INFECTION PROTECTION   Prevention and early detection of infection in a patient at risk

Injury, perioperative positioning: risk for

POSITIONING: INTRAOPERATIVE   Moving the patient
or body part to promote surgical exposure while reducing the risk of discomfort and complications
SKIN SURVEILLANCE   Collection and analysis of patient data to maintain skin and mucous membrane
integrity

Injury, risk for

ELECTRONIC FETAL MONITORING: INTRAPARTUM
Electronic evaluation of fetal heart rate response to
uterine contractions during intrapartal care
FALL PREVENTION   Instituting special precautions
with patient at risk for injury from falling
LABOR INDUCTION   Initiation or augmentation of
labor by mechanical or pharmacological methods
LATEX PRECAUTIONS   Reducing the risk of a systemic
reaction to latex
MALIGNANT HYPERTHERMIA PRECAUTIONS   Prevention or reduction of hypermetabolic response to
pharmacological agents used during surgery

Knowledge deficit (specify)

TEACHING: DISEASE PROCESS   Assisting the patient to
understand information related to a specific disease
process
TEACHING: INDIVIDUAL   Planning, implementation,
and evaluation of a teaching program designed to
address a patient's particular needs
TEACHING: INFANT CARE   Instruction on nurturing
and physical care needed during the first year of
life
TEACHING: PERIOPERATIVE   Assisting a patient to understand and mentally prepare for surgery and the
postoperative recovery period
TEACHING: PRESCRIBED ACTIVITY/EXERCISE   Preparing
a patient to achieve and/or maintain a prescribed
level of activity

TEACHING: PRESCRIBED DIET   Preparing a patient to correctly follow a prescribed diet

TEACHING: PRESCRIBED MEDICATION   Preparing a patient to safely take prescribed medications and monitor for their effects

TEACHING: PROCEDURE/TREATMENT   Preparing a patient to understand and mentally prepare for a prescribed procedure or treatment

TEACHING: PSYCHOMOTOR SKILL   Preparing a patient to perform a psychomotor skill

TEACHING: SAFE SEX   Providing instruction concerning sexual protection during sexual activity

TEACHING: SEXUALITY   Assisting individuals to understand physical and psychosocial dimensions of sexual growth and development

Loneliness, risk for

FAMILY INTEGRITY PROMOTION   Promotion of family cohesion and unity

SOCIALIZATION ENHANCEMENT   Facilitation of another person's ability to interact with others

VISITATION FACILITATION   Promoting beneficial visits by family and friends

Management of therapeutic regimen, community: ineffective

ENVIRONMENTAL MANAGEMENT: COMMUNITY   Monitoring and influencing of the physical, social, cultural, economic, and political conditions that affect the health of groups and communities

HEALTH POLICY MONITORING   Surveillance and influence of government and organization regulations, rules, and standards that affect nursing systems and practices to ensure quality care of patients

Management of therapeutic regimen, families: ineffective

FAMILY INVOLVEMENT   Facilitating family participation in the emotional and physical care of the patient

FAMILY MOBILIZATION   Utilization of family strengths to influence patient's health in a positive direction

FAMILY PROCESS MAINTENANCE   Minimization of family process disruption effects

Management of therapeutic regimen, individual: effective

ANTICIPATORY GUIDANCE   Preparation of patient for an anticipated developmental and/or situational crisis

HEALTH SYSTEM GUIDANCE   Facilitating a patient's location and use of appropriate health services

Management of therapeutic regimen, individuals: ineffective

BEHAVIOR MODIFICATION   Promotion of a behavior change

SELF-MODIFICATION ASSISTANCE   Reinforcement of self-directed change initiated by the patient to achieve personally important goals

Memory, impaired

MEMORY TRAINING   Facilitation of memory

Mobility, impaired physical

EXERCISE THERAPY: AMBULATION   Promotion and assistance with walking to maintain or restore autonomic and voluntary body functions during treatment and recovery from illness or injury

EXERCISE THERAPY: JOINT MOBILITY   Use of active or passive body movement to maintain or restore joint flexibility

POSITIONING   Moving the patient or a body part to provide comfort, reduce the risk of skin breakdown, promote skin integrity, and/or promote healing

Noncompliance (specify)

HEALTH SYSTEM GUIDANCE   Facilitating a patient's location and use of appropriate health services

SELF-MODIFICATION ASSISTANCE   Reinforcement of
   self-directed change initiated by the patient to
   achieve personally important goals

Nutrition, altered: less than body requirements

EATING DISORDERS MANAGEMENT   Prevention and
   treatment of severe diet restriction and overexercising or binging and purging of food and fluids
NUTRITION MANAGEMENT   Assisting with or providing a balanced dietary intake of foods and fluids
WEIGHT GAIN ASSISTANCE   Facilitating gain of body
   weight

Nutrition, altered: more than body requirements

EATING DISORDERS MANAGEMENT   Prevention and
   treatment of severe diet restriction, as well as
   overexercising or binging or purging of food and
   fluids
NUTRITION MANAGEMENT   Assisting with or providing a balanced dietary intake of foods and fluids
WEIGHT REDUCTION ASSISTANCE   Facilitating loss of
   weight and/or body fat

Nutrition, altered: risk for more than body requirements

NUTRITION MANAGEMENT   Assisting with or providing a balanced dietary intake of foods and fluids
WEIGHT MANAGEMENT   Facilitating maintenance of
   optimal body weight and percent body fat

Oral mucous membrane, altered

ORAL HEALTH RESTORATION   Promotion of healing
   for a patient who has an oral mucosa or dental
   lesion

Pain

ANALGESIC ADMINISTRATION   Use of pharmacologic
   agents to reduce or eliminate pain
CONSCIOUS SEDATION   Administration of sedatives,
   monitoring of the patient's response, and provision
   of necessary physiologic support during a diagnostic or therapeutic procedure

PAIN MANAGEMENT   Alleviation of pain or a reduction in pain to a level of comfort that is acceptable to the patient

PATIENT-CONTROLLED ANALGESIA (PCA) ASSISTANCE   Facilitating patient control of analgesic administration and regulation

Pain, chronic

ANALGESIC ADMINISTRATION   Use of pharmacologic agents to reduce or eliminate pain

PAIN MANAGEMENT   Alleviation of pain or a reduction in pain to a level of comfort that is acceptable to the patient

PATIENT-CONTROLLED ANALGESIA (PCA) ASSISTANCE   Facilitating patient control of analgesic administration and regulation

Parent/infant/child attachment, altered: risk for

ATTACHMENT PROMOTION   Facilitation of the development of the parent-infant relationship

ENVIRONMENTAL MANAGEMENT: ATTACHMENT PROCESS   Manipulation of the patient's surroundings to facilitate the development of the parent-infant relationship

PARENT EDUCATION: CHILDBEARING FAMILY   Preparing another to perform the role of parent

TEACHING: INFANT CARE   Instruction on nurturing and physical care needed during the first year of life

Parental role conflict

CRISIS INTERVENTION   Use of short-term counseling to help the patient cope with a crisis and resume a state of functioning comparable to or better than the pre-crisis state

FAMILY PROCESS MAINTENANCE   Minimization of family process disruption effects

ROLE ENHANCEMENT   Assisting a patient, significant other, and/or family to improve relationships by clarifying and supplementing specific role behaviors

Parenting, altered

ABUSE PROTECTION: CHILD   Identification of high-risk, dependent child relationships and actions to prevent possible or further infliction of physical, sexual, or emotional harm or neglect of basic necessities of life

ATTACHMENT PROMOTION   Facilitation of the development of the parent-infant relationship

DEVELOPMENTAL ENHANCEMENT   Facilitating or teaching parents/caregivers to facilitate the optimal gross motor, fine motor, language, cognitive, social and emotional growth of preschool and school-age children

FAMILY INTEGRITY PROMOTION   Promotion of family cohesion and unity

Parenting, altered, risk for

ABUSE PROTECTION: CHILD   Identification of high-risk, dependent child relationships and actions to prevent possible or further infliction of physical, sexual, or emotional harm or neglect of basic necessities of life

ATTACHMENT PROMOTION   Facilitation of the development of the parent-infant relationship

DEVELOPMENTAL ENHANCEMENT   Facilitating or teaching parents/caregivers to facilitate the optimal gross motor, fine motor, language, cognitive, social and emotional growth of preschool and school-age children

FAMILY INTEGRITY PROMOTION   Promotion of family cohesion and unity

NORMALIZATION PROMOTION   Assisting parents and other family members of children with chronic illnesses or disabilities in providing normal experiences for their children and families

Peripheral neurovascular dysfunction, risk for

CIRCULATORY CARE   Promotion of arterial and venous circulation

EXERCISE THERAPY: JOINT MOBILITY   Use of active or passive body movement to maintain or restore joint flexibility

PERIPHERAL SENSATION MANAGEMENT   Prevention or minimization of injury or discomfort in the patient with altered sensation

Personal identity disturbance

DECISION-MAKING SUPPORT   Providing information and support for a patient who is making a decision regarding health care
SELF-ESTEEM ENHANCEMENT   Assisting a patient to increase his or her personal judgment of self-worth

Poisoning, risk for

ENVIRONMENTAL MANAGEMENT: SAFETY   Monitoring and manipulation of the physical environment to promote safety.

Posttrauma response

COUNSELING   Use of an interactive helping process focusing on the needs, problems, or feelings of the patient and significant others to enhance or support coping, problem-solving, and interpersonal relationships
SUPPORT SYSTEM ENHANCEMENT   Facilitation of support to patient by family, friends, and community

Powerlessness

SELF-ESTEEM ENHANCEMENT   Assisting a patient to increase his or her personal judgment of self-worth
SELF-RESPONSIBILITY FACILITATION   Encouraging a patient to assume more responsibility for own behavior

Protection, altered

ELECTRONIC FETAL MONITORING: INTRAPARTUM   Electronic evaluation of fetal heart rate response to uterine contractions during intrapartal care
ENVIRONMENTAL MANAGEMENT: VIOLENCE PREVENTION   Monitoring and manipulation of the physical environment to decrease the potential for violent behavior directed toward self, others, or environment
INFECTION CONTROL   Minimizing the acquisition and transmission of infectious agents

INFECTION PROTECTION   Prevention and early detection of infection in a patient at risk

POSTANESTHESIA CARE   Monitoring and management of the patient who has recently undergone general or regional anesthesia

SURGICAL PRECAUTIONS   Minimizing the potential for iatrogenic injury to the patient related to a surgical procedure

SURVEILLANCE: SAFETY   Purposeful and ongoing collection and analysis of information about the patient and the environment for use in promoting and maintaining patient safety

Rape-trauma syndrome

CRISIS INTERVENTION   Use of short-term counseling to help the patient cope with a crisis and resume a state of functioning comparable with or better than the pre-crisis state

RAPE-TRAUMA TREATMENT   Provision of emotional and physical support immediately following an alleged rape

Rape-trauma syndrome: compound reaction

COUNSELING   Use of an interactive helping process focusing on the needs, problems, or feelings of the patient and significant others to enhance or support coping, problem-solving, and interpersonal relationships

RAPE-TRAUMA TREATMENT   Provision of emotional and physical support immediately following an alleged rape

Rape-trauma syndrome: silent reaction

COUNSELING   Use of an interactive helping process focusing on the needs, problems, or feelings of the patient and significant others to enhance or support coping, problem-solving, and interpersonal relationships

RAPE-TRAUMA TREATMENT   Provision of emotional and physical support immediately following an alleged rape

Relocation stress syndrome

COPING ENHANCEMENT   Assisting a patient to adapt to perceived stressors, changes, or threats that interfere with meeting life demands and roles

DISCHARGE PLANNING   Preparation for moving a patient from one level of care to another within or outside the current health care agency

HOPE INSTILLATION   Facilitation of the development of a positive outlook in a given situation

SELF-RESPONSIBILITY FACILITATION   Encouraging patient to assume more responsibility for own behavior

Role performance, altered

ROLE ENHANCEMENT   Assisting a patient, significant other, and/or family to improve relationships by clarifying and supplementing specific role behaviors

Self-care deficit, bathing/hygiene

BATHING   Cleaning of the body for the purposes of relaxation, cleanliness, and healing

SELF-CARE ASSISTANCE: BATHING/HYGIENE   Assisting patient to perform personal hygiene

Self-care deficit, dressing/grooming

DRESSING   Choosing, putting on, and removing clothes for a person who cannot do this for self

HAIR CARE   Promotion of neat, clean, attractive hair

SELF-CARE ASSISTANCE: DRESSING/GROOMING   Assisting patient with clothes and makeup

Self-care deficit, feeding

FEEDING   Providing nutritional intake for patient who is unable to feed self

SELF-CARE ASSISTANCE: FEEDING   Assisting a person to eat

Self-care deficit, toileting

ENVIRONMENTAL MANAGEMENT   Manipulation of the patient's surroundings for therapeutic benefit

SELF-CARE ASSISTANCE: TOILETING   Assisting another with elimination

Self-esteem disturbance

SELF-ESTEEM ENHANCEMENT   Assisting a patient to increase his or her personal judgment of self-worth

Self-esteem, chronic low

SELF-ESTEEM ENHANCEMENT   Assisting a patient to increase his or her personal judgment of self-worth

Self-esteem, situational low

SELF-ESTEEM ENHANCEMENT   Assisting a patient to increase his/her personal judgment of self-worth

Self-mutilation, risk for

ANGER CONTROL ASSISTANCE   Facilitation of the expression of anger in an adaptive nonviolent manner
BEHAVIOR MANAGEMENT: SELF-HARM   Assisting the patient to decrease or eliminate self-mutilating or self-abusive behaviors
ENVIRONMENTAL MANAGEMENT: SAFETY   Monitoring and manipulation of the physical environment to promote safety

Sensory/perceptual alterations: visual

COMMUNICATION ENHANCEMENT: VISUAL DEFICIT   Assistance in accepting and learning alternate methods for living with diminished vision
ENVIRONMENTAL MANAGEMENT   Manipulation of the patient's surroundings for therapeutic benefit

Sensory/perceptual alterations: auditory

COMMUNICATION ENHANCEMENT: HEARING DEFICIT   Assistance in accepting and learning alternate methods for living with diminished hearing

Sensory/perceptual alterations: kinesthetic

BODY MECHANICS PROMOTION   Facilitating the use of posture and movement in daily activities to prevent fatigue and musculoskeletal strain or injury

Sensory/perceptual alterations: gustatory

NUTRITION MANAGEMENT   Assisting with or providing a balance dietary intake of foods and fluids

Sensory/perceptual alterations: tactile

PERIPHERAL SENSATION MANAGEMENT Prevention or minimization of injury or discomfort in the patient with altered sensation

SURVEILLANCE: SAFETY Purposeful and ongoing collection and analysis of information about the patient and the environment for use in promoting and maintaining patient safety

Sensory/perceptual alterations: olfactory

NUTRITION MANAGEMENT Assisting with or providing a balanced dietary intake of foods and fluids

WEIGHT MANAGEMENT Facilitating maintenance of optimal body weight and percent body fat

Sexual dysfunction

SEXUAL COUNSELING Use of an interactive helping process focusing on the need to make adjustments in sexual practice or to enhance coping with a sexual event/disorder

Sexuality patterns, altered

SEXUAL COUNSELING Use of an interactive helping process focusing on the need to make adjustments in sexual practice or to enhance coping with a sexual event/disorder

Skin integrity, impaired

INCISION SITE CARE Cleansing, monitoring, and promotion of healing in a wound that is closed with sutures, clips, or staples

SKIN SURVEILLANCE Collection and analysis of patient data to maintain skin and mucous membrane integrity

WOUND CARE Prevention of wound complications and promotion of wound healing

Skin integrity, impaired, risk for

PRESSURE MANAGEMENT Minimizing pressure to body parts

PRESSURE ULCER PREVENTION Prevention of pressure ulcers for a patient at high risk for developing them

SKIN SURVEILLANCE   Collection and analysis of patient data to maintain skin and mucous membrane integrity

Sleep pattern disturbance

SLEEP ENHANCEMENT   Facilitation of regular sleep/wake cycles

Social interaction, impaired

SOCIALIZATION ENHANCEMENT   Facilitation of another person's ability to interact with others

Social isolation

SOCIALIZATION ENHANCEMENT   Facilitation of another person's ability to interact with others

Spiritual distress (distress of the human spirit)

SPIRITUAL SUPPORT   Assisting the patient to feel balance and connection with a greater power

Spiritual well being, potential for enhanced

SPIRITUAL SUPPORT   Assisting the patient to feel balance and connection with a greater power

Suffocation, risk for

AIRWAY MANAGEMENT   Facilitation of patency of air passages

ENVIRONMENTAL MANAGEMENT: SAFETY   Monitoring and manipulation of the physical environment to promote safety

RESPIRATORY MONITORING   Collection and analysis of patient data to ensure airway patency and adequate gas exchange

Swallowing, impaired

ASPIRATION PRECAUTIONS   Prevention and minimization of risk factors in the patient at risk for aspiration

SWALLOWING THERAPY   Facilitating swallowing and preventing complications of impaired swallowing

Thermoregulation, ineffective

TEMPERATURE REGULATION   Attaining and/or maintaining body temperature within a normal range

TEMPERATURE REGULATION: INTRAOPERATIVE   Attaining and/or maintaining desired intraoperative body temperature

Thought processes, altered

DELUSION MANAGEMENT   Promoting the comfort, safety, and reality orientation of a patient experiencing false, fixed beliefs that have little or no basis in reality

DEMENTIA MANAGEMENT   Provision of a modified environment for the patient who is experiencing a chronic confusional state

Tissue integrity, impaired

WOUND CARE   Prevention of wound complications and promotion of wound healing

Tissue perfusion, altered: cerebral

CEREBRAL PERFUSION PROMOTION   Promotion of adequate perfusion and limitation of complications for a patient experiencing or at risk for inadequate cerebral perfusion

CIRCULATORY CARE   Promotion of arterial and venous circulation

INTRACRANIAL PRESSURE (ICP) MONITORING   Measurement and interpretation of patient data to regulate intracranial pressure

NEUROLOGIC MONITORING   Collection and analysis of patient data to prevent or minimize neurologic complications

PERIPHERAL SENSATION MANAGEMENT   Prevention or minimization of injury or discomfort in the patient with altered sensation

Tissue perfusion, altered: renal

FLUID/ELECTROLYTE MANAGEMENT   Regulation and prevention of complications from altered fluid and/or electrolyte levels

FLUID MANAGEMENT   Promotion of fluid balance and prevention of complications resulting from abnormal or undesired fluid levels

HEMODIALYSIS THERAPY   Management of extracorporeal passage of the patient's blood through a dialyzer

492

PERITONEAL DIALYSIS THERAPY   Administration and monitoring of dialysis into and out of the peritoneal cavity

Tissue perfusion, altered: cardiopulmonary

CARDIAC CARE: ACUTE   Limitation of complications for a patient recently experiencing an episode of an imbalance between myocardial oxygen supply and demand resulting in impaired cardiac function

CIRCULATORY CARE   Promotion of arterial and venous circulation

RESPIRATORY MONITORING   Collection and analysis of patient data to ensure airway patency and adequate gas exchange

SHOCK MANAGEMENT: CARDIAC   Promotion of adequate tissue perfusion for a patient with severely compromised pumping function of the heart

Tissue perfusion, altered: gastrointestinal

FLUID/ELECTROLYTE MANAGEMENT   Regulation and prevention of complications from altered fluid and/or electrolyte levels

GASTROINTESTINAL INTUBATION   Insertion of a tube into the gastrointestinal tract

NUTRITION MANAGEMENT   Assisting with or providing a balanced dietary intake of foods and fluids

Tissue perfusion, altered: peripheral

CIRCULATORY CARE   Promotion of arterial and venous circulation

INTRACRANIAL PRESSURE (ICP) MONITORING   Measurement and interpretation of patient data to regulate intracranial pressure

NEUROLOGIC MONITORING   Collection and analysis of patient data to prevent or minimize neurologic complications

PERIPHERAL SENSATION MANAGEMENT   Prevention or minimization of injury or discomfort in the patient with altered sensation

Trauma, risk for

ENVIRONMENTAL MANAGEMENT: SAFETY   Monitoring and manipulation of the physical environment to promote safety

SKIN SURVEILLANCE   Collection and analysis of patient data to maintain skin and mucous membrane integrity

Unilateral neglect

UNILATERAL NEGLECT MANAGEMENT   Protecting and safely reintegrating the affected part of the body while helping the patient adapt to disturbed perceptual abilities

Urinary elimination, altered

URINARY ELIMINATION MANAGEMENT   Maintenance of an optimum urinary elimination pattern

Urinary retention

URINARY CATHETERIZATION   Insertion of a catheter into the bladder for temporary or permanent drainage of urine

URINARY RETENTION CARE   Assistance in relieving bladder distention

Ventilation, inability to sustain spontaneous

ARTIFICIAL AIRWAY MANAGEMENT   Maintenance of endotracheal and tracheostomy tubes and preventing complications associated with their use

MECHANICAL VENTILATION   Use of an artificial device to assist a patient to breathe

RESPIRATORY MONITORING   Collection and analysis of patient data to ensure airway patency and adequate gas exchange

RESUSCITATION: NEONATE   Administering emergency measures to support newborn adaptation to extrauterine life

VENTILATION ASSISTANCE   Promotion of an optimal spontaneous breathing pattern that maximizes oxygen and carbon dioxide exchange in the lungs

Ventilatory weaning response, dysfunction (DVWR)

MECHANICAL VENTILATION   Use of an artificial device to assist a patient to breathe

MECHANICAL VENTILATORY WEANING   Assisting the
    patient to breathe without the aid of a mechanical
    ventilator

Violence, risk for: self-directed or directed at others*

ANGER CONTROL ASSISTANCE   Facilitation of the ex-
    pression of anger in an adaptive nonviolent
    manner
ENVIRONMENTAL MANAGEMENT: VIOLENCE
    PREVENTION   Monitoring and manipulation of the
    physical environment to decrease the potential for
    violent behavior directed toward self, others, or
    environment

*Since the development of these links by NIC, NANDA has split this
diagnosis into "Violence, risk for: self-directed" and "Violence, risk
for: directed at others."

Violence, risk for: directed at others

Bibliography

NANDA PROCEEDINGS

Gebbie KM, Lavin MA, eds: *Classification of nursing diagnoses: proceedings of the first national conference,* St Louis, 1975, Mosby.

Gebbie KM, ed: *Classification of nursing diagnoses: summary of the second national conference,* St Louis, 1976, Clearinghouse, St Louis University.

Kim MJ, Moritz DA, eds: *Classification of nursing diagnoses: proceedings of the third and fourth national conferences,* St Louis, 1982, McGraw-Hill.

Kim MJ, McFarland GK, McLane AM, eds: *Classification of nursing diagnoses: proceedings of the fifth national conference,* St Louis, 1984, Mosby.

Hurley ME, ed: *Classification of nursing diagnoses: proceedings of the sixth conference,* St Louis, 1986, Mosby.

McLane A, ed: *Classification of nursing diagnoses: proceedings of the seventh conference,* St Louis, 1987, Mosby.

Carroll-Johnson RM, ed: *Classification of nursing diagnoses: proceedings of the eighth conference,* Philadelphia, 1989, JB Lippincott.

Carroll-Johnson RM, ed: *Classification of nursing diagnoses: proceedings of the ninth conference,* Philadelphia, 1991, JB Lippincott.

Carroll-Johnson RM, Paquette M, eds: *Classification of nursing diagnoses: proceedings of the tenth conference,* Philadelphia, 1994, JB Lippincott.

Rantz MJ, LeMone P, eds: *Classification of nursing diagnoses: proceedings of the eleventh conference,* Glendale, Calif, 1995, CINAHL Information Systems.

AHCPR Agency for Health Care Policy and Research; a federal agency within the U.S. Public Health Service, U.S. Department of Health and Human Services, responsible for the multidisciplinary development of clinical practice guidelines for selected conditions (e.g., incontinence, pain, depression).

critical thinking/diagnostic reasoning The cognitive process of collecting information, interpreting and clustering information, naming clusters, and formulating nursing diagnosis.*

defining characteristics Signs and symptoms indicating the presence of a nursing diagnosis.

diagnostic label Terminology used to name/label a nursing diagnosis.

DSM IV The fourth edition of the American Psychiatric Association's *Diagnostic and Statistical Manual of Mental Disorders;* the official manual of mental disorders clinically useful for making treatment and management decisions in varied clinical settings.†

etiology Previous term for related factor.

expected outcomes Changes in patient behaviors resulting from nursing interventions.

functional health patterns Health patterns useful in assessing human functioning.

function level classification‡
   0 = Completely independent.
   1 = Requires use of equipment or device.
   2 = Requires help from another person for assistance, supervision, or teaching.
   3 = Requires help from another person and equipment device.
   4 = Dependent; does not participate in activity.

ICD-10-CM A clinical modification of the ICD-10 which serves as the official system in the United States for the classification of all diseases, injuries, impairments, symptoms, and causes of death.

life processes Events/processes occurring throughout the lifespan that are related to health status.

NANDA North American Nursing Diagnosis Association.

*Gordon M: From *Nursing diagnosis: process and application,* ed 3, St Louis, 1994, Mosby.
†From American Psychiatric Association: *Diagnostic and statistical manual of mental disorders,* ed 4, Washington, DC, 1994, The Association.
‡Code adapted from Jones E and others: *Patient classification for long-term care: users' manual,* HEW, Publication No. HRA-74-3107, November 1974.

nursing diagnosis   A clinical judgment about an individual, family, or community responses to actual and potential health problems/life processes. Nursing diagnoses provide the basis for selection of nursing interventions to achieve outcomes for which the nurse is accountable.*

patient goals/expected outcomes   Goals the patient will achieve fully or in part as a result of nursing interventions, along with the changes in patient behavior, function, cognition, and affect, indicating goal achievement.

potential nursing diagnosis   Now referred to as at-risk nursing diagnosis.

qualifiers for diagnoses†

Suggested/not limited to the following:

Acute: severe but of short duration

Altered: a change from baseline

Chronic: lasting a long time, recurring, habitual, constant

Decreased: lessened, lesser in size, amount or degree

Deficient: inadequate in amount, quality or degree, defective, not sufficient, incomplete

Depleted: emptied wholly or in part, exhausted of

Disturbed: agitated, interrupted, interfered with

Dysfunctional: abnormal, incomplete functioning

Excessive: characterized by an amount or quantity that is greater than necessary, desirable, or useful

Increased: greater in size, amount or degree

Impaired: made worse, weakened, damaged, reduced, deteriorated

Ineffective: not producing the desired effect

Intermittent: stopping or starting again at intervals, periodic, cyclic

Potential for enhanced: (for use with wellness diagnoses) made greater, to increase in quality, or more desired

related factors   Factors contributing to an actual nursing diagnosis.

risk factors   Predisposing factors that increase vulnerability to the development of a nursing diagnosis (used with at-risk nursing diagnoses).

signs and symptoms   Objective manifestations and subjective sensation, including perception and feelings.

taxonomy   The science of classification (i.e., the study of the general principles of scientific classification).

---

*Approved at the Ninth Conference on Classification of Nursing Diagnoses.

†From North American Nursing Diagnoses Association (NANDA): *Nursing diagnoses: definitions and classification 1997-1998,* Philadelphia, 1996, The Association.

Glossary

Classification of nursing diagnoses by human responses patterns*

Exchanging

Altered nutrition: more than body requirements
Altered nutrition: less than body requirements
Altered nutrition: potential for more than body requirements
Risk for infection
Risk for altered body temperature
Hypothermia
Hyperthermia
Ineffective thermoregulation
Dysreflexia
Constipation
Perceived constipation
Colonic constipation
Diarrhea
Bowel incontinence
Altered urinary elimination
Stress incontinence
Reflex incontinence
Urge incontinence
Functional incontinence
Total incontinence
Urinary retention
Altered tissue perfusion (specify type), (renal, cerebral, cardiopulmonary, gastrointestinal, peripheral)
Fluid volume excess
Fluid volume deficit
Risk for fluid volume deficit
Decreased cardiac output
Impaired gas exchange
Ineffective airway clearance
Ineffective breathing pattern
Inability to sustain spontaneous ventilation
Dysfunctional ventilatory weaning response (DVWR)
Risk for injury
Risk for suffocation
Risk for poisoning
Risk for trauma

*From North American Nursing Diagnoses Association (NANDA): *Nursing diagnoses: definitions and classification 1997-1998,* Philadelphia, 1996, The Association.

Risk for aspiration
Risk for disuse syndrome
Altered protection
Impaired tissue integrity
Altered oral mucous membrane
Impaired skin integrity
Risk for impaired skin integrity
Decreased adaptive capacity: intracranial
Energy field disturbance

Communicating

Impaired verbal communication

Relating

Impaired social interaction
Social isolation
Altered role performance
Altered parenting
Risk for altered parenting
Risk for altered parent/infant/child attachment
Sexual dysfunction
Altered family processes
Caregiver role strain
Risk for caregiver role strain
Altered family process: alcoholism
Parental role conflict
Altered sexual patterns

Valuing

Spiritual distress (distress of the human spirit)
Potential for enhanced spiritual well-being

Choosing

Ineffective individual coping
Impaired adjustment
Defensive coping
Ineffective denial
Ineffective family coping: disabling
Ineffective family coping: compromised
Potential for enhanced community coping
Ineffective community coping
Family coping: potential for growth
Ineffective management of therapeutic regimen
    (individuals)

Noncompliance (specify)
Ineffective management of therapeutic regimen: families
Ineffective management of therapeutic regimen: community
Effective management of therapeutic regimen: individual
Decisional conflict (specify)
Health-seeking behaviors (specify)

Moving

Impaired physical mobility
Risk for peripheral neurovascular dysfunction
Risk for perioperative positioning injury
Activity intolerance
Fatigue
Risk for activity tolerance
Sleep pattern disturbance
Diversional activity deficit
Impaired home maintenance management
Altered health maintenance
Feeding self-care deficit
Impaired swallowing
Ineffective breastfeeding
Interrupted breastfeeding
Effective breastfeeding
Ineffective infant feeding pattern
Bathing/hygiene self-care deficit
Dressing/grooming self-care deficit
Toileting self-care deficit
Altered growth and development
Relocation stress syndrome
Risk for disorganized infant behavior
Disorganized infant behavior
Potential for enhanced organized infant behavior

Perceiving

Body image disturbance
Self-esteem disturbance
Chronic low self-esteem
Situational low self-esteem
Personal identity disturbance
Sensory/perceptual alterations (specify) (visual, auditory, kinesthetic, gustatory, tactile, olfactory)
Unilateral neglect
Hopelessness
Powerlessness

Knowing

Knowledge deficit (specify)
Impaired environmental interpretation syndrome
Acute confusion
Chronic confusion
Altered thought processes
Impaired memory

Feeling

Pain
Chronic pain
Dysfunctional grieving
Anticipatory grieving
Risk for violence: directed at others
Risk for self-mutilation
Post-trauma response
Rape-trauma syndrome
Rape-trauma syndrome: compound reaction
Rape-trauma syndrome: silent reaction
Anxiety
Fear

Classification of nursing diagnoses by functional health patterns*

Health-perception—health management

Health-seeking behaviors (specify)
Altered health maintenance
Ineffective management of therapeutic regimen (individuals)
Effective management of therapeutic regimen: individuals
Ineffective management of therapeutic regimen: families
Ineffective management of therapeutic regimen: community
Noncompliance (specify)
Risk for infection
Risk for injury
Risk for trauma
Risk for perioperative positioning injury
Risk for poisoning
Risk for suffocation
Altered protection
Energy field disturbance

Nutritional-metabolic

Altered nutrition: more than body requirements
Altered nutrition: risk for more than body requirements
Altered nutrition: less than body requirements
Ineffective breastfeeding
Interrupted breastfeeding
Effective breastfeeding
Ineffective infant feeding pattern
Impaired swallowing
Risk for aspiration
Altered oral mucous membrane
Fluid volume deficit
Risk for fluid volume deficit
Fluid volume excess
Risk for impaired skin integrity
Impaired skin integrity
Impaired tissue integrity

*Modified from Gordon M: *Manual of nursing diagnosis, 1997-1998,* St Louis, 1997, Mosby.

Risk for altered body temperature
Ineffective thermoregulation
Hyperthermia
Hypothermia

Elimination

Colonic constipation
Perceived constipation
Constipation
Diarrhea
Bowel incontinence
Altered urinary elimination
Functional incontinence
Reflex incontinence
Stress incontinence
Urge incontinence
Total incontinence
Urinary retention

Activity-exercise

Activity intolerance
Risk for activity intolerance
Fatigue
Impaired physical mobility
Risk for disuse syndrome
Bathing/hygienic self-care deficit
Dressing/grooming self-care deficit
Feeding self-care deficit
Toileting self-care deficit
Diversional activity deficit
Impaired home maintenance management
Dysfunctional ventilatory weaning response (DVWR)
Inability to sustain spontaneous ventilation
Ineffective airway clearance
Ineffective breathing pattern
Impaired gas exchange
Decreased cardiac output
Altered tissue perfusion (specify type)
Dysreflexia
Disorganized infant behavior
Risk for disorganized infant behavior
Potential for enhanced organized infant behavior
Risk for peripheral neurovascular dysfunction
Altered growth and development

Sleep-rest

Sleep pattern disturbance

Cognitive-perceptual

Pain
Chronic pain
Sensory/perceptual alterations (specify: visual, auditory,
    kinesthetic, gustatory, tactile, olfactory)
Unilateral neglect
Knowledge deficit (specify)
Altered thought processes
Acute confusion
Chronic confusion
Impaired environmental interpretation syndrome
Impaired memory
Decisional conflict (specify)
Decreased adaptive capacity: intracranial

Self-perception—self-concept

Fear
Anxiety
Risk for loneliness
Hopelessness
Powerlessness
Self-esteem disturbance
Chronic low self-esteem
Situational low self-esteem
Body image disturbance
Risk for self-mutilation
Personal identity disturbance

Role-relationship

Anticipatory grieving
Dysfunctional grieving
Altered role performance
Social isolation
Impaired social interaction
Relocation stress syndrome
Altered family processes
Altered family processes: alcoholism
Altered parenting
Risk for altered parenting
Parental role conflict
Risk for altered parent/infant/child attachment

Caregiver role strain
Risk for caregiver role strain
Impaired verbal communication
Risk for violence: directed at others

Sexuality-reproductive

Altered sexuality patterns
Sexual dysfunction
Rape-trauma syndrome
Rape-trauma syndrome: compound reaction
Rape-trauma syndrome: silent reaction

Coping—stress-tolerance

Ineffective individual coping
Defensive coping
Ineffective denial
Impaired adjustment
Post-trauma response
Family coping: potential for growth
Ineffective family coping: compromised
Ineffective family coping: disabling
Ineffective community coping
Potential for enhanced community coping

Value-belief

Spiritual distress (distress of human spirit)
Potential for enhanced spiritual well-being

Index

Italic entries indicate corresponding nursing care plans.

Index

Index

513

Index

T